The Playful Life

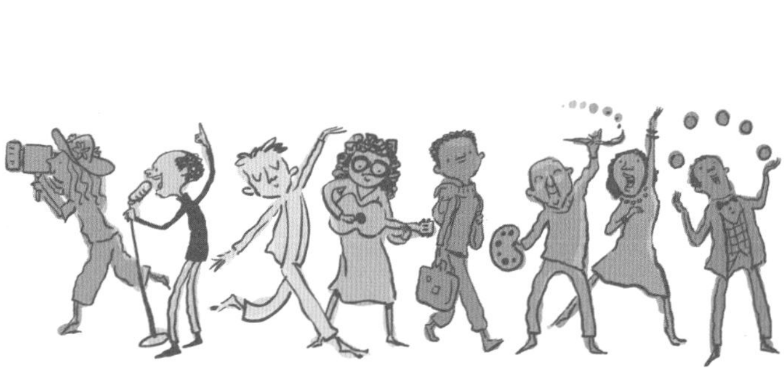

The Playful Life

THE POWER OF PLAY IN OUR EVERY DAY

Julie P. Jones, PhD

Jed Dearybury

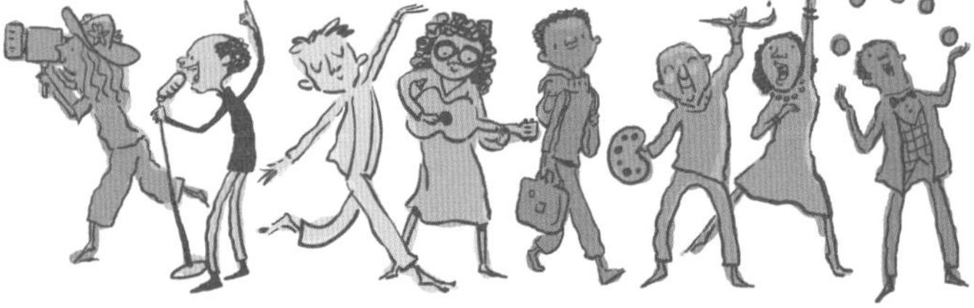

JOSSEY-BASS™
A Wiley Brand

Published by John Wiley & Sons, Inc., Hoboken, New Jersey.
Published simultaneously in Canada.

For general information on our other products and services or for technical support, please contact our Customer Care Department within the United States at (800) 762-2974, outside the United States at (317) 572-3993 or fax (317) 572-4002.

If you believe you've found a mistake in this book, please bring it to our attention by emailing our reader support team at wileysupport@wiley.com with the subject line "Possible Book Errata Submission."

Wiley also publishes its books in a variety of electronic formats. Some content that appears in print may not be available in electronic formats. For more information about Wiley products, visit our web site at www .wiley.com.

Library of Congress Control Number is Available:

ISBN: 9781119882008 (paperback)
ISBN: 9781119882015 (ePDF)
ISBN: 9781119882022 (ePub)

Cover Artwork & Design: *New York Times* bestselling author Peter H. Reynolds

SKY10036126_092722

PRAISE FOR *THE PLAYFUL LIFE*

This book feels like you're having a conversation with two friends while simultaneously learning an immense amount in the process Jed and Julie's playful candor helps you take in all that you're reading and digest it. And boy, did we eat it up. Highly recommend this book to anyone looking to educate themselves on the importance of play, the importance of self, and the importance of the curious world around them.

—**PJ and Thomas McKay**, bloggers and influencers, *The Property Lovers*

As an educator and public speaker across the nation, it's my job to engage people with laughter and learning. At the heart of that work is the power of play. After reading Jed and Julie's book, I now understand all the more just how important playfulness is to life. Read this ASAP. You won't regret it!

—**Gerry Brooks**, lifetime educator and national public speaker

The Playful Life is a gem, with so many practical and easily implemented ideas to make every day more joyful and fun! Julie P. Jones and Jed Dearbury have struck the perfect balance of providing inspiring and meaningful anecdotes alongside tons of actionable things we can do immediately to make life more playful. The book is timely, practical, and a must-read!

—**Adam Bellow**, CEO and cofounder, Breakout EDU

In their first book, *The Playful Classroom*, Jed and Julie demonstrated how play could lead to deeper thinking, improved creativity, and better social-emotional skills. In their second book, *The Playful Life*, they build on that foundation by sharing how play can be an end rather than a means to an end. While the style is playful and approachable, the book is a deep reading, proving that play is actually a very serious topic. The book offers a more expansive view of play, including both as a behavior and as a mindset. Play is collecting things. Play is building and making. Play is imagination. Play is creative risk-taking. The authors provide practical ideas and strategies you can implement tomorrow.

—**John Spencer**, professor and author

Play is more important and more necessary than ever, and Julie and Jed are experts on the subject. They are expert guides to help us all cultivate a more playful approach to life. Stop what you're doing and READ THIS BOOK. I guarantee your future, more playful self will be grateful you did.

—**Jarrett Lerner**, author and illustrator

We have evolved to play. It is in our DNA. It has been part of our human story since the beginning of time. Without it, our lives long for fullness. As someone who walked away from two decades of a playless life to fully embrace my playful spirit, I strongly encourage you to read this book and join me in living a playful life.

—**Darryl Edwards**, founder and CEO, Primal Play

This book expertly and joyfully allows the reader to engage and learn the benefit of having a "playful brain and mindset" to face our challenges and overcome obstacles. Being better at play may be the antidote that lifts folks out of an exhausted existence and into the space of fun, humor, laughter, and showing life who is living it.

—**Dr. Janet Taylor**, psychiatrist and author,
The Courageous Classroom

What a fun read (which I suppose is to be expected from a book about the art of play, but one never knows)! No matter who you are, this humorous and informative book will remind you of the importance of play and of the wide-eyed, childlike enthusiasm for life we adults tend to forget. This is the first book I've read that told me to stop reading and go do a spontaneous activity that brings me joy, which inspired me to go do said spontaneous thing, but then immediately return to the book to see what other wonderful advice it held.

—**Michael Judson Berry**, actor and writer

Play connects us. Play heals. Play helps us learn. But in modern life, play is a forgotten art, a casualty of our test- and work-obsessed culture that isolates us from what makes us human. *The Playful Life* is an ode to play, written as a heartfelt romp that models playfulness itself. Julie and Jed teach us that play isn't simply what we do; it's a mindset we hone, a skill that we sharpen, a habit that we build, and so much more. And whether we're looking to engage with life or avoid burnout, it all begins with the relationship we explore with our own inner child.

—**Takeru "TK" Nagayoshi**, 2020 Massachusetts Teacher of the Year

Julie and Jed's new book, *The Playful Life*, inspires the reader to go beyond the bounds of societal expectations and engage the world joyfully, expressively, and eagerly, returning to us the eyes of a child. With rejuvenated vision, we can see our experiences and communities with a sense of wonder and curiosity about the possibilities, allowing us not just to think, but dream big . . . AGAIN!

—**Natalia Rosario**, urban planner

Hopelessness is chronic and stress is a silent killer. Due to such painful realities in life, intentionality in healthy mental hygiene has become more imperative now than ever before. In *The Playful Life*, Julie Jones and Jed Dearybury serve us up heaping and happy doses of cheerful perspectives, brimming with life-applicable lessons and amusing dashes of hilarity. I felt my world destressing with each and every word and I became more playful with every jot and tittle!

—**Marvin Rogers**, author and wine industry executive

Playfulness doesn't make hard things, big feelings, or problems go away, but it can help us grow through them and connect more fully with others around us. This book outlines the tangible, accessible ways to become more playful in life along with the many benefits supported by research. Bonus: it's playfully written! Kudos to the authors and all those on the mission to live playfully.

—**Alison Hughey, MT-BC,** music therapist

CONTENTS

HEY Y'ALL

How y'all doing?

It's been a tough few years since our last book, right? Who knew when *The Playful Classroom* was sent to press that it would be released during the global shutdown that came as a result of COVID-19? While it wasn't the best-timed release for a book about playful teaching because schools were in survival mode at the time, it certainly reminded us both about the need for play in our everyday lives more than ever before.

Now, over two years removed from that initial shuttering of so much of the world, we are starting to emerge on the other side only to find rumors of another variant, reports of war, and the continued widening of political divides around the globe.

Almost daily since the release of our first work about the power of play, someone has said to us, "We love learning about play in the classroom, but we really need a book about how to bring more playfulness into our everyday lives." At the heart of each request was someone seeking permission to play. They were weighed down by the worry, grief, and fear of the past two years, coupled with the reality that life was moving on whether we were ready or not. The enormity of the anxiety we all faced—albeit different for everyone, depending on a variety of social, economic, and community factors—is overwhelming to think about. Sadly, not enough people are talking about how to help us recover from the emotional toll the pandemic has had on our lives.

Enter us, Julie and Jed, Jed and Julie—two educators who love our students, love our profession, love our community, and love people—who desire to make the world better with everything we do. Our world is different now from when *The Playful Classroom* was launched . . . the world pre-2020. Eyes have been opened to an interconnectedness in such a way that we can never go back to "the way it used to be." At the same time the pandemic was taking over, the murder of George Floyd by police officers forced the world to face a deeply oppressive system that disproportionately hurts Black people. Seeing the hurt the world was facing on multiple fronts, coupled with the desire coming from our readers of our previous work, *The Playful Life* was born.

We believe play, as both a behavior and a mindset, is a key to change. The empathy it builds, the friends it makes, the wounds it heals, the memories it makes, the walls it destroys. We need more play, and we needed it yesterday. Y'all hear us?

Admittedly, we don't always get it right. We are both white people: one of us a member of the queer community, the other an LGBTQ+ ally who is heterosexual. We were raised in the Deep South, in small towns that often jaded our worldview by the whiteness that surrounded us. Our entire adult lives have been spent moving away from a single, and often warped, view of the world to embracing all the beauty that is humanity around the globe. We recognize that play looks different for everyone based on religious, cultural, and community values. At the heart of this work are shared benefits we all need as we move through time to the next generation of people.

As you read, consider the words of our grannies as they sent us out into the backyard: "Play purdy," they'd say. At the heart of those words was their desire for us to get along, be nice, work together, treat others with respect, value others as ourselves, love one another, talk through our differences, and to join together in play because it is good for our lives.

Play purdy, y'all.

FOREWORD

It is *there* in each of us. Our own play nature. And it has been refined over millions of years as an integral part of each of us. If sufficiently triggered by life opportunities, that nature shapes how we experience ourselves, shapes how we see the world, and can color how we see and experience others. This may seem surprising, as play is not generally viewed as a necessary inclusion for an overall balanced and fulfilling life. However, as you read *The Playful Life*, you will see elements of yourself you may not have recognized, but which add authenticity, fulfillment, sustained motivation . . . and more *fun* to your daily and hourly traverse wherever you live, and whatever your life setting or circumstances.

Is yours a life with too little play? Or have you, like most responsible citizens, relegated play as something you engage in when all other "responsibilities" are completed?

You are about to embark on a book, grounded in the life experiences of the authors and reflecting good science, that will comprehensively allow you, if you heed its directions, to prompt you, with solid guidance, *to see and experience yourself as, among your other attributes—yes, you are—a PLAYER*. And in this recognition and this embrace of your own playfulness, you can reap its many benefits that would otherwise elude you.

I can say this from the perspective of one who was fortunate to be grounded in a playful secure family, and who later as a research physician–psychiatrist discovered that violent antisocial men—murderers—and others whose lives demonstrated extreme deficiencies in play differed substantively from those whose play was sufficient. From this research base, I have had the opportunity to review the play backgrounds of thousands, in highly varied settings, over a 50+ year play-focused journey. I have also met and learned from animal and human play scholars as well as laboratory-based basic scientists that, indeed, there is an emergent play science. So whether it is observing bear play in Alaska, or convening scholars to better understand the neuroscience of play, or today finding personal joy in a romp with my dog, my long and rich play odyssey is enriched by this life-changing book, Julie and Jed's *The Playful Life*.

What does it mean to be a playful person? What are the varieties of playfulness available but not necessarily incorporated actively and regularly into *your* life? And if being playful eludes you, how do you find it, revel in its manifold benefits, personalize it so it fits the reality of your current life? This search, and guidance to achieve more play, which are the themes of this book, provide not only individual resources that include personalized fun, innovativeness, and creativity, but also wisdom to find and participate in play-enhanced communal activities.

In our polarized culture, a playful life has greater capacity for tolerance and problem-solving than one without play! Play, as depicted so well, is an antidote for a society needing tolerance and compassion for it to function and survive.

So, reading this book can and will be a life-changer. *(And maybe a cultural changer also?)*

The following pages provide an enticing, readable entrée into the world of playfulness. They contain plenty of "southernisms" that, nonetheless, provide the wisdom and practicality to overcome the usual barriers that prevent most of us from becoming fully (and playfully) what is our common, waiting-to-be-fully activated, human endowment.

This book is written by two educators who have both traveled personal and professional routes to discover and prioritize, understand and enact, this essential and—from my seasoned viewpoint—instinctively necessary (and at its core a survival necessity) component of our shared human nature.

Their classroom educator experience and personal travels have grounded them in the need for play. *The Playful Life* brings into reach more play for all of us.

What a gift!

So this Foreword is prompted by my respect for Julie and Jed, whose life experiences and play-based scholarship have produced this accessible book. It well describes and solidifies the long, more scholarly research-based journey into play science that I have enjoyed.

And, this is a *fun* book to read. Beyond that, reading it shows—in virtually every page—the need for all of us to recognize the importance of our play natures, and to prioritize and activate them as our essential play design dictates.

—Stuart Brown

ABOUT THE AUTHORS

Since starting her career in 1999, **Dr. Julie Jones** has had an exceptional journey in education. She has taught 4th, 5th, 7th, 8th, and 9th through 12th grades in both general and special education, as well as teacher education courses at the University of South Carolina and Converse University. As an innovative educational development professional, she maintains an active research agenda with interests including instructional technology and pedagogy, always with a mix of creativity and play. She is an educational consultant for the Hub City Writers Project, spearheading the Books as Mirrors program, which ensures children see themselves in the books they read. Before working on the *We Are Playful . . .* series, she was the editor of the *Teacher Education Journal of South Carolina*, and past president of the South Carolina Association of Teacher Educators. Follow her on Twitter @JuliePJones, and view her full curriculum vitae at www.juliepjones.com.

Jed Dearybury began his education career in 2001. During his 13-year early childhood classroom tenure, Jed received numerous honors. He was featured in *GQ* magazine as Male Leader of the Year, met President Obama as the South Carolina winner of the Presidential Award for Excellence in Math and Science Teaching, and was named as a top 5 finalist for South Carolina Teacher of the Year. While working on the *We Are Playful . . .* series, Jed has been leading professional development across the country, as well as training the next generation of educators through his work in higher ed. Since August 2019, he has been the Director of Creativity and Innovation at MrDearybury.com LLC. His mission: Equip, Encourage, Empower the teaching profession using creativity, laughter, and hands-on fun! Connect with him online on Twitter @mrdearybury or www.mrdearybury.com.

ACKNOWLEDGMENTS

Dearest Reader,

Thank you for picking up this book. If not for you reading these words, the message and your inclination to play might not have had the chance to ignite. Let that fire burn! This journey could not have happened without several key players, listed here in no particular order.

1. New walking shoes, which provided the bounce for idea percolation.
2. Peter and Paul Reynolds, for helping us to be happy dreamers.
3. The caffeine, whether hot or cold, provideth stimulation and sustenance.
4. Those pimento cheese biscuits: 'nuff said.
5. Melissa Walker . . . forever and always our continuous guide.
6. Tabitha Brown . . . and Donna . . . for the laughter and moments of truth.
7. Life changes that force us to confront trauma and write our experiences.
8. Coffee shops that are open on Sundays.
9. Google for always being present with answers to our random questions:
   a. 100 ways to cook an egg
   b. The domestication of the potato
   c. What is a Peter Pan's age?
   d. How much money does Dabo make?
   e. How to you spell kumquat?
   f. Is cornhole one word or two?
10. Trisha at the pottery place for the stroke and coat.
11. Landa and the couch. Laina for the appointment booking.
12. Matt Matt . . . because he is ever so patient with both of us.

13. Amy Fandrei and the people in that room who continue to believe in us and the work we do.
14. The small humans in our lives who keep us humble.
15. Our cool glasses that help us see the world through a playful lens.

Julie and Jed

SECTION 1

Meaning

Evidence of play goes back to the beginning of humanity. A spinning top was discovered in an ancient Egyptian tomb, a baby's rattle was unearthed in Turkey, and a doll's head was found in the ruins of a hut on the Italian island of Pantelleria. The toys are estimated to have been between four and six thousand years old. While those "play purdies" (what our grannies used to call toys) are extremely old in age, the Strong National Museum of Play, also known as *The Strong*, named after its founder, Margaret Woodbury Strong, has named one toy the oldest of all: the stick. Yep, y'all read that right . . . a stick. Just a plain ol' stick laying in the yard right outside.

There are lots of ideas in our world of what play is, and most of them have to do with objects. Play is more than the stick. Play isn't the toy or the (insert object of choice).

Play is the opportunity for creativity and innovation.

Play is the spontaneous act resulting from curiosity or wonder.

Play is both free and structured, both behavior and mindset.

The top, the rattle, and the doll are all objects that allow children to be creative and invent new ideas and explore concepts,

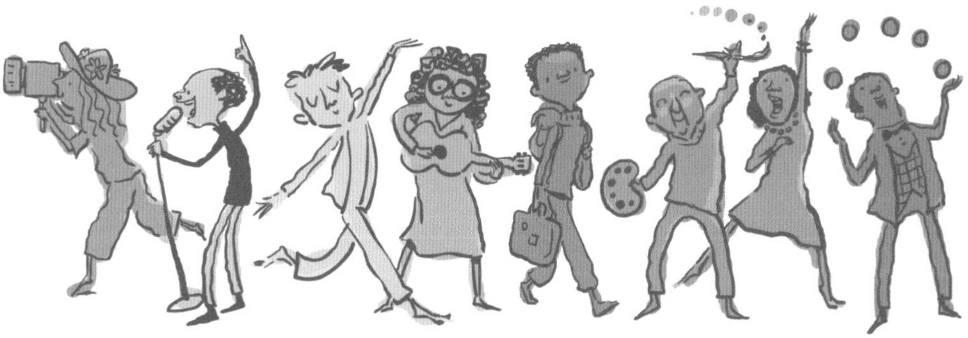

that allow for their users to be curious, and invite them to play and be playful.

In this section, we break down the meaning of play. In starting with a conversation on meaning, we're ensuring that we're all talking about the same thing. But before we do, let's chat about that stick for a minute. Take a gander at this bit from The Strong regarding their selection. Sticks:

> Promote free play—the freedom to invent and discover. They encourage playing outside instead of inside. Sticks are all around us; they are natural and free. And playing with sticks isn't just for children and animals. Adult artists, crafters, decorators, and architects all make use of sticks in sculptures, wreaths, furniture, and building design. Few adults or children can resist simple play with sticks—from drawing in the sand on the beach, to building a campfire and then toasting marshmallows. Sticks are not only possibly the oldest toys, they're possibly the best! (The Strong, 2021)

Here's the thing, y'all . . . like they said, play is not just for kids! So many people say to us some variation of—*oh you wrote a book on play! I'd love to buy that for my grandkids*. Bless their hearts. Play is so much more than toys and running around the yard. The origins of the word play include old English—*plegian* (exercise)/*plega* (brisk movement)—and middle Dutch—*pleien*—meaning to leap for joy, dance (*Definition and Etymology of Play*, n.d.). Our hearts are full just reading it and we cannot wait for you to dig into the power of play for your every day.

CHAPTER 1

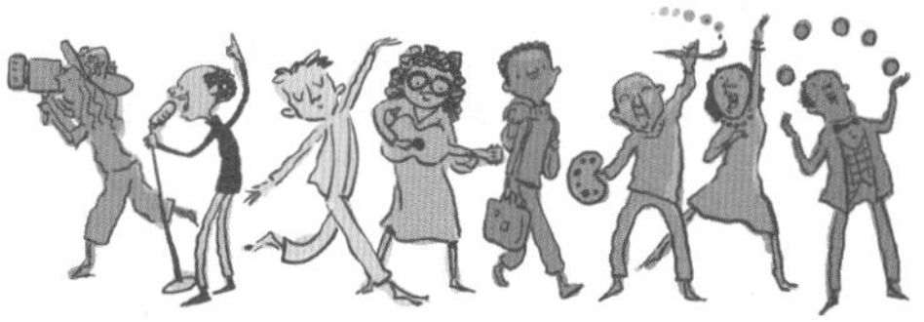

Wanna Play?

So we've gotten you excited and now you wanna be playful, do ya?

A lot of us have *want* in our lives. We want abs, to own a big mansion, to travel around the world to exotic places, etc. etc., but we don't always wanna reckon with the work that it takes to get there. All these aren't always easy for the average person to achieve. They take a lot of time and effort, and often money that many of us don't have.

I (Jed) confess that I have wanted nice abs as bad as a mule wants a pickle patch for my whole life. I have always had this adorable little spare tire around my waist, and I would love to be able to do yoga without my belly gettin' in the way, but I have done literally nothing in my life to get them. Julie and I had a great laugh as we talked about my stomach prohibiting my doing advanced yoga. We know many of you will relate. I am not sure why my girthy abdominal area has always been such a nuisance for me, but alas it has. Even when I was at the peak of my own personal fitness journey from 2009 to 2018, a flat stomach eluded me. I ran almost every day during those years. Some days I ran one mile, some days 26. I put in the training to run seven full marathons over that time period, but not once did I ever lay in the floor (in the South we say "in the floor") and do crunches or planks. All of the books I read about running said that a strong core would help me. I knew that the abs I always dreamed of were in that floor. But alas, I never got down there to get them. I guess I don't want those abs so bad after all, do I? Of course I want them, but the reality is this: their importance wasn't/isn't significant enough to drive me to the floor to work out and get them. Maybe one day.

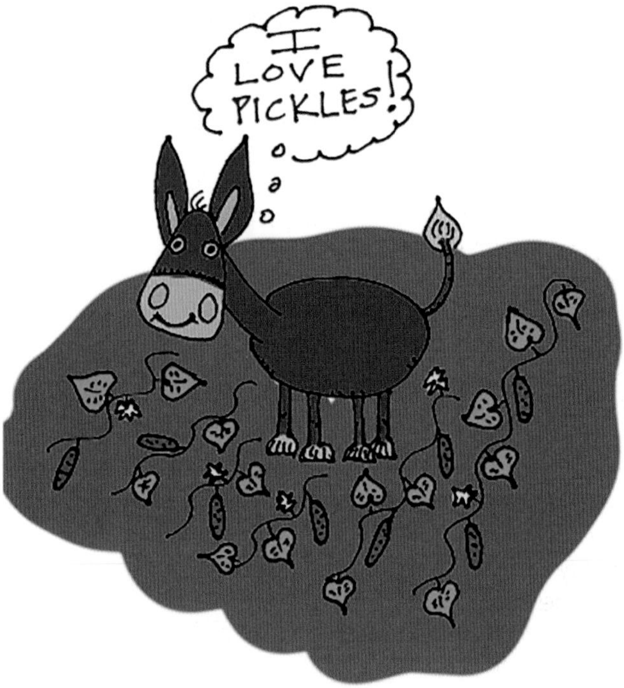

Why am I talking about abs in a book about becoming more playful? This is why:

A playful life takes work, y'all.

> "Wait! I need life to be more fun and peaceful, not more work and stress."

We hear y'all yellin' that at us. We agree. You do need play in your life—we all do. But to get it takes some intentional work and reflection on the things in our lives that are keeping us from fun and peace.

Julie and I have to work at being more playful every day. Sometimes we get to our coffee shop and the world is caving in on us. Writing deadlines, work ridiculousness, financial stress, family drama . . . all the things you deal with, too. The exhaustion of it all can be overwhelming. The instinctive reaction that many of us have when life brings All. The. Heaviness. is to curl up in a ball and pull the covers over our head while we ignore the world.

Sometimes, that is exactly the best thing to do.

When we began to research the effect playfulness had on our brains (that's coming in Section Two), things began to change for us. When the woes of life tried to interfere with our days, we would seek out moments of play to help us through. Some days we would walk on our local rail trail. Some days we would go to Target. Some days we would play rock, paper, scissors just for the fun of it. Our favorite thing? Doodlin'. Many days we get out our bullet journals (Leuchtturm 1917, size A5, if anyone wants to know) and doodle. Yes, doodle—not draw. Draw is a word that can be intimidating to many folks. "I can't draw" is a common phrase we hear. But have you ever heard anyone say "I can't doodle"? No way. Anyway, we'd start doodlin' and things would start to turn around in our day. We love to do collaborative doodles too. Julie will draw something, then I'll add to it. Her turn, then my turn again. We do this in our journals, on scrap paper. Lawd, we've even used small beverage napkins. After just a few minutes, we have a fun page of art. Y'all know what else we created? A moment of playfulness that helped us forget about the heaviness for a bit. Notice I said "a bit." It is not that playfulness made the hard things go away. It didn't solve all of our problems by any means. The angst that we brought into the coffee shop was/is still there, but what did go away was the unfocused mind, the overwhelmed heart, the anger, the bitterness—all the emotions that were holding us back from figuring out how to live in that moment.

What came from the doodlin?

A better mood.
A bit of clarity.
A bit of strength.
A bit of courage.

The energy we needed to help us face the challenges of the day arrived as we giggled at the fun that came to life before our very eyes because we took a moment to play. Imagine if we had just sat there sulking, pouting, fussing, whining. . . . Our moods would have worsened, headaches would have likely arrived, and the problems still would have needed our attention. All the while we would be in pain and in a pissy mood.

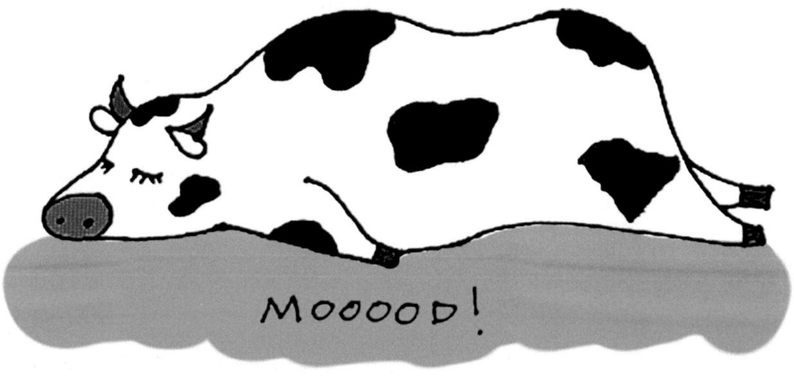

Think of all the people who could be negatively impacted by our unchecked mood (moooooed, we do love a cow!) that day had we not found some playfulness. The drivers we encounter on the roads, the clerks at the stores we visited, the strangers we stand beside in line at the grocery store, those we text, call, or email, our friends, our family. As I think about interrupting someone's good day with my bad attitude, I think of my friend Tabitha Brown. Yes, I call her a friend even though I don't know her very well. She and I did speak at the same conference one year, and she does follow me on Instagram, so that makes us besties, right? Anyway, she has the best saying when it comes to this very topic. She says, "Have a good day, and if you can't . . . don't go messing up nobody else's." She's so wise, y'all. If you don't know her, look her up right now. Seriously, put this book down and find her. She embodies a playful life. When we watch her, listen to her, read her book, or engage with her on social media, we always feel that she is taking a playful approach to life. Julie and I both read her book *Feeding the Soul (Because It's My Business): Finding Our Way to Joy, Love, and Freedom* while writing this book. Her work impacted us both and we were texting constantly about the inspirational words she was sharing. We loved it so much that we began to listen to the audio version so that we could hear her voice. Even the way she speaks is playful. It must be our Southern bond that attracts us to her fun speaking voice. She mentions that she was often made fun of professionally because of her Southern twang, and Julie and I both relate to that deeply. But the way Tab handles it exudes the playful life. She doesn't run from her accent—she embraces it. In fact, the way she embraces every trial and tribulation that comes her way has an element of playfulness to it. She looks for ways to press on through the heaviness with laughter and fun. Don't mishear us here, though. Tears are absolutely gonna happen, and sometimes the heartaches will still be bigger than we can handle. As Adele said in her recent interview with Oprah, sometimes you gotta sit in those feelings (of course, she said this in a British, not a Southern, accent) (CBS, 2021). It boils down to this: a playful spirit will pull us through.

The gift that Tabitha's work brings to the world and how it connects to the power of play in our lives is this: *feed your soul, honey*. Play feeds every part of who you are. Playfulness and the positive effect it has on us as humans is so deeply intertwined in our DNA that our brains have adapted to release all the feel-good chemicals we need to thrive as a species while we play. It's true. Catecholamine, dopamine, norepinephrine, anandamide, serotonin . . . all of that floods our minds when we experience moments of play (Basso & Suzuki, 2017). And one of them, serotonin, even helps you poop (GI Society, 2022)! Who isn't happier when they are having good poops?

Julie: Lawsy, Jed! Y'all, the last time we talked about serotonin and poop was in a restaurant. That's not proper. Not at all.

Jed: Julie, who cares about properness? Why isn't poop proper? We all poop. It is a necessity of life, and if we don't poop there is no way we can live a playful life.

Julie: Um . . . you can talk about poop with your mama, but not here. This is not the place. Y'all, just excuse him.

Jed: I love to poop. I feel better after I do. I will not apologize. That is all.

Julie: While Jed has run to the potty (bless his heart), I'm taking over. Julie here.

As you are about to read in the next chapter, there is a framework of developing a playful mindset that will help us look into the nooks and crannies of our lives. The places that could use a pick-me-up. Right now there may be cobwebs there. Maybe a speck or two of dust. Possibly a dead possum if it's been a while since we looked into these spaces of life. But in these spaces lies lots of potential for us to experience playfulness. To do that, we must first become aware of their presence and the possibility that they have. Becoming aware often starts with reflective questions.

Before we get to that part (we see some of you skipping ahead—stop that. Get back here!), we want a bit of a disclaimer here. We are very intentional in our writing about saying "we and us" instead of you, you, you. Sometimes books talk *at* you instead of *with* you. They feel a bit preachy. A bit off-putting.

We need you to know that we are in this with you. We're trying to figure out how to make our lives more playful right alongside you. But for this next little bit we want to use the upcoming questions to reflect on ourselves. We acknowledge that we are not all in the same boat, and that many of us have privileges far above others to create a playful life. The fact that we're writing and you're reading these words shows privilege for us both. How?

We're sitting at a table writing these words on laptops with a hot beverage beside us.

We bought that beverage with money we earned.

We have money in our bank account (not much, mind you . . . we are educators in the United States).

We have the freedom to carve boundaries and creative time in our day.

We have access to playful spaces, playful people, and playful ideas.

Because of all these resources, we recognize our privilege and we know that our readers may or may not relate.

Please hear this: no matter the resources in our lives, we all have access to our minds, moods, and mojo. A bit of self-reflection will help us all to focus on what we *do* have and how these personal resources can help or hinder our individual playful lives.

Like Tabitha says, "Get into it, y'all."

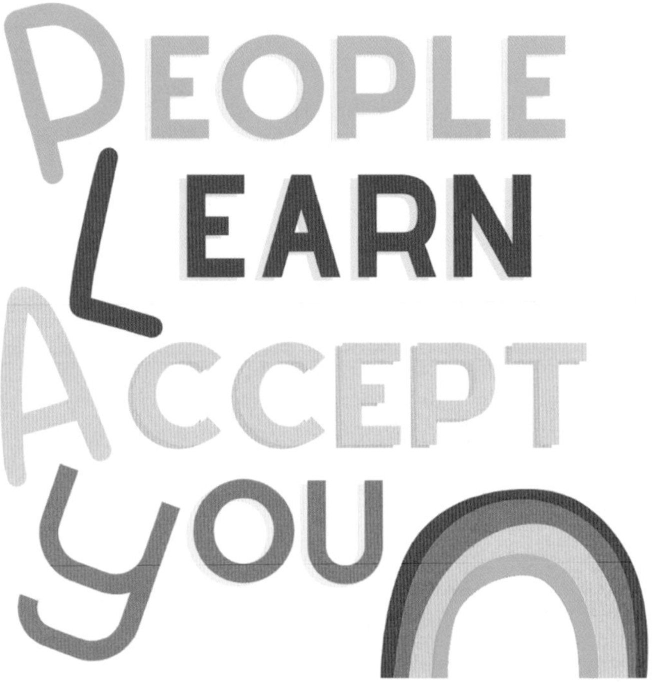

As we mentioned, the nooks and crannies need some attention first. Let's consider the following questions together. We'll answer them honestly. Write your answers here if you want, or maybe even grab some paper and doodle your thoughts as you read. Right now is a great time to create a playful moment.

People

- Who are the people around **you** most?
- How do they inspire **you** to be more playful?
- Do they wanna play with **you,** or do they think it's silly?
- Are they keeping **you** in a box or helping you transform the box into a really cool homemade rocket ship so that you can zoom to the stars?

Learn

- Are **you** willing to learn new things?
- Are **you** willing to apply new learning to multiple areas of your life?
- Are **you** willing to help others around you learn what you are learning?
- Are **you** willing to unlearn all that you have been taught about the way grownups should "behave" in regard to playing?

Accept

- Can **you** accept people for who they are?
- Can **you** accept that this journey may be uncomfortable at times?
- Can **you** accept that we all play differently, and that this difference is beautiful?
- Can **you** accept that what you have always been taught about play may be wrong?

You

- Have **you** noticed that all of the questions here have something to do with **YOU**?

Being playful, whether you are at work, at home, or out with your friends, has everything to do with you. Your mindset, your mood, your mojo, your mates (like they say down under)—YOU.

And guess what, it's different for everyone. That's what's so jazzy about it. (Jed here—Jazzy? I'm picturing you singing in Rose Apothecary alongside Moira and the Jazzagals right now. Those ladies were the epitome of the playful life!)

<<pause for silent stare>>

<<proceeds to type>>

Jed and I play differently, but there's enough overlap that we enjoy a lot of time together. Enough differences that we bicker like siblings.

We all play according to our personalities because we are all uniquely designed, playful individuals. We've got a lot of ground to cover, a lot of diggin' to do. We're gonna get real personal.

We hope you're honest with yourself.

We're gonna lead you to water, but doggone it you gotta put your head down in it and take a big ole ~~drink~~ drank (Yes, drank.)

<<Julie cuts eyes at Jed.>>

<< Jed nods his head and sips his herbal tea.>>

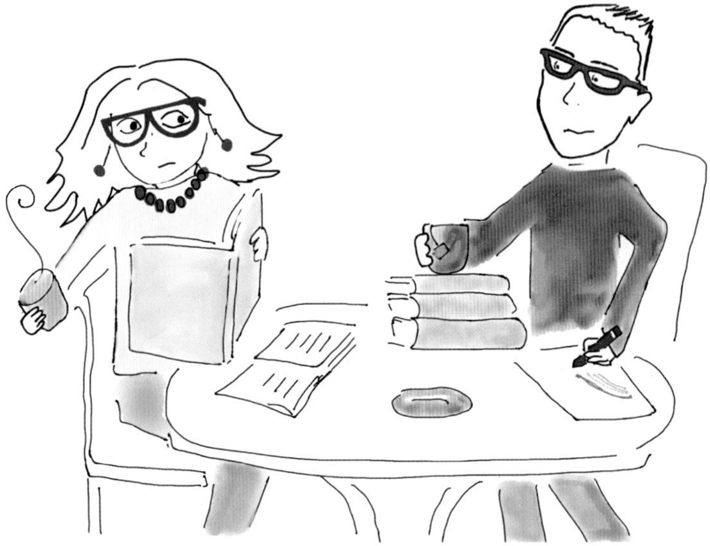

CHAPTER 2

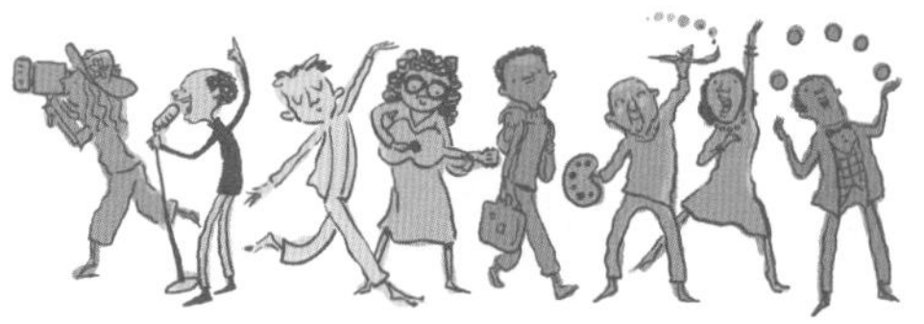

Defining Play

All of us have played, we hope. Despite our location, our culture, and our socioeconomic status, life brings us moments of play whether we seek them out or they seem to manifest randomly.

A funny noise. (Tell us a poot doesn't make you giggle.)

Tension broken by a chuckle. (We always seem to get tickled during a prayer.)

That little dance you do at a door if you leave when someone else tries to enter a room. (Imagine if you really dance while doing it.)

The sudden smell of fried chicken in your office at 8 a.m. (Gimme a biscuit, y'all.)

The times where laughter erupts, where smiles are big, where hearts are tingly, where our minds are distracted from the conundrums of life. (Have you played the game *Taco, Cat, Goat, Cheese, Pizza*?)

Regardless of what we all know about the definition of play, it's safe to say most of us could describe the feeling of it rather than wordsmith an actual definition. Before we get too deep here, we must tell you—academics have yet to agree on a definition of play. Some say it is merely the work of the child. Some say it's all fun and no rigor. Some say that it has to come after the "serious work." Some even think that it's just a bunch of toys and games (you read that intro, right?). We've got opinions about all these definitions and those will come out more as you continue to read this book.

As we were writing this work, we stopped to ask people on the streets of our hometown how they define play.

Here's what we got:

- Having fun.
- Board games with friends.
- What you do at recess.
- What kids do.
- What is that? (laughs)
- I can't define it but I know I'm too tired to do it.
- Something I used to do when I was little.
- Something kids these days don't know how to do.
- Something you don't do in the street. LOL.
- Dressing up a Barbie.
- Building a sandcastle at the beach.

Even Google has an opinion. The first definition offered in our quick search says play is "an activity engaged in for enjoyment and recreation, especially by children." Another definition in these results implies that play is an activity for enjoyment and recreation rather than for a serious or practical purpose.

Y'all. We've clearly got some work to do. We'll go ahead and step a toe up on our soapbox. Play is definitely is these answers, but gosh it's so much more. Play can be free. But play can also be calculated.

Play. Can. Be. Rigorous.

Have you ever experienced a chess match? That experience is most definitely playing, but think about the amount of brain power it takes to win a round of that game. We get a bit fired up when someone tells us that play isn't for the intellectual. You can guarantee we'll make eye contact with each other across the room and silently bless your heart. Not to be snooty here, but we are talking to those of you who are so high in the ivory tower that you've forgotten the true power of play in your own life. That's why we have a whole section titled "Memory." Way too many of us have forgotten all we learned from play and its benefits in our lives.

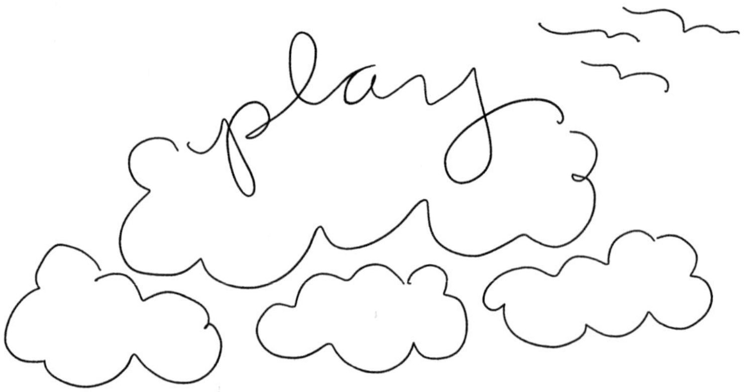

Regardless of what the doubters, the naysayers, the uppities, the misinformed say about the actual meaning of the word, the connotation of "play" we all tend to agree on is the resulting feeling of lightness, both in attitude and in work. Read that again—we did not say the work is light. Rather, the feeling of engagement is light. Play and work can be synonymous, and for those who love their jobs, play and work are often the same. *Play* is definitely one of the most elusive words out there. In English, we use it in so many ways, there's no wonder we are so confused. We don't know whether to scratch our watch or wind our butts (yes, that's a nod to Dolly Parton as Truvy—we're big fans). Let's take a look at some of the possible meanings of play we've heard.

- "Y'all wanna play?" (a behavior).
- "Stop that playin' now! Straighten up" (acting up, being silly).
- "Oh, that's nothin'. I was just playin'" (joking).
- "They play guitar pretty well—you should take a listen" (making music).
- "She plays first base" (a position in a game).
- "Let's take a play break" (a moment of respite).
- "Let's go watch a play tonight" (a theater performance).
- "You best not be playin' with me" (messin' around).
- "He made the game-winning play" (sports move).
- "He played the peacemaker in that meeting" (assume a role/act as).
- "They play the races" (bet on).
- "How did that play out?" (happen).
- "He played his cards right" (handle a situation well).
- "That was a play for sympathy" (an attempt to obtain).

It's no wonder the definition of play is so elusive. We seem to use the word to mean so much, yet the responses from our simple question are focused on childhood behaviors.

When most people hear play, they think of the behavior—check back to the list of answers we got on the street. They think of monkey bars and swings.

Hide-and-seek and Red Rover. Red light, green light, and Doggie Doggie Who's Got the Bone?

Four square.
Freeze tag.
Mother, may I?
A tisket, a tasket.
Sardines.
Pickle.

Yes, they're right. But let's expand this concept—there's *play*. Then there's *playful*. One describes a behavior, the other a mindset. We're going to talk about both.

Play is throwing a frisbee in the yard or painting what you see or reading for pleasure.

Playfulness is the tendency to smile or laugh during all of these activities.

Play is looking through 3D glasses.

Playfulness is the way we see the world.

Play is skipping or frolicking.

Playfulness is the inclination to do so.

Play is a behavior—the act of singing or competing in a race.

Playfulness is a mindset—an approach to each situation with intentional fun.

Jed and I each have a need to put more movement in our days. The pandemic has added some girth to our frames that we're trying to say goodbye to. We also get really chatty when we meet, and need to work through life events before we start the writing process. We found that starting our days on the rail trail, a paved path through the trees that follows a retired railroad track in town, is actually a crucial part of our writing—it gets the ideas flowing and puts us in a creative space. Through walking this path side by side, we get our heads on straight. Writing a book is playful for us in general, but sometimes it gets a bit heavy. The walks we take allow us to share stories and giggle about life. There are fun little games posted along the trail—hopscotch, spot-a-shape, etc. Squirrels scare the mess out of us with their sneakiness. We look for pareidolia in the cracks of the asphalt and the bark of the trees. We don't walk long, maybe 30–45 minutes, but the payoff of that small amount of time playing along the trail is exponential.

The walk is our form of morning play.

The act of making this a part of our routine is purposefully inviting playfulness into our lives.

While *playfulness* and *play* are two separate concepts, both are needed and reap maximum benefits. Read on.

CHAPTER 3

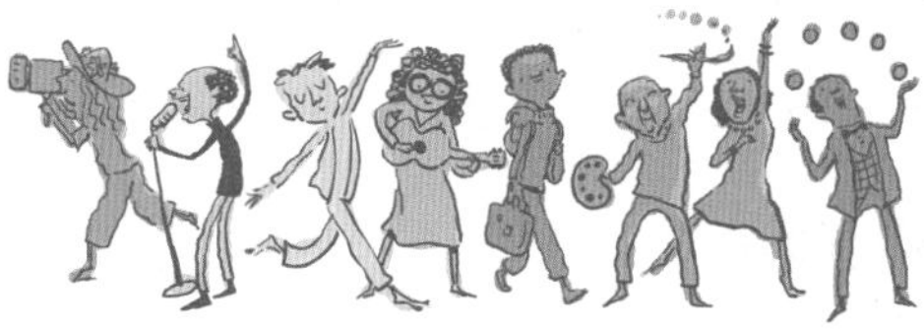

Play as a Behavior

If you're a *write-in-the-book* kind of person, we'd like you to circle the images below that show play. If you're a *writing-in-the-book-are-you-kidding?!* kind of person, just touch the images below that show play.

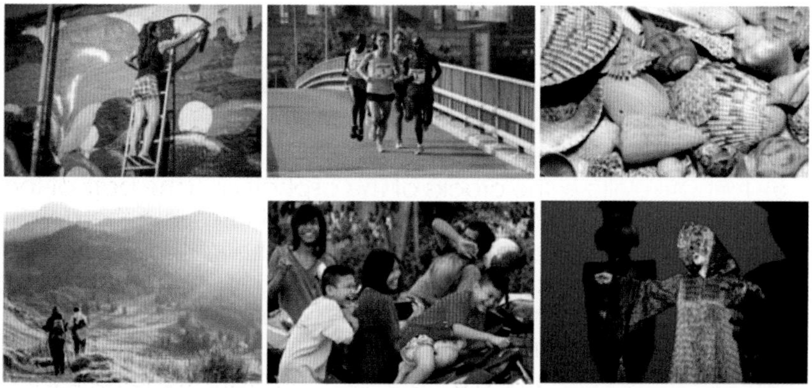

Okay, that was a trick. The answer is that all of these represent play—yes, even collecting seashells!—as do making art, exploring, storytelling, and cracking jokes with your friends. As Julie and I write this section, there are strangers all around us. It's a Saturday morning in May and the weather is beautiful. We're sitting at an outside table by our favorite coffee shop and bookstore. One day, we hope y'all can join us here. We had a deep discussion with each other about what the people around us assumed the definition of play was. We started assuming they would say things like walking in the park, chatting with friends, reading a book, doodling in a journal, coffee dates, etc., but then we realized . . . most of them probably didn't think of play as that kind of behavior because of the way our society as a whole defines and understands play only as frivolous activity. Think back to some of the definitions we shared ". . . especially by children." That perspective couldn't be more wrong. Yet, we are told to "act like grown-ups," and it discourages us adults from thinking that play could or should be a part of our everyday lives.

So, after a mutual pep talk for social courage, we got up and asked them. You've already read the results of that question, in Chapter 2. Their responses are all behaviors. This aspect of play is one we all clearly understand. Play as *doing*.

Although their responses were not as holistic as we hoped, we felt empowered and validated in our quest to help our fellow humans better understand play. We knew, based on their responses, that we had met our audience in real life. These are the people we are writing to. The popular opinion of play from everyone we talked to on the street, and in our daily lives, simply mirrors the need for this book—the work that needs to be done. In looking around, we see so many examples of play. And all of them are playful behaviors.

Sit with us a minute and take a look around right here on Main Street, USA. There are teams dressed in fun costumes—red, orange, and green tutus—running around holding clipboards on a scavenger hunt as part of their day of team building with a local organization. Friends are crowded around cafe tables filled with steaming cups of joy and pastries, laughing and telling stories. A couple walks by with their dogs on leashes and others stop to give the canines a little rub. They wave to someone on a bike riding by. Another friend strolls up be-bopping to whatever is playing in their headphones. A group walks out of the nearby bookshop with a bag of delightful hardbacks—they're clearly excited to get started on a reading adventure. At the table next to us, a man in a suit makes careful notes on his paper. He's not distracted at all by the busy-ness that surrounds us. (He's in flow—more about this later.)

Play as a behavior—these experiences—they're us making memories. We are all in the act of doing something we enjoy. Our behaviors are playing a vital part in making those memories and creating these moments of happiness. They are acts of play.

Across the time it took us to write this work, when we had conversations with friends, they were all unanimous: the experiences they remember are the ones where they played. The ones with cardboard boxes in the backyard. The ones in the treehouse. The ones where they kicked the can down the street. The ones where they didn't have the toys they wanted so they made things to play with using whatever they had.

The behaviors in which they had FUN.

Jed and I have a list of favorite words, and *neotenous* is one of them—it means retaining juvenile traits as adults. Now, we have a playful perception of this term . . . if you feel like taking a gander at the search results for this word, you might go down a rabbit hole of scientific-what-in-tar-nation? Don't do it. Don't look this word up. There's just too much. We recommend our basic definition shared here.

How many of the behaviors of childhood actually make it to adulthood, though?

Building a mud pie
Asking why
Splashing in puddles
Dancing in the rain
Chasing a butterfly
Catching lightning bugs
Giggling for no reason
Daydreaming alternate realities
Digging in the dirt
Examining wooly worms
Skipping to the mailbox
Coloring outside the lines
Making silly faces

Cutting cartwheels (okay . . . we know this one is stretch. God bless our aging bones.)

When we reflect on behaviors that are fun, the answer is different for each of us. Play for me (Julie) is often reading, sketching, creative writing, and sometimes even cleaning my house. But that might make you feel like you just licked honey off a briar. Play for Jed is creating, doodling, playing the piano, and going for a walk. Someone reading this book might find jumping out of planes to be their fave form of play.

(sharp intake of breath)

Whatever cranks your tractor, whatever gets you going—that is likely your go-to form of play.

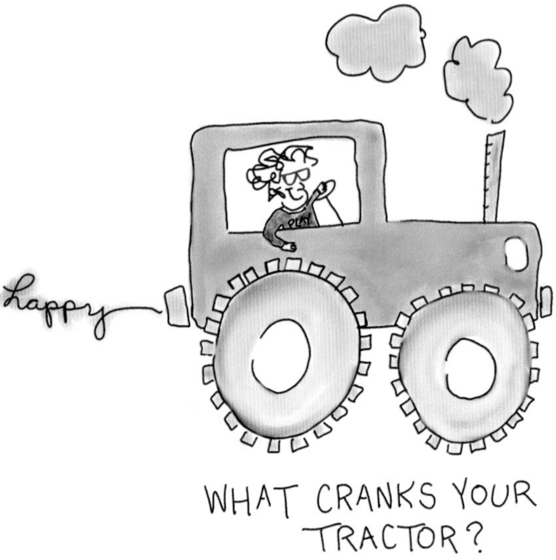

Play as a *behavior* is a *verb*. It's the doing. So how about play as a mindset?

CHAPTER 4

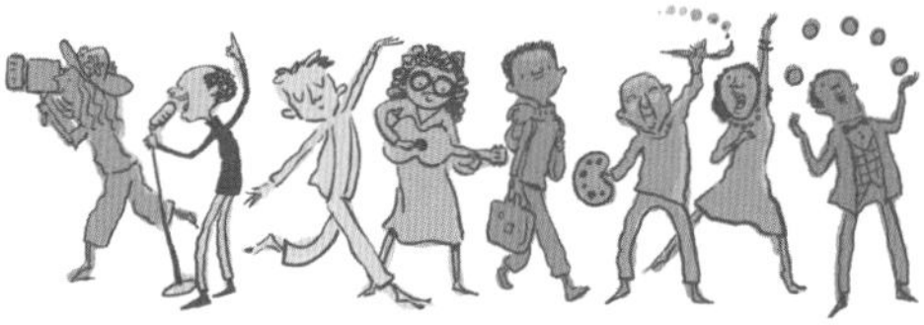

Play as a Mindset

Play can also be a state of mind. To keep it clear, we'll refer to this quality as "playful," an adjective to describe your approach to life; your mindset, if you will. How does your mind tell your body to react if there is a traffiic jam on your way to an important event? What does your brain tell you to do if you get caught in the rain? How does your perspective dictate your reaction to broken car windows as you leave class for the day? Admittedly, all of those things can be absolutely frustrating. Especially if they all happen on the same day. But the right mindset can help you through these kinds of events without sky-high blood pressure and an erupting temper. We will fully confess that we sometimes yell at the traffic, scream at the downpour, and cuss the guy who broke our car windows. (Julie here. I find myself talking at traffic in my fake British accent. It doesn't feel so bad then.) We ain't perfect. But because we, like you, are works in progress, we aim to look for moments where play can save us. Traffic jam ahead? OOH, fun detour to new places or extra time for a car dance party. Caught in the rain? YASSSS jump in the puddles and pretend you are Gene Kelly. Busted-out car windows? Be thankful you are safe and get excited about new windows sans bug guts. YAHOOO! All of the moments here have the possibility to derail the day, but those who have a playful mindset tend to make it through a bit easier than those who yell, scream, and cuss. (Although sometimes cussin' can sure make you feel better.)

Dr. Anthony DeBenedet, our friend and a medical doctor just outside Detroit, Michigan, wrote a book that inspired our previous work on play in the classroom and continues to inspire us here. We met him at the US Play Coalition Conference just before the whole world shut down from COVID-19. Anthony was the guest

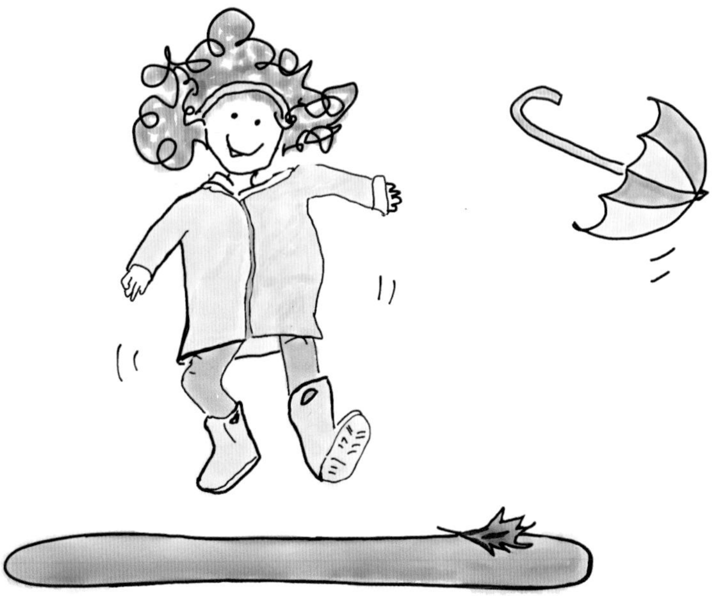

speaker, and his talk inspired many subsequent conversations among the three of us. His book *Playful Intelligence* explains the analysis of hundreds of interviews, and the resulting qualities that manifested across playful adults. The five attributes that influence a playful mindset are sociability, wonder, imagination, spontaneity, and humor. When these key areas of our playful intelligence are intentionally cultivated, the ripple effect into our playful mindset is exponential.

According to DeBenedet, playfulness is not a new concept—not a radical new form of intelligence. Rather, it's an extension of the work done by Dr. Howard Gardner, a cognitive psychologist who is known for his theory of multiple intelligences (Gardner, 1983) showing how we are all more than our IQ.

Anthony DeBenedet's work extends the work of Howard Gardner as it applies to play. These ideas didn't just fall off the turnip truck yesterday. They've been around since Moses was a baby—but his work aids in our synthesis because it extends our understanding of social relations. It helps us reflect on the qualities in our own lives that indicate a level of playfulness. Let's dig into Anthony's work here—it will help us understand how we currently handle what life throws our way.

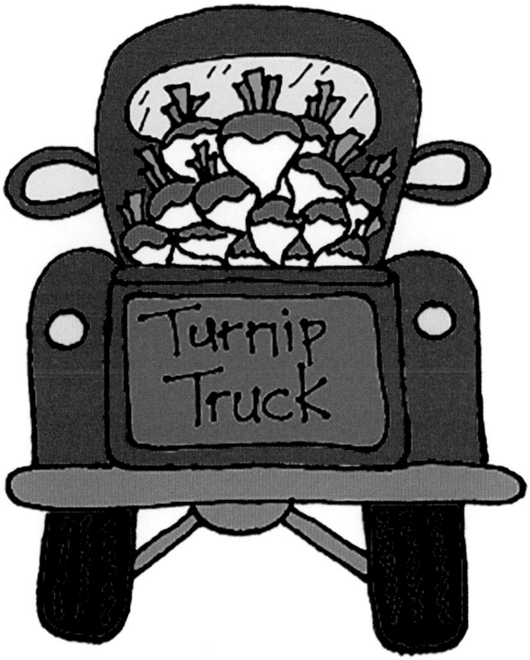

Jed: Wait a second, Julie. . . . What does that mean, we are more than our IQ? I have heard that the IQ test is biased as well. Help me understand.

Julie: Oh, wow. Okay . . . soapbox alert. Simply put, IQ tests are based on the belief that a person's intelligence can be represented with a score from one paper-and-pencil test. Yes, just one score from one day. You can see how problematic that is, right? So much room for a mess of judgment. But that's not all, folks. These tests have a history of bias and racism. According to Ibram X. Kendi (2019), author of *How to Be an Antiracist*, "Standardized tests have become the most effective racist weapon ever devised to objectively degrade Black and Brown minds and legally exclude their bodies from prestigious schools." If you wanna read more about IQ tests, check out the history lesson we've included for your reading pleasure.

History lesson: In 1905, Alfred Binet, a distinguished-looking fella with a pointy mustache, was commissioned by the French government to create an assessment that would identify which students in France might experience difficulty in school. Binet and his buddy, Theodore Simon (both of whom I'm sad to tell you have no playful photo results in any of our searches) thus published the Simon-Binet IQ test in 1908. We Americans got interested, and popped in this assessment convo in 1916 when Stanford psychologist Lewis Terman standardized Binet's original tests using a sample of American participants. So, like your MS Word file that's revised and renamed 100 times, this test continues to be used in schools today. Thank heavens this isn't the only huckleberry on the bush.

Dr. Howard Gardner got all in a tizzy about IQ tests early in his career. For those of you outside the education world, Gardner is known for seven (now eight) established multiple intelligences synthesized in the early 1980s. His seminal work, *Frames of Mind,* refutes the idea that one score represents human intelligence. Instead of one score,

Gardner established eight categories of intelligence: musical/rhythmic, visual/spatial, linguistic/verbal, bodily/kinesthetic, interpersonal, intrapersonal, existential, and naturalistic. Before you read on thinking that a frog's butt is watertight, let's pause. As with any theory, there is agreement and disagreement, flaws and success. There is also the lens to be questioned. From what lens is Gardner working when he identifies these eight intelligences? Of course, when we question, we dig to find our answers. This quote from Gardner's work summarizes what we've found: "I recognize that the ideal of what is valued will differ markedly, sometimes even radically, across human cultures, with the creation of new products or posing of new questions being of little importance in some settings. The prerequisites are a way of ensuring that a human intelligence must be genuinely useful and important, at least in certain cultural settings" (Gardner, 1983, p. 61). Although we are currently satisfied, we continue to read these works knowing that human bias is ever-present.

I was puzzled over the connection between the intelligences and play personalities (which you'll read about toward the end of this section) during a recent trip Jed and I took to Harvard. I emailed Dr. Gardner about the connection between the two—I know there is one. After some pedantic back and forth, he and I have come to agreement that personalities and intelligences are different constructs. We also agree it is futile to try to determine which comes first—it's really a chicken-and-egg question. But that's not important here. Just know we believe playful intelligence exists (DeBenedet, 2018), multiple intelligences exist (Gardner, 1983), and we are here to show how both work together to build a playful life.

Sociability

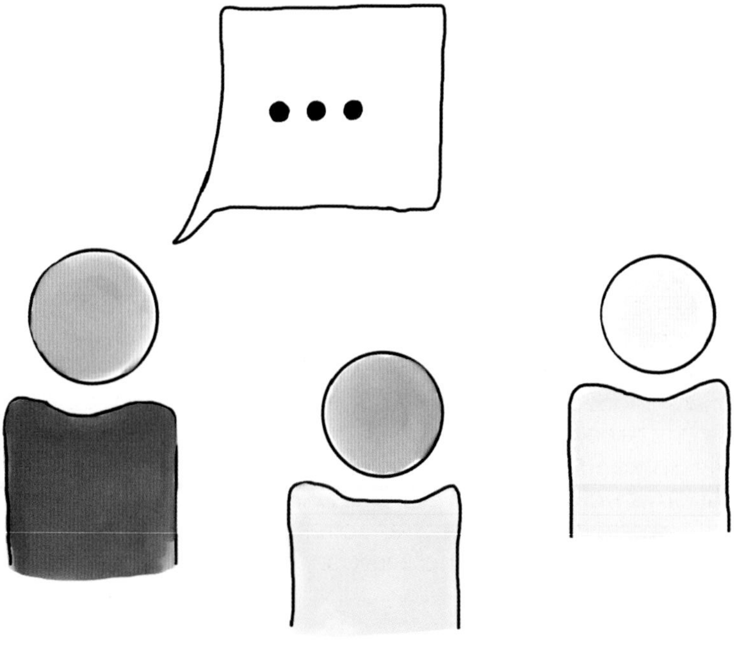

Have you ever been to a gathering/meeting/party where it was very clear who was friends with whom? Where you could actually feel the social division in the room? Yes, a middle school dance is a great example and likely your work holiday parties as well. Now, imagine that someone from one of those groups walks over to another group and strikes up a conversation. People are no doubt watching; there's likely tension. What will happen? Laughter. Glee. Inclusion. Sociability. This kind of person—the one who rejects the *them-versus-us* mentality—embodies this first trait in our list. Not because they build bridges, but because they actually see humanity in the room rather than cliques of people—it's the initial perspective, not the solution. Their sense of egalitarianism is strong. This means they ascribe to the belief that all people are equal and deserve equal rights and opportunities. They don't look for the power struggle because they only seek to connect through humility.

How often do we listen to people in conversations—really listen, not just wait to talk?

We love Parker Palmer's (2017) explanation of listening. He writes that being listened to is what the human self most yearns for. When we are listened to, we feel received, heard, known, and in the process of being honored. When we listen deeply, we offer each other the chance for personal and social change. Often, listening is done for the purpose of being polite, and not for connection. Part of having a playful mindset includes listening for the sake of understanding. This latter practice builds relationships and trust between us all.

My (Jed) niece plays soccer. It is definitely something that brings her joy, and she is really great at it. She wants to score in every single game because she loves the idea of being the one who shot the goal that led to the win. But sometimes that's not always possible. The coach gives instructions and places her where she is needed most. Her teammates call out directives that benefit the group and not her seasonal goal tally. She doesn't always get what she wants and her ability to listen to others is key to her sociability on the team—her ability to be a part of the cohesive unit. We know you've heard the cliché "Take one for the team." This is what she's doing. Have you ever played with someone who doesn't have this skill? Who chooses to ignore the warnings from friends during a game? Someone who is more me, me, me and less team, team, team. Or someone who has created division between players—some worthy and some not? How do you like them? Are they your bestie? Do you want to invite them over for game night? We are guessing the answer is no. There is room for growth. **Awareness** is where we begin.

Wonder

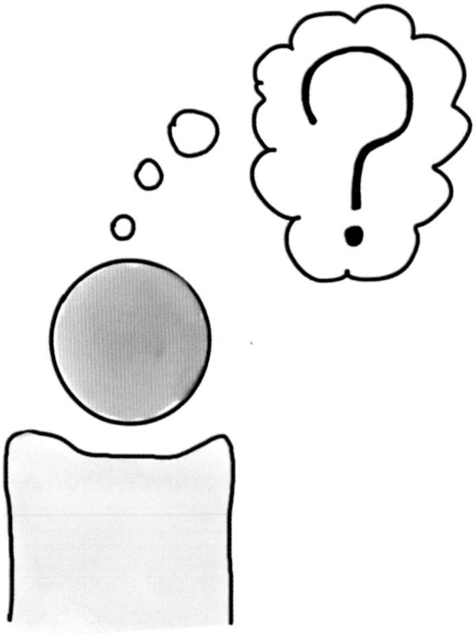

No, not "I wonder" as in "I'm curious." This is different. This is the sense of wonder. As in awe. The emotion we allow ourselves to have in the small moments.

Focus here on the *how* rather than the *what*. How do we *perceive* our environment? Are our eyes open to beauty?

We don't need to go *big* and create carnival-like experiences (although we all love a vacay). We just need to practice experiencing the wonder in our world.

How often do we seek beauty in small moments?

In the book *A Shadow Passes* (1919), English author and playwright Eden Phillpotts writes of looking at a buckbean through a microscope: "The universe is full of magical things, patiently waiting for our senses to grow sharper." Sometimes the wonder isn't obvious. We have to look for it.

I (Julie) am an early riser. I wasn't always, but now that my quiet time is limited with my two teenage daughters and my efforts to be present with them while I have them at home, I intentionally get up early to capture moments alone. I slide out of bed, grab my robe, and get into my house shoes. I put them in the same place every night so I can find them in the dark. After a quick brush of my teeth, I walk down the stairs. There is a large window in my foyer that lets in light from the moon. Sometimes, if it has rained the night before (like this morning), I can see the sparkles of water droplets clinging to the window pane. It's like holiday lights—the sheer beauty of light coming through each droplet is awe-some.

Jed interrupting: When I have a moment like that I think about how far the light has traveled, coming from the sun, bouncing off the moon, finally landing on my window to create magic with water molecules that have been around since the beginning of time and in that moment my eyes are the lucky ones that gets to see them meet. Talk about WONDER!

Julie: In my defense, it's too early yet to think that hard, but it sure is pretty.

Imagine how many opportunities we miss when we don't **intentionally** look for the beauty in the cracks all around us.

Imagination

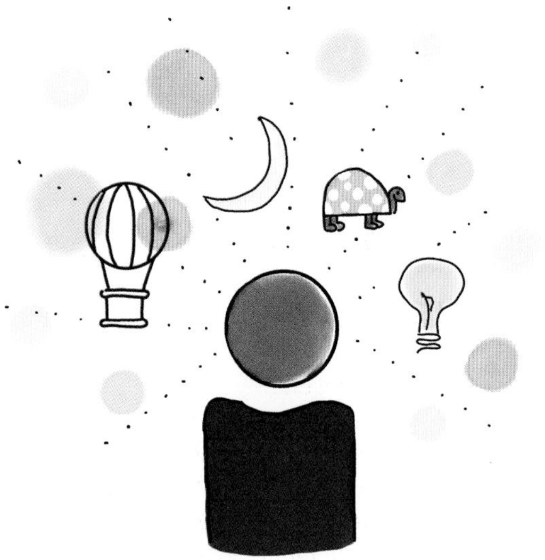

While artists and musicians are often credited with this quality, we want to take it a bit deeper. Imagination is the ability to take whatever situation we have, reimagine it for what we hope it to be, and take the necessary steps to move forward.

The key to imagination here is the hope.

What do we have now that didn't exist 20 years ago? This is easy—just look at your phone. What clickable squares are present that meet your needs? My phone has Etsy, Instacart, Libby, and Calm. Jed's phone has The Weather Channel, Hulu, BuzzFeed, and SoundHound.

These are all examples of how someone saw a need and embraced their imaginative spirit to rise to the challenge. They answered the call of hope. Now, we don't have to invent the next Wow Wow 3000 to be considered imaginative. But we must confess, we are now imagining what the Wow Wow 3000 is (that's here for all you Wow Wow Wubbzy fans), and how fun it might be in the swimming pool. Since we are encouraging you to live a playful life, why not doodle an image of what you think the Wow Wow 3000 is? Share your art with the world on social media #ThePlayfulLife.

How often do we reframe problems to seek solutions?

I had always wanted a room filled with books. There is something about holding a book, smelling a book, that calms me. I could only imagine what it feels like to be surrounded by them. In my new home (we moved at the height of the 2020 pandemic), I created such a room. I sit in there with my feet up holding a book and breathing in the aroma of paper. It's so wonderful, I am looking to other spaces in my home that could be transformed to give peace. Lately, I've been eyeing my bedside table. I don't need a table there. I need a low bookshelf. Matching ones on each side. I read in bed All. The. Time. It makes sense. Combined with my love of thrifting and repurposing, I am now on a mission. I share this story here because this quality doesn't have to be elaborate and complicated. This is a simple example of imagination—seeing my space and imagining what it could be. Trusting the **process** of discovery. I analyzed my current situation, imagined what it could be, and took the step of creating a space that fills me up.

Spontaneity

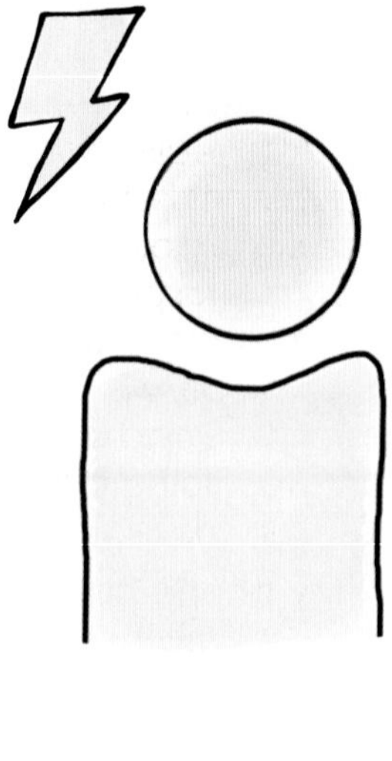

Being spontaneous is incredibly difficult in the busy days we live in. We live and die by our calendars, alarms, schedules, and time clocks. We do this so much that many of us can barely function when we go off-script. Spontaneity is the quality of embracing unexpected experiences at a moment's notice. It's the habit of doing this so often, we are not rattled when change comes our way.

How do you react when unexpected opportunities rearrange your schedule for you?

Hi. Julie here. I'm a planner. I have two digital calendars and at least two paper calendars. Each has its own purpose.

Jed interrupts (again) Lists, don't forget your lists. The day we met, you literally had three grocery lists for three locations on three different days. I am anxious just typing that.

Julie pauses. (Grins) You're right.

But what we're talking about here is not planning, but rather the willingness to go "off plan." As I type these words, it's December and the forecast is for clear skies and a high of 75. If my kiddos get in the car this afternoon and want to go for a walk or do something—anything—to enjoy this sunshine, how inclined am I to embrace the unexpected change despite what's on the calendar? That's spontaneity. I get that we have responsibilities in life, but consider your gut reaction to a curveball in your carefully planned life. If our gut reaction is negative, we need to work on our openness to spontaneity.

Researchers in Italy and Austria recently published findings that proved a causal relationship between spontaneity and psychological well-being (Testoni et al., 2016). Citing Moreno and Freud (who to me look like the Godfather and George Carlin, respectively), they discuss the challenge of living creatively—if we are co-creators of our own universe, we must also be flexible and adaptive if we want to create reality from our dreams.

Jed doesn't know I'm typing this, but he modeled this concept beautifully earlier this week. The past few months for us both have been full. He has traveled a lot, speaking and training in school districts across the country. In other words, he has been "on" a lot, and he needed an escape. As we were working, he took a minute to scroll his Instagram and saw that one of his favorite celebrities, Leslie Jordan, was doing a live show at the Ryman in Nashville. Within minutes, Jed looked at his calendar, saw that it was empty on the date of the event, bought tickets, booked a hotel, and even made a reservation for a fun dinner. I watched in awe (and a bit of jealousy, if I'm honest). He did this without knowing if anyone would go with him. He bought two tickets just in case he found a friend who wanted to join, but he was totally willing to go it alone because he knew his brain needed some playful down time. Talk about spontaneity.

When we are open to new experiences, we invite opportunities for growth. The more we embrace these unexpected moments the practice of spontaneity becomes a **habit**.

Humor

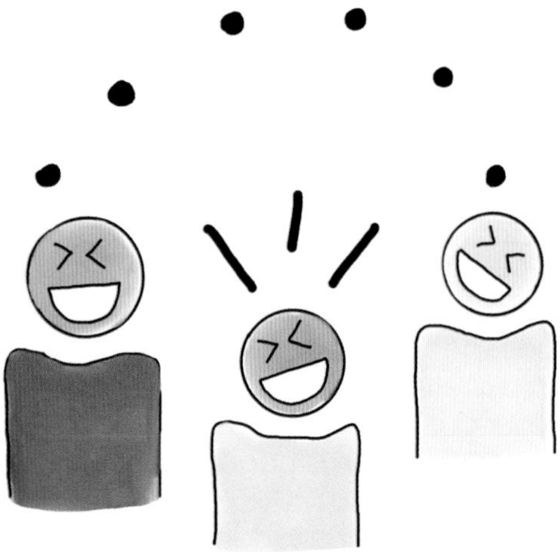

LOL. LM*O. HAHAHAHA. Snort. Humor is the easiest trait to recognize because we all associate it with laughter. Did you know that when we laugh—when we experience joy—the brain releases dopamine (the pleasure chemical)? At the same time neurons are firing for new thoughts in the front of the brain, these happy chemicals are pushing up from the back. These neural connections join in the happiest of *Fantasia*, Mickey-directing symphonies ever. When our brains make these connections, we build *resiliency*—one of the main benefits of humor.

So that's what happens in the brain, but what about that part we can feel from humor? You know, the part you feel in your heart. It's human connection. And it's just as important in our lives as anything else. When humor is used to put others at ease, amuse, and improve relationships, we are allowing ourselves to open up and engage honestly with others.

How often do we invite laughter into our lives to build community and grow the bonds of friendship?

According to the US Department of Veterans Affairs (2020), the benefits of laughter and humor are immense. You'll want to check out their website for more information, but here are just a few to tide you over:

- Laughter increases heart and respiratory rates as well as oxygen consumption over a short period. After these initial changes, a person moves into a state of relaxation. While these effects may not be equivalent to aerobic exercise, as some claim, that is not to say that laughter is entirely without benefit as a physical activity. Ten to 15 minutes of laughter per day may burn 10–40 extra calories.
- Laughter affects heart function. It increases stroke volume and cardiac output, and it dilates blood vessels.
- Watching humorous videos revs up the sympathetic nervous system (SNS), without increasing blood pressure.
- Laughter lowers levels of the stress hormone cortisol.
- Laughter activates the mesolimbic dopaminergic reward system in the brain.
- Laughter raises levels of beta-endorphins (the feel-good chemicals of the body) and increases human growth hormone

(Jed here). Julie mentioned my spontaneous trip to see Leslie Jordan in Nashville a while back, and if there is ever a time to tell you all about the fun I had at his show, it is in this section about humor. When I tell y'all I laugh 'til I peed, that is not a hyperbole. Ask my friend Max, who joined me that night. We cried laughing more than once. Leslie Jordan is someone who fully understands the power of humor to build community and grow the bonds of friendship. And he does it through the art of storytelling with the most authentic heart. What makes his work even more special is that he shares so openly and honestly about deeply personal events from his life that it draws you in and makes you feel as if you've known him forever. If you aren't familiar with him, a few need-to-knows are that (1) he is an actor/comedian, (2) he grew up in a conservative Southern evangelical church, and (3) he's an openly gay man. Why are those the important things to know? As an openly gay man myself who also grew up in a conservative evangelical church in the South, I can tell you first-hand that those two groups of people, the gays and the evangelicals, are not always the best of friends. In fact, I'd say it is very rare for them to get along at all. But at Leslie's show, his humor and authenticity somehow brought them together for more than two hours. One minute he's telling a funny story about his youthful days as a gay guy, and the next minute he's singing a hymn.

Out of nowhere he randomly cracks a joke about the weather and the whole audience—both the conservative evangelicals and the gays—was laughing hysterically, as one in the same room.

Humor helps relieve tension, reassure people, and draw them together. Imagine the positive **results** on society if we would all embrace laughter just a bit more.

CHAPTER 5

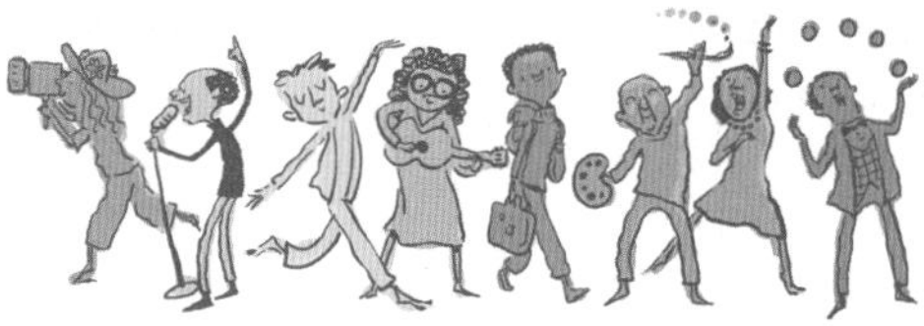

Cultivating a Playful Mindset

"Oh my gosh—I just love you guys! You're so fun!" We've heard that. And sometimes we feel playful. Especially when we have people over, and we're all sociable.

We smile.
We laugh.
We take all the selfies.

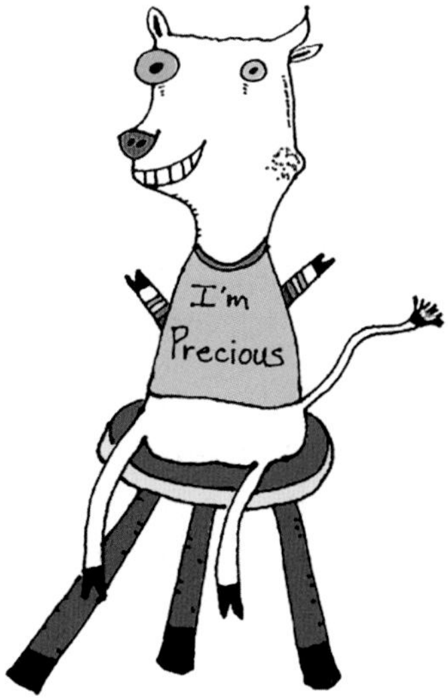

But we also feel playful when we're sitting alone at home with a book. We feel it when we're doodling and are all warm and fuzzy from the *precious* cow who now appears on the page before us. Yes, he's sitting on a stool. Aren't all cows? We sometimes even feel it when we are walking down the street and see a pretty sunset, a fluffy cloud, or even a crack in the sidewalk that looks like a friendly creature smiling at us.

After considering our own playful process, and many, *many* conversations with our playful friends, we penned what we believe are steps that help us define a playful mindset. It's important to note here that this is a process, not a destination. Just like yoga is a practice, play is something we actively work toward. Every day. Did you see those hidden gems we hid in the previous chapter? Did you notice the bold words? Yep, that was intentional. Keep reading to see the connection!

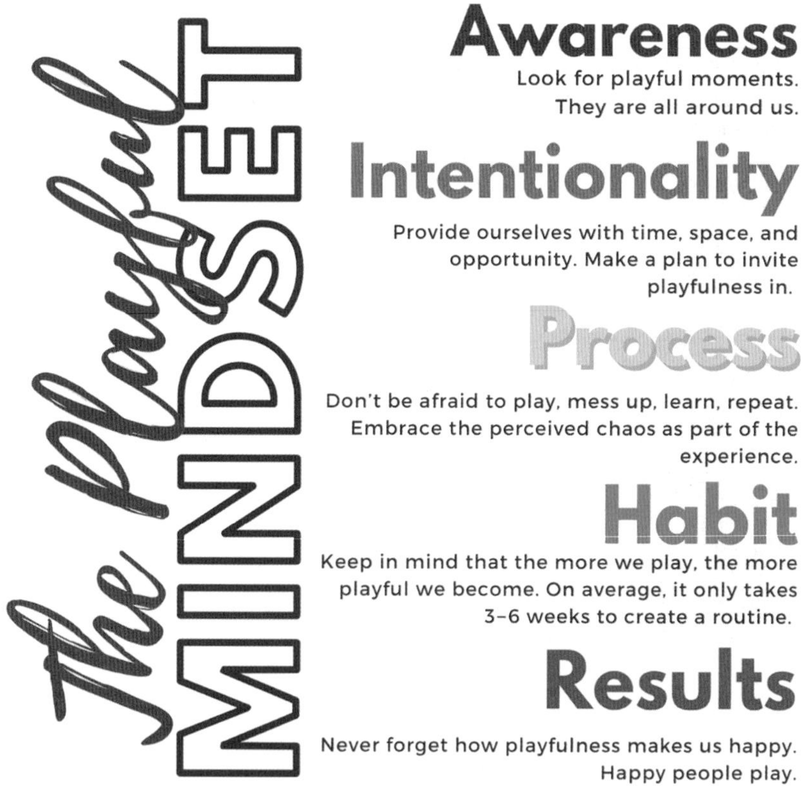

Awareness

Look for playful moments. They are all around us.

Speaking of cows on a stool, let me (Julie) tell you something funny. Every morning, as I take my girls to school—a 20-minute drive through the country—we pass several fields and farms. We all love the colors of the sunrise, and since we leave the house at 7 a.m. (my oldest is rather punctual), we have the opportunity to capture the sunrise daily. Yes, we have a collection—see the following.

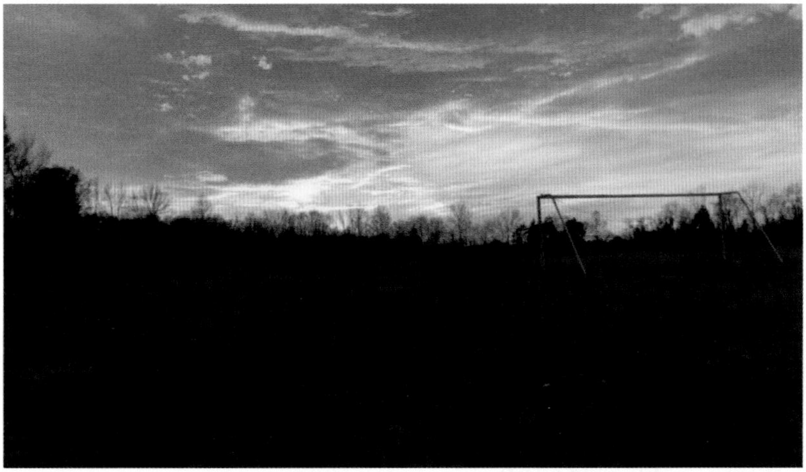

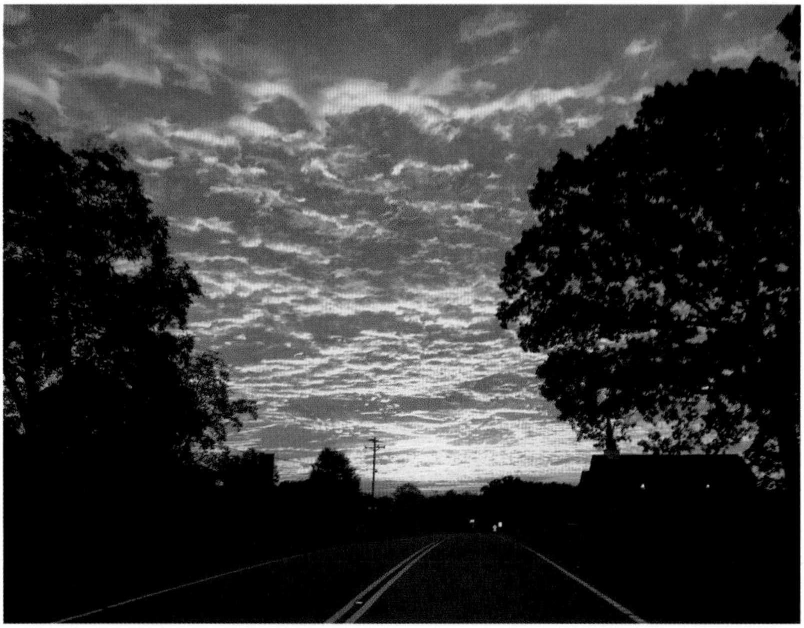

We also pass two fields of cows—one of which has a large pond, and recently *many* baby cows to complete the picture. Each day, I say, "Awww, look at those cows," and they both say, "Mooooo." Or at least one of them does. Sometimes middle schoolers are too cool for that. I digress. This morning, I missed the cows. Why? Because on the other side of the road, I saw a horse. It was the blackest, most beautiful creature. On its face was a white spot, right where we'd say his forehead was. So the conversation went like this—

Me: What a pretty horse. . . . What should its name be? There is a white spot right here—did you see it? How about Moon?

Them: Sure, Mom.

Me: Moony?

Oldest: No. Mooney is in *Harry Potter*.

Me: Okay, so just Moon?

Them: Yes.

Me: What about Dr. Moon? (chuckles to self). See, it's all alone. Those other horses keep calling him a smart-horse (rude because they really calling him a smart*ss, but he's a horse, not a donkey). He's done with them. Dr. Moon needs some new horse friends. Bless him. . . . Oh, look! More cows!

Them: Mooo.

This story is true. It is exactly how our morning went.

I didn't spend money to make it happen. It wasn't a complicated ordeal. It was our ordinary morning drive. I just happen to actively look for playful moments everywhere. Maybe it's become a coping mechanism for me—a way to balance all the worries of the world. So far, it helps.

Intentionality

Provide ourselves with time, space, and opportunity. Make a plan to invite playfulness in.

Are you a planner? Do you have your life scheduled minute by minute on a digital calendar? I do. I know, I mentioned this before. I have a work calendar and a home calendar (sometimes Google and iCal are nice and actually do the merge they are supposed to do). I also have a kitchen calendar on the fridge, and a hand-stenciled calendar in my notebook. But I also juggle the schedules of middle schoolers, teach at the university, and try to create a life in between. I have to have the calendar. Here's what I'm aiming to be better at—not letting the work of daily life dictate each and every minute. Stephen Covey (1990) tells us, "Don't prioritize your schedule. Schedule your priorities." I want to be proactive, not reactive, to my calendar because I know if I wait for the "leftover" time to focus on what's important to me, it will never happen.

So, I plan for play. Play as a behavior. That kind of play. We have one of those advent calendars with the doors—you know the kind. Each day of December, you open a door and there's a surprise inside. Tonight's experience is to make paper snowflakes to hang. I love it because it gets to stay up long past December when the traditional holiday decorations come down. But as I write this to you, I am reflecting. I do not (yet) plan a play calendar for the other months. Why not? It only takes about an hour or so to sit down and pencil in an event in each box. For our advent calendar, some of the experiences are simple, such as watch a holiday movie with hot cocoa. These planned experiences don't have to be elaborate. They simply serve as something to look forward to. How often are we giving ourselves daily treats (tangible or not) to look forward to?

Process

Don't be afraid to play, mess up, learn, repeat. Embrace the perceived chaos as part of the experience.

Y'all. I wanna be an artist so bad. I mean, so bad. Like a painter. I want my work hanging on a wall in a hipster coffee shop, a children's bookstore, or some posh museum filled with trendy art. But quite frankly, my art isn't all that great. Truly, it's subpar. Julie is such a great painter. I am confident that one day her work will hang somewhere cool while mine goes to die alone in my home office's closet. I won't even hang most of it on the walls of my own house. While it sounds like self-deprecation here, I am not feeling sorry for myself one bit. In fact, I am ready to leave this place and get home to my acrylics and brushes. Why did writing about my poor art skill make me want to paint? Because I am never gonna get any better if I don't respect the process and do the work to cultivate my artistic skills. I haven't always been so eager to hone those skills. Truthfully, I was/am afraid to paint a lot of times. I am terrified of messing up. I have at least 20 blank canvases in my supply stash right this minute because I am scared to death of ruining them. Paint? Yep. I have all kinds. Acrylic, oil, watercolor, gouache, tempera, and finger. (Julie here . . . I just spit my drink.) LOL. Yes . . . finger paint. I am scared of that too. Fear aside, I do find my courage from time to time and create a masterpiece. Okay, maybe not a masterpiece, but definitely a tried-my-best-erpiece. Recently, I found some courage to try a new technique with paint using palette knives. Without getting into an art lesson here, it's basically smearing the paint on the canvas. I decided to smear a rainbow on top of another rainbow. I was scared to do it. But I did it. Guess what? It turned out to be a hot mess. But, I learned some things, and I will try again soon because I trust the process. Try. Fail. Try Again. Repeat as needed.

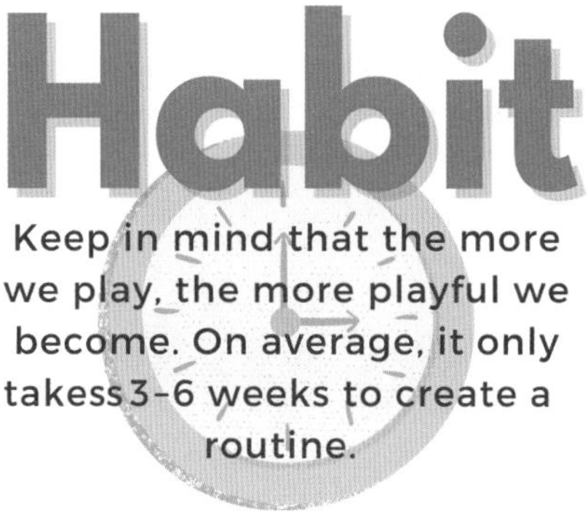

What we have talked about so far is intentional moments of play that we plan, schedule, and prepare for. But once the habit of play sets in, the moments just happen regardless of location, date, time, etc. Even now we are sitting in a coffee shop dancing and singing to the music playing. This wasn't a planned dance party. We didn't curate the perfect playlist, invite our friends, or eat hors d'oeuvres. A fun song came on and we started chair-dancing. The baristas joined in. It was a blast. Were people staring at us? Of course they were. But what a sad feeling to merely stare at a dance party when we have an opportunity to join in. Those who did join understand the power of the playful mindset. The baristas needed a pick-me-up to get through their workday, and we needed a jolt to our mojo to get us moving toward our writing goal for the day. Guess what . . . we passed our goal. I am convinced that the habit of playfulness integrated into our work/life flow helped make that happen. That, and some caffeine.

Now, how much play is needed? I get it: you want a prescription—a formula for the playful life. Y'all. That formula ain't gonna happen. It's different for us all. You might be inclined to have more play in your week than I do. You might have noticed an ebb and flow of focus or concentration during your time playing. During these experiences, you might have even lost your sense of time: *Have you ever been so engrossed in a task that you forgot to eat?*

If so, you have been one of the lucky individuals to experience a state of flow. This is what Diane Ackerman calls *deep play* (2000). Deep play can happen if you're creating, and deep play can happen as you play checkers with a buddy. Deep play is easy to see in children as they play on the playground in what many of us know as free play: the play in which we are free to choose our path without instructions or guidance from someone else. Those experiences of free play during which you collaborated with your teammate to strategize and win a board game—that is play.

The exhilaration you experienced when you decided to go for it (whatever it was), taking a risk knowing you might fail, but trying anyway—also a result of play.

We need to cultivate a habit of play—whether free or structured play throughout the week—heavens, every day if possible!

Results

Never forget how playfulness makes us happy. Happy people play.

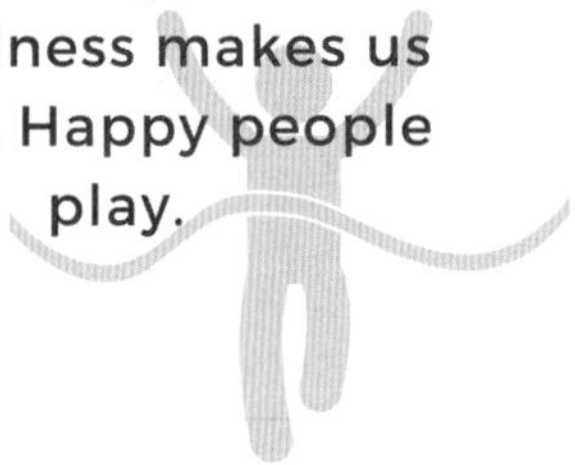

Have you ever watched a teenager with a new video game?

They play to figure it out.

What about a toddler with a new toy?

They play to see what happens.

A mechanic with a new project?

They play to see how it works—to find what might be going wrong.

A mathematician with a puzzle to solve?

They play as they look for patterns—a sequence that leads to a solution.

The joy—y'all, the sheer joy. These are just a few examples of how play leads to results, and these results bring happiness. (Jed here) I promise you I feel joy while I paint even though it's not that great. I like to think like this about my paintings, even the not-so-great ones. Never before in all of humanity has that piece of art existed until that very moment in time. I gave it life, y'all! That's so exciting to me. Can you fathom? "All of time" is a long time, and my effort brought forth this new thing! Okay, maybe I am a bit hyperbolic, but you feel me, right?

I (Julie) feel joy as I close a book cover and return it to its home on the shelf, the story now living in my mind. What do I do? I scan the shelves. Pulling my fingers along the spines of the book's friends, seeing which one wants to be read next. Eventually, I pull another one down and begin another adventure. I read daily. Nonfiction in the morning, fiction at night. I'm intentional—getting up at 5:15 to have coffee and words on the page. Sometimes, I love the book, and sometimes it's not the right season for me and that particular work. I trust the process and keep on. It's a habit that brings me comfort and joy. Because I read, I have ideas. Because I have ideas, I write. The creative process continues.

When we are aware of the opportunity to play, and intentionally make time for play, respect the process of play, and cultivate a habit of play, the result is life!

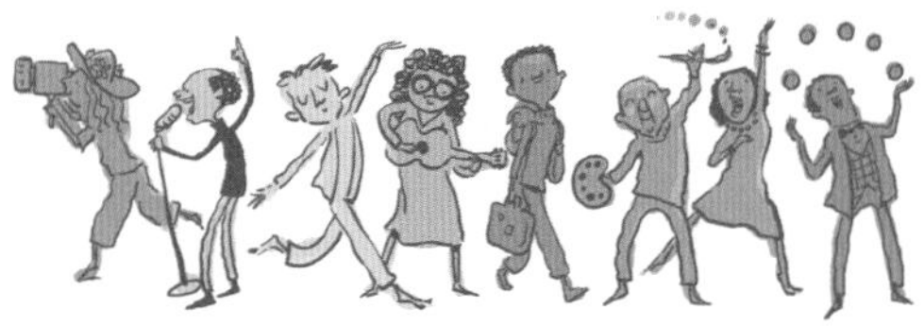

Play & Ponder

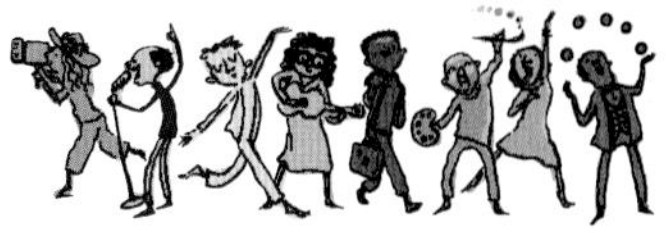

At the end of each section you will find an opportunity for you to play and ponder. Ponder means to think about something carefully, especially before making a decision or reaching a conclusion. Use these questions and playful experiences to guide you to reflect about your lived experience and how you can take action to create a more playful life.

- Be spontaneous. Right now, put down this book and do something that brings you joy. Don't make a plan. Don't worry about the other things on the to-do list. Get up. Go do it. Seriously. *Go!* When you get finished with whatever you decide to do, think about how it made you feel, then tell a friend about your experience. Next time, take them with you.
- Discovering who *you* are as a playful being is vital to the playful life. If you don't like something, you shouldn't do it. Focus on things you do enjoy. What are those things? We often encourage students to doodle a page of pictures that captures their thoughts. Why not take a moment and do that now? Don't like to doodle? Then maybe create a vision board of your playful desires using pics from magazines. You could make a digital version too. :)
- Are there opportunities in your day to be playful?

The answer to this question is a big ol' yes! Even if your job is high-stress, like a neurosurgeon or astrophysicist, you are likely to use the restroom at some point during the day. Why not have a dance party in front of the mirror while you are in there? Even if it's only a brief moment of silliness making faces while you wash your hands, a little bit of play goes a *long* way. Other ideas are to:

Skip to your next destination if you are walking. Who cares if people laugh? You will feel better and get in a bit of cardio while you work!

Listen to a funny podcast while sitting in traffic. We love NPR, but sometimes the news is a bit heavy. Why be stuck in traffic adding to the misery with the day's news when you can literally have a moment of laughter during the middle of the madness?

Okay. You are in your cubicle. Life is being sucked out of you with every passing minute. There is a coworker on the other side of the partition feeling the same way. Write a silly word on a piece of paper and toss it over. Listen to their guffaw. It is contagious. Yes, I just did this with Julie and it totally worked. My word? . . . kumquat. HAHAHAHAHA

SECTION 2

Memory

Your play history is made up of all the things you ever did in the past connected to playing. A cardboard box in the backyard, coloring at your granny's, climbing trees with your cousins, your first middle school party, the prom, etc. See how those experiences cover the span of your life? Have you ever reflected on your own play history and how it has impacted your life? While we hope that you were coloring at your granny's well into your teen years, the reality is you probably colored around age 5 and the prom was much later. Regardless of the time period of your life, all of these experiences make up your play history. In essence, what role did play/playfulness serve in the years of your life prior to the moment you picked up this book? Take a moment here to do some thinking. Maybe call a family member or friend and have a chat about the times when . . .

We all have different play histories. Some of us had very privileged lives growing up. Trips to Disney and the petting zoo are far more common for some than others. Privilege doesn't

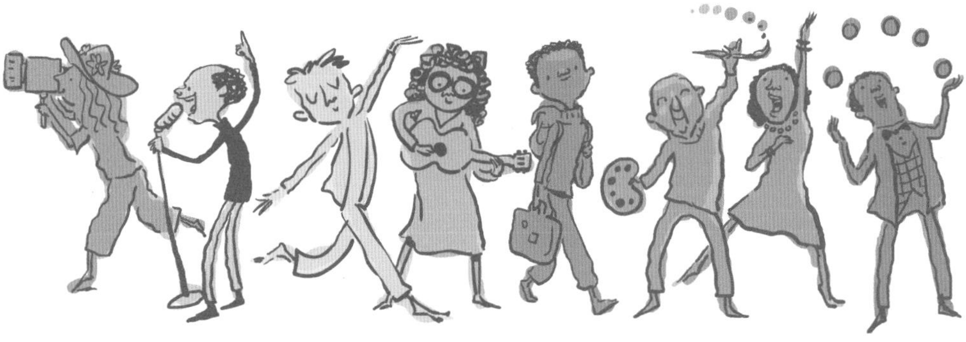

always have to do with financial means, though. Skin color, religious beliefs, gender, and heterosexuality often provide benefits for some that are not granted to all. Some folks were privileged with safety and stability in their families that allowed for a much different type of play history than others. I (Jed) grew up in a home that was a bit tumultuous. My play history was not the same as some of my friends. Don't mishear me. My mom was/is *amazing* and provided so many playful moments in my life. One year we didn't have much money for Halloween decorations so she and I made a hundred or so bats, pumpkins, and ghosts out of construction paper and hung them from the ceiling with yarn to make the home a bit more festive. It was one of my favorite Halloweens ever because of the fun we had decorating the house. Mom was always creating moments (read memories) of play in spite of the difficult circumstances we often faced. I credit my mother with instilling in me the spirit of play that I carry with me today. I think it was because of the instability that she always found ways to guide my sister and me toward being more playful in our day-to-day routines because she knew even then that play would help us through the hardships. She was no scientist, nor researcher, but she was (and *is*) a good mama and she knew what we needed to make it through.

I am no scientist, either, but I am able to read the work of scientists—the research—(put your fur down, you academic folks like Julie—that research is in the next chapter) and see the impact that our play histories have on us adults. You will read later about specific research regarding animals and play, but a sneak peek of the results of that research is that we all have a biological predilection to play. It's part of our DNA. And because it is part of our DNA, we strive to cultivate this inherent playful nature. Isn't it amazing how my mama knew? Was it her own biological predilection that was leading her to create those moments? Maybe. I like to think her instincts were aligned with a biological need to protect her children from the "danger that lurked" beyond the cave, nest, home. She protected us by honing our natural survival instincts. She gave us a play history that would follow us into adulthood and remind us of the need for playful living as we faced the trials that were sure to come as we aged.

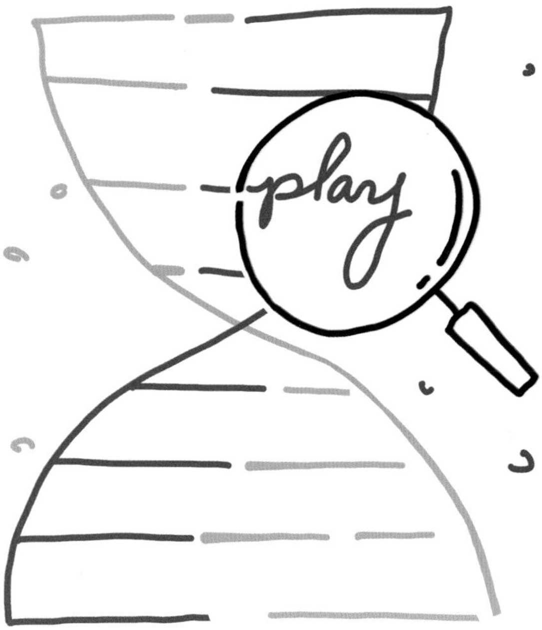
play

CHAPTER 6

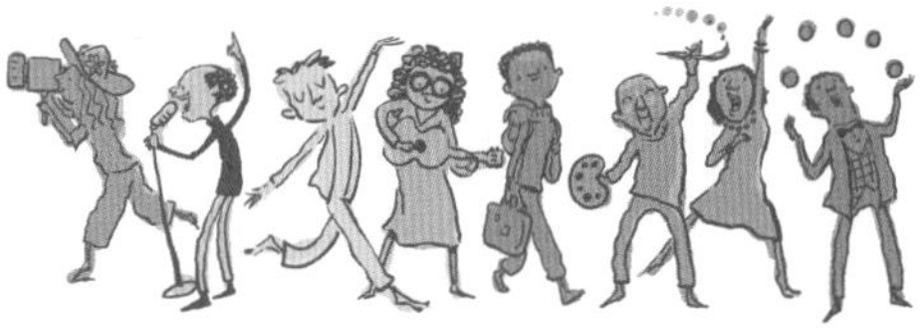

Things We Learned from Playing

Think back to a playful experience you had as a child. Picture it (thank you, Sophia Petrillo) . . . a play memory in your head.

Where are you?
What time is it?
What are you doing?
Who is with you?

Most times, what brought us joy as children will give a special kind of joy to us as adults.

The beauty of having a few more years on us is the benefit of experience. But, we have to be careful not to let that experience keep us from doing something new. There is a concept called the novice advantage. Jonathan Eckert (2016) wrote an entire book about it. The promise is this: when we are new to something, we have questions. We seek out support. We take risks and try new things because we have no baseline for how this will go. We are motivated by a passion to know more. Play and playful experiences can bring us comfort, but they can also open our minds to new ways of thinking; new ways to connect with others.

We asked our friends and social media connections what they learned from play as a child. Take a look at their responses.

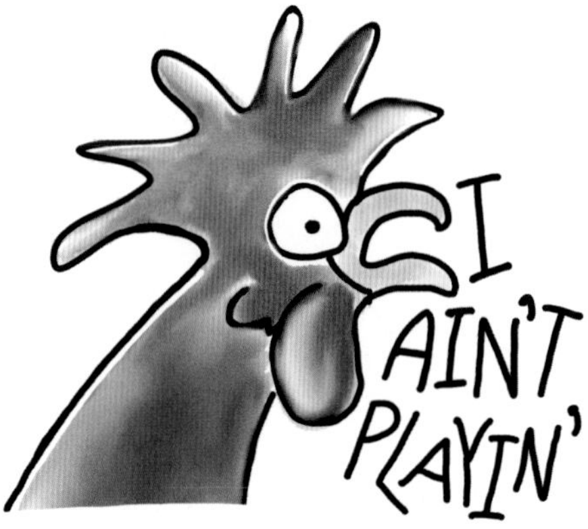

Generally:

- How to share.
- How to divide into teams.
- How to solve problems.
- How to use the materials I have.
- How to work with someone with different ideas.
- How to handle conflict.
- How to use my imagination.
- How to read body language.
- How to be fair.
- Life isn't fair.
- How to take a joke.
- How to be patient.
- How to entertain myself.
- How to engage in life with other people.
- How to be alone.
- How to organize things.
- How to try new things.
- How to love old things.
- What I like.
- What I don't like.
- How to use time wisely.
- Determination/Tenacity.
- Healthy aggression/competition.
- How to speak up.
- When to be quiet.
- Following directions.
- Empathy.
- How to make friends.
- How to handle enemies.
- We all make mistakes.

Specific stories:

- Gravity always wins.
- It's okay to get dirty.
- The mess is worth it.
- Sometimes I win.
- Sometimes I lose.
- Everyone isn't good at the same thing.
- Some people are better than me at things.
- I am not always the best.
- Sometimes you get hurt.
- Sometimes you need a plan.
- Sometimes you just go with the flow.
- Sometimes you don't get what you want.
- Roosters fight back.
- Climbing is difficult, but the view is worth it.
- That yellow stuff inside pecans isn't really cheese.
- Dog food isn't that bad.
- Mud pies really do taste like mud.
- Sometimes the kickball wins.
- The bottom of the lake is gross.
- Grass can cut.
- Tag is more than a game!
- Bees like to sting big toes.
- Mama bird is always nearby.
- Fire is hot.
- A crooked Christmas tree won't stand.
- Geese love a loose diaper.
- Worms poop.
- Brake means stop.
- Water doesn't always make a soft landing.
- Let the hot cocoa rest.

Let's get raw. Be honest with ourselves.

How often do you incorporate play in your life now? How much time do we intentionally dedicate to the experiences that bring us joy?

When did we stop playing?

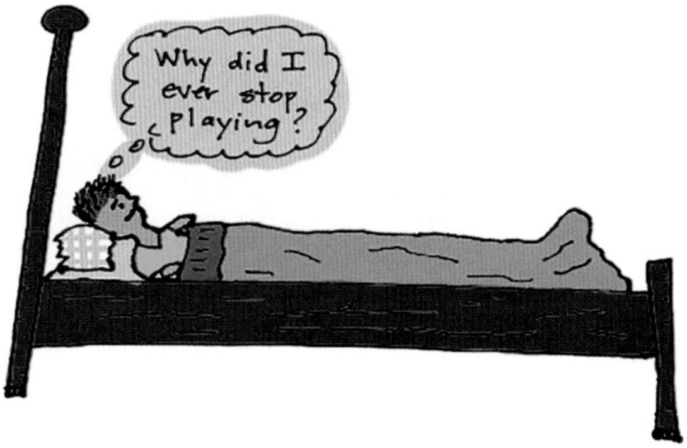

This question is one that haunts us as night falls. It keeps us awake when others are sleeping. Not really, but it does trouble us. Why, you ask? Because we know the answer. And sadly, we think much of the reason lies within our school system. Gosh, how it grieves us to type that, but we know it's true because we are both lifelong educators who have seen the negative impact school has had on playful living. We saw the effect so much so that we literally wrote a book called *The Playful Classroom* in the hope that we could bring play back to schools. The standardized testing culture coupled with the strings attached to funding for high scores on said tests led the way to the removal of play across the board. Kindergarten used to be full of playfulness, but it was replaced by "rigorous" academia so that students would be career-ready at the age of 5. Talk to any educator you know and they will confirm this to be the truth. There are experimental schools where play is valued, but for the masses, there is no time for play, only learning. The irony of that is not lost on us as play is *in fact* learning, regardless of the age.

Later, we begin to live how the world tells us is right. Get up, go to work, work hard, come home, check work email, check the news, eat dinner, work some more, sleep, repeat. Play? Fun? No. We're much too adult for that. As a culture, we've lost touch with the importance of playful living.

This week, I (Julie) was reading the news on my phone as I dried my hair. Weird, maybe. But that's my process. The article I saw can be accessed via the QR code here. The financial crisis in Lebanon was so grave that not even the children wanted to play. I cannot fathom in my privileged existence a world that allows things to be so bad that even the children have no impetus to play. I was affected. I texted Jed the article with the message. What can we do? This is awful. For now, we keep writing. Returning to this section in the first round of book edits, we have now seen Russia invade Ukraine and over the weekend in America, there were numerous racially motivated attacks by white supremacists. We find ourselves still asking . . . *what can we do?*

We clearly need this work in your hands. The world feels especially heavy these days, and the power of play can help lighten that load. In Section Three you'll read about how it can also heal and turn things around. In early 2022, I was reading Glennon Doyle's *Untamed* (2020). In that work she alluded to the words of Archbishop Desmond Tutu, who said we need to keep pulling the people from that river—in other words, keep saving them. However, at some point, we look up-river to find out who or what in the world is pushing them in the river in the first place. That is our advocacy work. Once you understand the benefits of play and why it's so very important, it might be your advocacy work as well.

CHAPTER 7

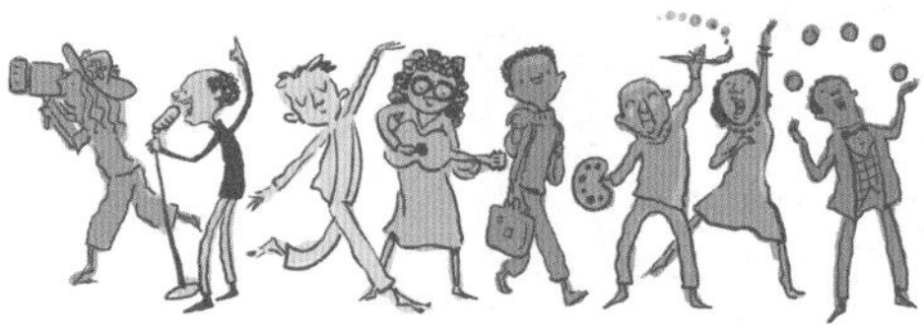

Cognitive Benefits of Play

There are a gozillion benefits of playful living—inside, outside, and beside. Seriously, there are more reasons to play than our grannies have shoes, and trust us. . . . That is a lot!

JULIE: Beside?
JED: Yes . . . all the people beside you.
JULIE: Yes . . . genius.

For you academics in the crowd (Julie, put your hand down), this chapter is for you. Some of you need these nuggets, these juicy research bits to support a change of thinking. Like that dollop of mayo in your cornbread recipe, this part makes the experience rich and tasty for you. You'll see a mix here of some classic (early research) and some more recent publications. If you're like me (Jed), all this research may feel a tad heavy. I will admittedly tell you that I skimmed over some of it. Not because I don't value the research or want it to be in my repertoire of knowledge, but because it gets all jumbled in my brain. I need real-world, concrete explanations of each one so that my brain can be full of BDNF and my DMN gets stronger (read on and you'll see what that means). Do you need the simple nuggets? Do you need to see a real-world connection for playful benefits? Check out this list of authentic lessons we compiled.

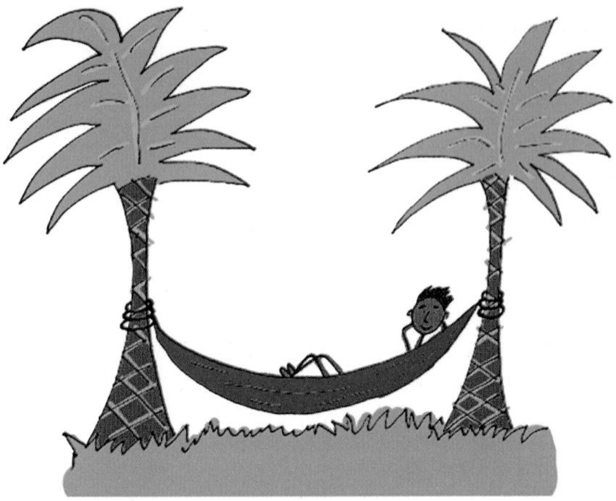

Repetition is the mother of learning. So who's the father? "Dad"ication.

Play Improves Attention and Cognitive Function

Beating your bestie at *Scrabble*, completing the *TV Guide* crossword puzzle (your Great-Aunt Ophelia probably still has a subscription), or engaging in other playful experiences that challenge your brain can help prevent memory loss and improve brain function. Recently, a dear soul in our life had brain surgery. Her doctor recommended *Sudoku* as a method of regaining brain function and sustaining brain activity during the recovery process. The social interaction of playing critical thinking games like *Settlers of Catan* and *Risk* with family and friends can also help ward off stress and depression. There was a time when early cognitive researchers ignored play, assuming it was disconnected from intellectual growth. They were wrong. In reality, play and play-oriented movements improve cognition (Guadagni et al., 2020; Silverman, 1993). The same is true for adults. We just mentioned board games as a way of lessening stress and depression. Check this out—in 2020, Drew M. Altschul and Ian J. Deary found that playing board games can also improve adults' cognitive function well into our seventies and eighties (Altschul & Deary, 2020). Y'all. This was no small study. Altschul and Deary used data from participants in the Lothian Birth Cohort of 1936. They followed these study participants from age 11 into their seventies! Participants were assessed at age 11, then again at 70 (game-playing behaviors), 73, 76 (game playing again), and 79, using a comprehensive cognitive battery of 14 tests. What about the variability across social class, gender, level of activity or education? Yeah . . . they thought of that. All models were controlled for early life cognitive function, education, social class, sex, activity levels, and health issues. Mic drop.

Does playing analog games protect against cognitive decline in older age? Yes. Yes it does.

Okay, what about video games? We got you. Some researchers have suggested that just 1 hour of gaming can improve attention—Dr. Nan Qiu of the University of Electronic Science and Technology of China and Dr. Weiyi Ma of the University of Arkansas found that undergraduate and graduate students who spent 1 hour playing the video game *League of Legends* experienced changes in brain activity (Qiu et al., 2018). What about those of us who wear reading glasses for function? Well, for us older adults, the benefits of games are even more stunning. Brain-training apps may prevent the natural cognitive decline that tends to happen as we age (Savulich et al., 2017). Computer games offer benefits just like those off-screen.

How does free play help when we shift to academics—those tasks that require lots of attention? You guessed it. When we take frequent, brief play breaks, we pay attention to academic tasks better (Bjorkland & Pelligrini, 2000; Kesslak, So, Choi, Cotman, & Gomez-Pinilla, 1998; Pellegrini & Holmes, 2006; Stevenson et al., 1990). No matter how we spin it, play *wins*.

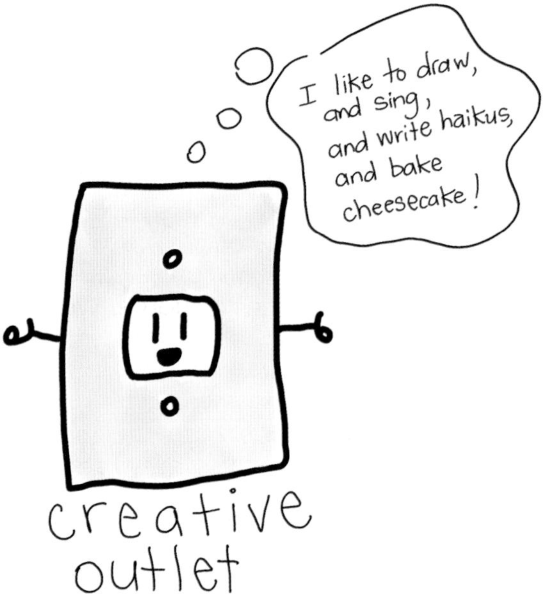

Play Enhances Creativity

In his TED talk "Tales of Creativity and Play," Tim Brown, CEO of the design firm IDEO, shares, "We think playfulness helps us to get to better solutions. Helps us do our jobs better and helps us feel better when we do them" (T. Brown, 2008). When we look at the traditional understanding of play, this makes sense. Play is fun—or the absence of work (not true!)—but when we really look at play and all it does for us, we realize it's the go-to way we begin to think. Play stimulates our imagination and inspires our creativity. No, not our ability to create art, as is a common misconception about being creative. Multiple research studies demonstrate how play engenders insightful, divergent thinking (Russ, 2003). Creativity is our ability to think, adapt old things into new things, and solve problems.

When we synthesize parts of our experience to create a new idea, this is the essence of what creativity is all about. Here are some examples of how your life has been impacted by the creativity of another person's *well, hot dang!* moment:

- You know, Alexander Fleming—the guy who discovered antibacterial properties of penicillin—was quite a playful character. His superiors scoffed at how he treated his research like one does a game, often explaining his work by saying, "I play with microbes," or "... it is very pleasant to break the rules and be able to find something that nobody had thought of."
- Mozart was notorious for his high-spirited pranks and jokes, which are also reflected in his music. His three-voice canon (KV559) has a nonsensical Latin part, which, when sung, sounds like risqué German.
- M.C. Escher wrote, "I can't keep from fooling around with our irrefutable certainties. It is, for example, a pleasure knowingly to mix up two- and three-dimensionalities, flat and spatial, and to make fun of gravity." Ahh, now those impossible staircases make sense.
- When Jim Watson and Francis Crick were uncovering the structure of DNA, they used colored balls—much like those you'd find in a kindergarten classroom. Watson wrote: "All we had to do was to construct a set of molecular models and begin to play." Their play resulted in the double helix we know today.
- We are told that in a famous encounter between Margaret Thatcher and Mikhail Gorbachev, Thatcher came to the table in a serious mood—she was determined to do ideological battle. Gorbachev reportedly brought a sense of fun and

lack of bitterness. The result? Diplomatic creativity. Well, hot dang (Bateson, 2015).

For those of you who want the brain science piece, Julie has added a little section here to crank your tractor. See the box below.

There is a protein in our brain called brain-derived neurotrophic factor (BDNF). I imagine it to be our brain's version of those sparklers kids play with on the Fourth of July. What does it do?

- Promotes the survival of nerve cells (neurons).
- Plays a role in the growth, maturation, and maintenance of nerve cells.
- Is active when cells communicate with each other.
- Regulates synaptic plasticity (important for learning and memory).

Why is this protein important? Y'all. Play and exploration trigger the secretion of BDNF. When we play, we grow brain cells! (Dewer, 2014; Gordon et al., 2003; Greenough & Black, 1992)

CHAPTER 8

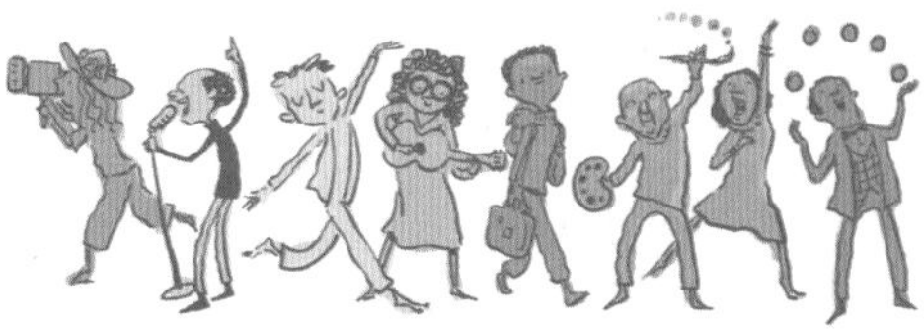

Social Emotional Benefits of Play

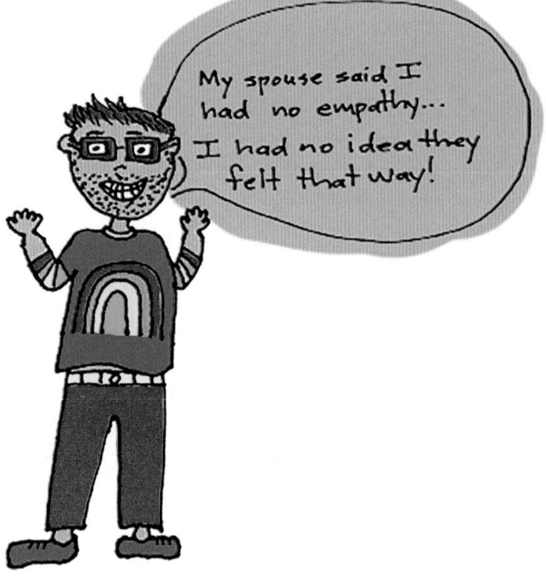

Play Develops Empathy

If ever there was a time our world needed more empathy, compassion, trust, and intimacy with others, it is now. Laughing, playing, or "cuttin' up," as we like to call it down here, can help strengthen all our abilities to see others with soft eyes. Grace, mercy, etc. Playing doesn't have to include a specific activity; as we have said many times already, it can also be a mindset. Having a playful mindset can help us loosen up, relax, and break the ice with strangers as well as get along a bit better with Uncle Frank, who sometimes likes to say the most inappropriate things at family gatherings. So, how do we work toward not being another Uncle Frank? How can we use play to enhance empathy?

- When you're in the game, be *in* the game. Be a part, not apart. Life is a contact sport—get involved, and model the behavior you would like to see from others.
- Consider all perspectives as you play with others. How does it feel to be on the other side?
- Oooh . . . be cautious with language. Avoid using the words "winners" and "losers," focusing instead on the people who won or lost. Winning and losing is an action, but it doesn't define us.
- Mama says, "If you ain't got nothing nice to say then don't say nothing at all." If you lose the game or if someone does better than you, say few words. If you win, you hush up. No one likes a braggadocious celebrant. Just because you are a rooster doesn't mean we want to hear you crow. Either way, compliment the opponent on a game well played.

While these tips focus on games where someone is winning or losing, they can also be applied to making art, telling jokes, or collecting poisonous dart frogs. No, we aren't anti-winners here, but we are definitely against defining a person based on their wins or losses. Not everyone makes the greatest art, tells the best jokes, or has the most adorable frog collection. We all need to be mindful that no one is perfect and we aren't the best all the time.

For some of us, reading is a form of play. We explore other worlds and new adventures through the power of story. Dr. Rudine Sims Bishop (1990) shares how these stories serve as a window (seeing another's life), a mirror (seeing ourselves reflected in the story), or a sliding glass door (through which our imagination walks and becomes a part of the story's world). When we routinely practice exploring through the lens of a character, our imagination builds empathy (Mar et al., 2006).

As 5- and 6-year-olds, we learned to read. At the same time, we were becoming aware of ourselves. Classical constructivist Jean Piaget tells us we are developing beyond our egocentric selves at this same time. This time in our lives is a beautiful symphony of development. The self-awareness we are cultivating in the first and second grade leads to empathy. As we are more aware of our own emotions, we can recognize them in others. The more we practice walking in the shoes of our neighbor, the stronger our sense of empathy becomes (Engelen, 2021).

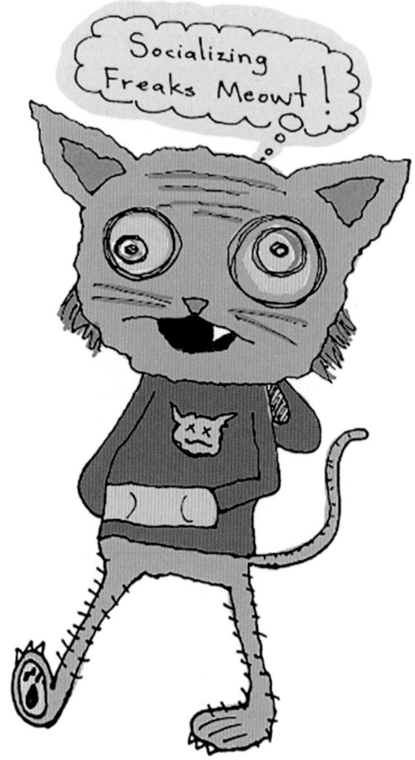

Play Enhances Our Social Skills.

JULIE: I have a friend with no social skills and a PhD in the history of palindromes.
I call him Dr. Awkward.

JED: I cannot believe people paid good money for that pun, Julie!

JULIE: (cannot reply, she's laughing so hard)

During the act of play, there is give and take. We have ideas, and so do those we play with. Through play, children are practicing the skill of communication—through oral and body language, cooperation, and teamwork. Even roughhousing establishes boundaries and builds trust. Our friend Dr. Anthony DeBenedet says rough play is good for our brains—in the amygdala and cerebellum (where our emotions live alongside language and logic) play stimulates neural growth (DeBenedet & Cohen, 2011). In fact, skills in a rough-and-tumble setting are linked to later academic performance. Kids, up to grade 3, who engage in intense physical play have higher cognitive and emotional intelligence than those who don't engage in physical play. I can remember my girls playing in the yard before they were school-aged. As they rolled in the grass play-fighting, they also read body language, facial expressions, and social cues that communicated when to keep going and when to stop. DeBenedet says, "It may be counter-intuitive, but (rough and tumble play) really helps kids develop."

As adults we continue to work on our skill of reading people through both play and playful communication. An NPR article (Yenigun, 2014) I read recently tells of an adult play group in San Francisco, California. On Friday nights, at the Taqueria San Jose on Mission Street, you might stumble upon small groups of grown-ups huddled around little figurines. This group, called SF Games, has been active for nearly 20 years. The premise? German-style board games. Unlike American games, such as *Monopoly*, this German-styles gaming ensures that there's always something to do. Instead of games in which you get to a certain point and somebody's knocked out with nothing to do for the next half-hour, this group of gamers teaches and includes all people, with little downtime. You'll find groups like this one all around the world.

These social groups are just one example of adult play that builds social skills. When we gather together, we give ourselves a chance to maintain social well-being. Whether that's through board games, soccer leagues, paintball, Zoom paint nights via live YouTube feeds, or book club chats—playing helps us connect.

Play Teaches Cooperation with Others

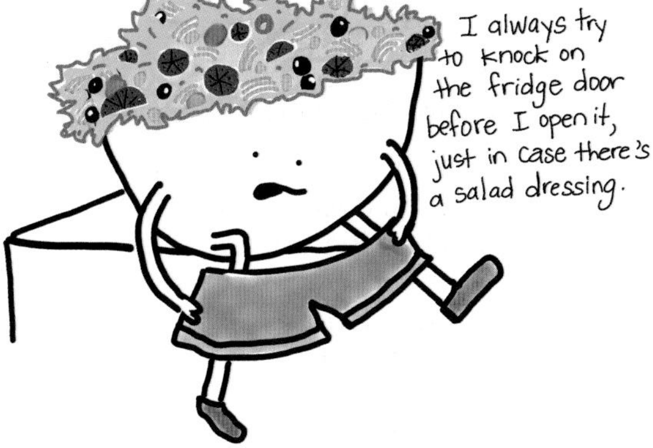

In the American South, the phrase "Y'all play purdy" is one ingrained in our childhood memory. Thanks to many a grandma we learned to "play nice" as we were coming up. Lawsy, if you didn't play nice on the playground at school, you had to sit out and no one wanted that. If you didn't play purdy at home, Granny likely had a hickory switch nearby. Because of that, we learned to work with each other, we created rules of play and followed them, and we socialized in what became our own miniature adult-like world.

Play is a powerful catalyst for positive socialization. As adults, we have the power to use a "play purdy" philosophy to break down barriers and improve our relationships with others. Remember the words of grannies, y'all! Let's dig into some deep thinking here.

Isabel Behncke (2015), a field ethologist who studies animal behavior in an effort to understand humans and our place in nature, explains play behavior as that of "a jester, a joyful shape-shifter, a biological wild card whose value and form changes according to context." Sadly, even in the animal kingdom, play often declines as a subject ages. Play is too often considered to be a developmental tool for a growing individual (in other words, play is too often viewed as the work of a child). Once the individual is an adult, play's perceived role as developmental scaffolding diminishes and play disappears. This realization was a sobering one, but not quite convincing for Behncke—enter the bonobos apes. This species uses adult play as a noteworthy part of their natural behavior—like humans, they are neotenous (say that out loud three times fast). That means they retain juvenile traits as adults. Why should that matter? Positive emotions motivate us (bonobos and humans alike) to interact with novel elements otherwise extraneous to our lives. Have you ever put googly eyes on your lampshade? What about needle-felting a squirrel? Please tell us you have at least made your own pot holder on one of those do-it-yourself looms! No? Well, you should try it. None of these is new to us, but they might be new to you. This novelty can be an entirely new experience or a new variation of a game previously known.

Here is the skinny, y'all. . . . Play makes individuals more adaptable—able to cooperate with others—because it makes us more social, and more successful in our sociability as a result of being more adaptable. Lifelong play, says Behncke, is a bridge between sociability and adaptability.

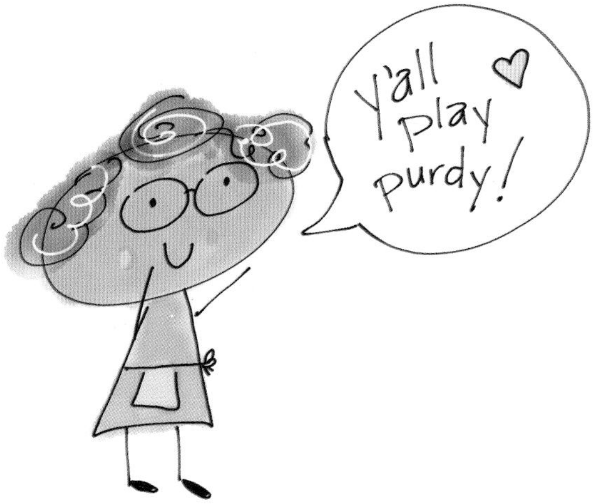
y'all play purdy!

CHAPTER 9

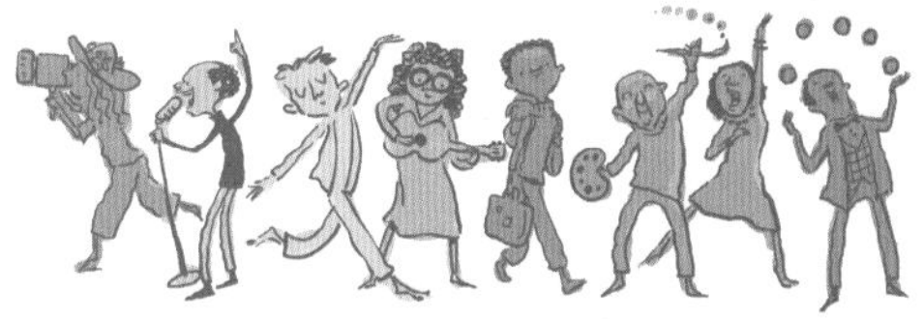

Physical Benefits of Play

Play Keeps Us Healthy, Young, and Happy

Ralph Waldo Emerson wrote these words in his journal on April 19, 1835: "It is a happy talent to know how to play" (Porte, 1984). This talent called play increases our energy and vitality and can even build up our resistance to illness. Take a gander at all the ways play influences our health:

- By strengthening bones, muscles, lungs, and the heart, play that includes movement helps decrease our chances of developing heart disease, diabetes, obesity, and high cholesterol, according to the Mayo Clinic (Kent, 2020).
- Play can even impact dementia (memory loss) (Harvard Medical School, 2020).
- Play slows the aging process, increases energy, and prolongs life (Harvard Medical School, 2020).
- Movement fuels the brain with oxygen, and it also feeds it neurotrophins, which increase the number of connections between neurons (Jensen, 2005).
- Play and movement may increase catecholamines (brain chemicals such as norepinephrine and dopamine), which generally serve to energize and elevate mood (Chaouloff, 1989; Jensen, 2005).
- Play helps build confidence—think of the rush we got as kids when we went down the big slide or went higher than the trees while swingin' (Harvard Medical School, 2020).
- Play teaches us to problem solve.

- Physical play, like sports and exercise, reduces stress hormones and triggers the release of endorphins.
- Laughter, a natural result of play, releases those same feel-good hormones (Yim, 2016).

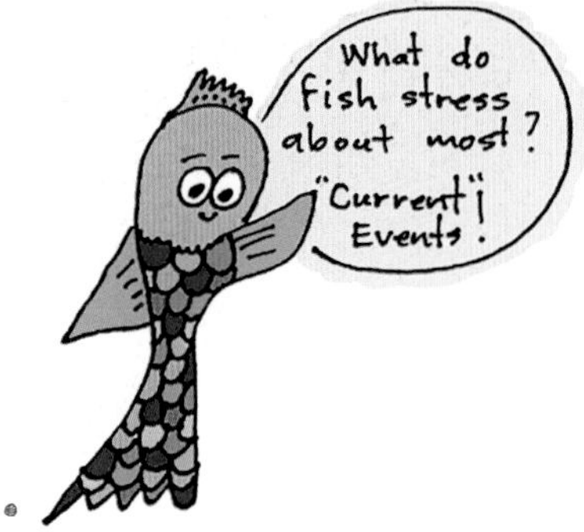

Play Relieves Stress and Helps Us Cope

What do you do after a long day of work? Some of us run home to our comfy clothes, "soft clothes" like our friend JoAnn says, and tune in to our latest streaming binge. Others make their way with friends to a local waterin' hole for happy hour. We do this instinctively because of the way playful moments trigger the release of endorphins, the body's natural feel-good chemicals. Endorphins promote our well-being and can even temporarily relieve pain. Have you ever had sore feet after work, but then go out dancing with friends that evening only to realize the pain of the day had faded away a bit? Thank your endorphins.

Did you know that soccer star David Beckham controls stress by playing with Legos? Surely you've seen Ellen DeGeneres dancing with and later pranking her TV show guests (Wallace, 2017). Oprah starts her day by walking the dogs and if it is just her and Steadman, she likes to cook to wind down later in the day (Schwantes, 2021). David Cameron played *Angry Birds* as a way to chill after a long day at the Prime Minister's office. Michelle Obama plays cards and enjoys puzzles with her family (Hao, 2022).

This section feels like one of those *no-*&%$ Sherlock* parts of a book. We all know playing helps us relax and de-stress. But what does the research say?

In 2011, two friends at Pennsylvania State University had read a great deal of research on leisure and found that no one had yet studied how playfulness might impact the process by which we all cope with stress. Xinyi Lisa Qian and Careen Yarnal surveyed 195 adult participants about their psychological stress, playfulness, emotions, and quality of life. Results suggest that being more playful leads us to seek companionship through play and that our mood is likewise enhanced (Yarnal & Qian, 2011).

Two years earlier and 600 miles away, two researchers at the University of Illinois wondered about the benefits of playfulness to the individual. Do playful people experience less stress? Can they cope better with all the things? Scientists don't make assumptions, no matter how obvious the connections might seem. So, they conducted a study to investigate the interrelationship among playfulness, stress, and coping styles (Magnuson & Barnett, 2013). In this investigation across nearly 900 university students, they found that playful individuals reported lower stress levels than their less playful buddies. The playful folk also had more flexible, more positive coping strategies.

What does this mean for us? Playfulness and play help us cope and connect with each other, making us happier and more open to life's opportunities.

CHAPTER 10

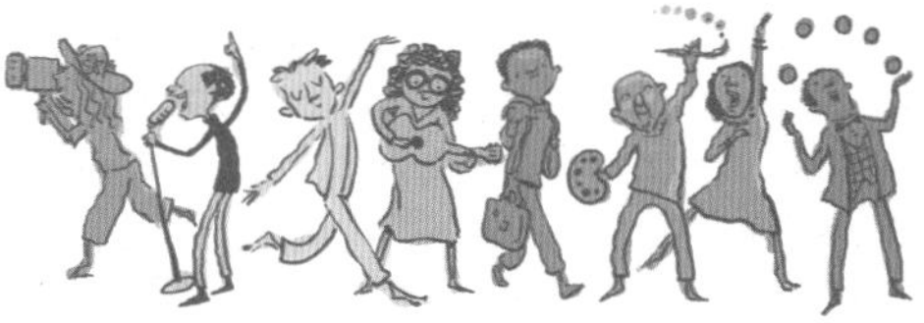

Play Personalities

We dabbled a bit in Chapter 3 with expressing how people play differently—while Jed and I both like to doodle, read, and play outdoors, our variations make us unique. I sketch architecture and nature scenes. Jed paints gay pop art. I enjoy mysteries and historical fiction, but never an unreliable narrator (I feel lied to, and that's no fun). Jed enjoys dystopian fiction and memoirs. Jed is a beach guy, but I prefer the lake. We didn't arrive at the understanding of these nuances easily. In fact, knowing what we like and what we enjoy has become a real benefit for living a playful life. We got there through a life of exploration and reflection—a life of intention and habit. Knowing this gives us direction. I can be intentional about my calendar and the experiences I seek because I know what I enjoy or what I might not. This is not the case for so many people. I have a dear friend who has no idea of his passion. It is akin to Gatsby's green light . . . something he constantly seeks, but feels just outside his grasp.

I have always been a reader. My mom tells me stories of finding me awake late at night with a flashlight under the covers with a Nancy Drew novel. My memory includes Sweet Valley Twins and the original Baby Sitters' Club in that list. Either way, I always had a book in my hand. When leaving the house, I was more likely to grab a book for the ride than I was to grab my wallet (thankfully, the wallet part has changed). I always asked for books as gifts and even today I delight in my Book of the Month subscription. It's a rarity when I can walk in my local Hub City Bookshop and not leave with some new treasure. Even my Instagram feed includes my latest joys of reader-escapism—most recently a light beach read set in Nantucket and a nonfiction text for urban planners. Reading is clearly a form of play for me. Nothing brings more joy than the thought of curling up in a big chair with a book and a cup of spiced tea beside me. Even better if it's cold outside. But I realize this is not the picture of happiness for everyone. Even in our circle of buddies, there is so much variety in what we consider to be playful. (Correct, no spiced tea for me—Jed.)

- Sarah and Melissa are readers too—we three love to leave book surprises on each others' porches.
- Katy enjoys listening her body and answering with yoga poses and recovery in deep meditation.
- Kennerty lives in Belgium and is traveling every weekend by train or foot to explore dark beer and delicious food.
- Matt is a huge sports fan and loves board games. His most favorite is *Catan*.
- Rebecca organizes marketing for her own business—carefully planning promotional events to align with what her customers want and need.
- Gen is a creator—she finds a way to paint or sketch daily. She takes special delight in designing her kids' Halloween costumes using cardboard boxes cut and painted to professional-grade style.
- Jed loves to collect things . . . travel experiences, books he's read, art supplies, rainbow things, and lots and lots of writing utensils. He even creates his own pen holders out of tin cans because he collects those, too.

I illustrate these few examples to make our next point. Play and playfulness are based on the individual. What is playful to me may confound you. What you enjoy might be what I adamantly avoid. My discovery of play types or play personalities was one of the most defining moments for me in my play trajectory. I can remember it vividly. We were sitting at a round table at the front of a large room at Clemson University's Madren Center. Jed was sitting beside me, taking up two chairs with himself and his bag. (This was over three years ago and she still recounts this like it was yesterday. She still has beef with me—Jed.) His journals, the carefully placed bag of colored pencils, and rows of Papermate InkJoy Gel pens aligned already in rainbow order. "I don't care for the Flair pens," he said, as if he were disgusted by their existence in front of me. I was a bit distracted by Jed's preparations, and annoyed at my discombobulated feeling because (I mean . . . *The Stuart Brown* was talking!) The lighting was turned down so the audience could see both the presenter (Stuart

Brown) and his slides—projected on two screens at either side of the stage. He clicked the button and the slide on the screen changed to display a graphic similar to the one you see next.

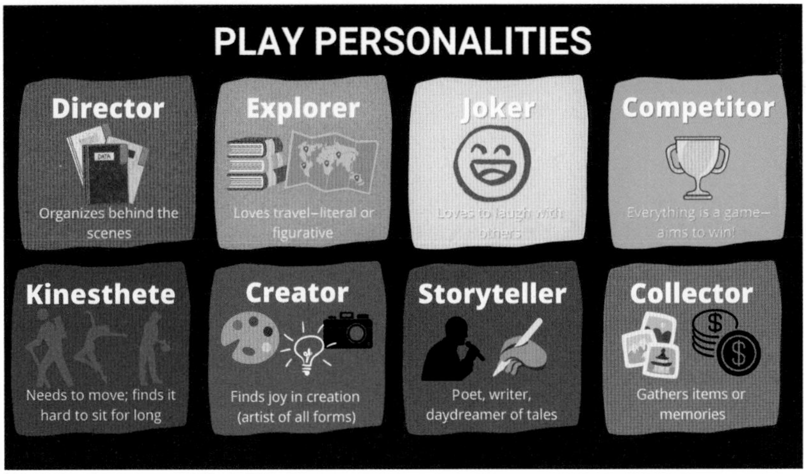

If you consult the internet with "play personalities" as your search terms, you'll get varied results. But the core eight play personality types Brown discussed in his keynote and in his book are summarized for you in the following sections.

The Joker

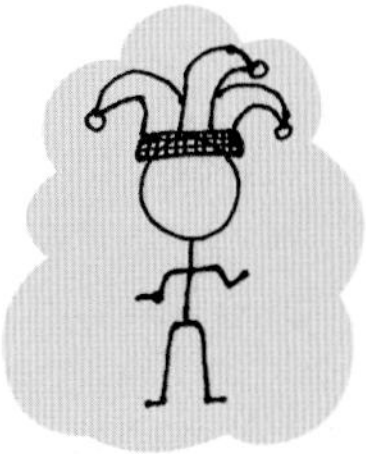

Giggle giggle. Har har. Whether or not you are this person, you no doubt know someone who enjoys entertaining the crowd. Jokers love to put on a show (big or small) with laughter. They are always pulling pranks. Puns bring a chuckle. They scroll and share the silliest of memes. I (Julie) am guilty of this. Sometimes I crack myself up. This one time, I was driving on the highway, and the truck in front of me swerved. I say, "Hey!" Guess why he swerved? Yep. A bale of hay was in the road. Get it? I said hey and it was hay! I died laughing, y'all. I'm still laughing.

Why did Adele cross the road? To say hello from the other side.

Why can't the bicycle stand on its own? It's too tired.

Did the grape cry when you stepped on it? No, It just let out a little wine.

I made a pun about the wind but it blows.

Have these puns made you laugh? Maybe? Maybe not? (Not me, says Jed. *Lame dad jokes* as Julie guffaws in the background.) I bet they've *groan* on you. Hahahahahaha.

Jed—Julie, enough already.

Jokers love to make people laugh, and their creativity in doing so is always under construction—growing ever stronger with practice.

The Kinesthete

First of all, you need to know that our buddy Stuart totally made this word up. We thought it . . . then we asked him. Yep. Made. It. Up.

But it's because there simply wasn't a word for it. Yesss, Stuart! Rock on, you neologist. You creator of words.

The kinesthete has difficulty staying still.

JED: Ken NUH steet? Ken NUS teeth? Kenneth—steet?
JULIE: No, thet.
JED: Lord, Julie. You don't say kenes-thetic.
JULIE: Yes you do. You say ken-es-the-tic.
JED: No. The th is silent!
JULIE: I say it that way.
JED: (eye roll)
JULIE: I'm done here.

After multiple attempts to Google this word and get an audio pronunciation, we failed. The only results are references to Stuart Brown's research.

The kinesthete has to move to think.

They won't be lounging on a Saturday morning. Instead you'll find them walking, swimming, mowing the lawn—whatever kind of movement strikes them. If you find yourself dancing, hiking, or constantly puttering about, this play personality type might be your cup of tea. Caution, though—this type is focused on movement, not competition. That's another play personality type. If you're likely to be found outside clearing land, turning the garden, playing football, or any other active situation, you might be a kinesthete.

The Explorer

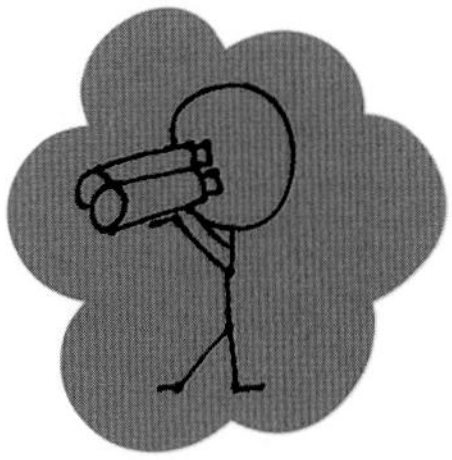

Whether you consider this category literally or figuratively, the explorer play personality type uses exploration as a tool for provoking their imagination and growing creatively. You might scroll online to secure your next travel experience, or you might lose yourself in reading a novel set in another place. We aren't definite on this, but we are pretty sure Dora and her fans are a part of this group. If you love the new and different—whether it's music, art, feelings, ideas, beliefs, perspectives, or places—you might be an explorer at heart. Dr. Brown tells us, "Each of us started our lives by exploring the world around us. Some people never lose their enthusiasm for it" (S. Brown, 2009).

That love of reading I mentioned earlier? Yep, this one is me.

The Competitor

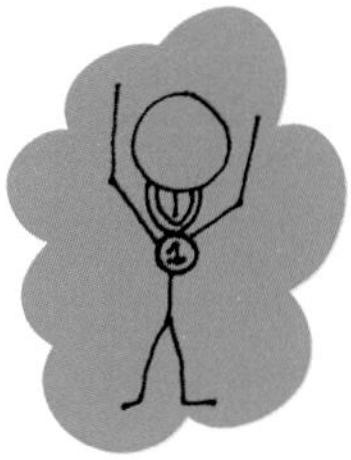

If you find comfort in rules—if you love playing games (especially when you win), this type might describe you. I live with one of these people. She's 14 years old. She's my daughter. When she was younger, she entertained us every night at dinner with "Guess my number" or "Would you rather . . ." Being told to brush her teeth before bed became a race with her sister. Now that she's older, I enjoy the fact that I can quickly and easily lure her away from screens with an announcement of "game night!" She almost always wins, but I'm okay with that. We all know people like this, and maybe you are *won* of them. (Stop it, Julie—this is not the Joker section.) I like games, but this is different. Living with a competitor helps me know this is not my personal play type. It's fun, but not all the time. All. The. Time. She wants to be a PE teacher and swim coach when she grows up. What a great choice!

The world needs competitors because they develop games noncompetitors would never think of. Take a moment and look up Walter Camp, the Father of American Football. No doubt this man was a competitor play type. Just look at his impact on our culture! Competitors will work toward mastery of any game that has specific rules—no matter if it's team-based or *Solitaire*. The skill to create, implement, tweak, and replay those rules is quite a level of intelligence. When given the choice to play for fun, or play and keep score, they *always* default to the latter. Why even play if you're not keeping score?

The Director

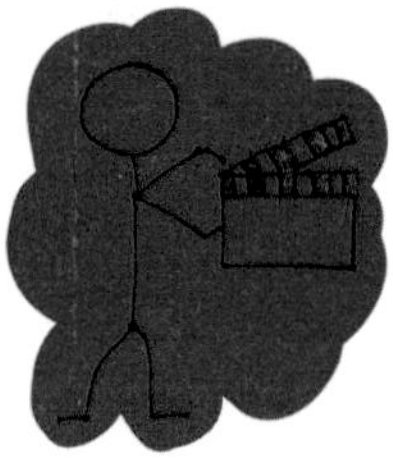

Directors are the great planners. They are the ones who love to organize the celebration—baby shower, wedding, class party, field trip, tailgate refreshments—you name it. They love to make order out of chaos. Because this scene always involves people, directors are often charismatic, affable folk who instigate fun. They may not outwardly like titles like, "Director of . . .," but they secretly love the power and control that allows them to improve all kinds of situations.

Do you catch that? The director isn't the loud, bossy one in the room. The real director is the one in the kitchen, working behind the scenes without recognition. The director doesn't need recognition—it's all about the end result: an organized event where all people leave feeling like it was the best day ever.

The Collector

Our state parks department has a challenge on their website: "Visit 47 parks to become the Ultimate Outsider!" Once you have collected 47 stamps, you can turn your guidebook in to a park ranger and get a free T-shirt. Does this kind of program appeal to you? Let's talk personal. What's on your refrigerator? Is it covered in magnets and photos? Do you have a drawer of every letter and card you've ever received? What about your walls? Do you display treasures you've gathered along life's way? If any of these are true for you, you might be a collector.

Collectors gather memories.

These friends collect experiences.

There's generally some kind of theme, and whatever it is, they can't get enough. You might wonder about the difference between a collector and an explorer—especially if a person likes to collect experiences. Well, first of all, you can be both. There's nothing that says you have to pigeonhole yourself. But there is a clear distinction. Brown shares an example: "One person I know travels the world to see solar eclipses—which might seem like the action of an explorer, except that he has to see every single one and methodically collects evidence of each eclipse" (S. Brown, 2009). This guy is a collector at heart.

The Artist/Creator

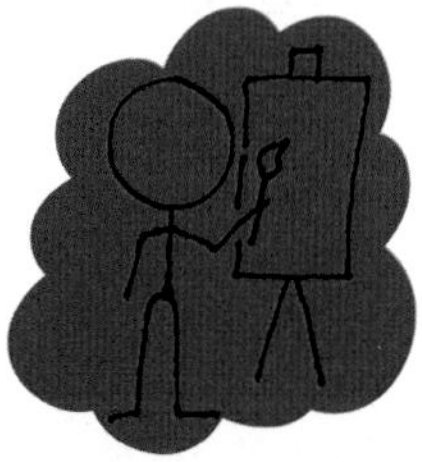

Painters!
Sculptors! and
Scribblers! oh my.
Potters!
Printmakers! and
Photographers! Say hi.

This is your space. Notice we didn't say "those with their own studio" or "those who are published." Anyone who finds joy in the act of creation is an artist or creator. In starting from scratch or joining disparate materials to build a product. In fixing something that was broken or improving something already made.

Do you know how many years we sat together over hot beverages, typing our ideas and scribbling our thoughts in journals together before we took the leap to send some chapters to Wiley/Jossey-Bass? The fact that we published a book and that you're now holding the second work in your hands still seems a miracle to us, but it makes us no more of an artist or creator than you. We just kept on in the joy of the work until we were brave enough to share it. "The point is to make something—to make something beautiful, something functional, something goofy. Or just to make something work" (S. Brown, 2009). This play personality type is clearly where Jed and I both like to be. Raise your hand if you feel happy in this space too.

The Storyteller

You are a storyteller if you are jotting down poems on napkins or crafting a novel in your spare time. Does reading inspire you to write? Does going to the theater or the movies make you chatty at dinner with tales of your own (or another's) adventures? Yep. This is your space then. Storytellers often play out scenes in their minds—whether it's daydreaming or their way of improving their afternoon chores. Did you have to slay dragons with your broom while sweeping your porch? Did you have to explain to the books why dusting the shelves was important for their health? Are you making up silly tales to tell those around you? Are you singing, dancing, narrating? You're a storyteller at heart.

In Section Five of this book, Mojo, we'll explain how to increase playful opportunities for each play personality type. For now, consider which type(s) you might be. If you're unsure, we've created a little quiz to help you out.

Play Personality Type Quiz

Directions: Circle or highlight the response that best represents you.

1. Which of these could you do for hours?
   a. Build a city from Legos
   b. Beat your high score
   c. Make party treats
   d. Perform in local theater
   e. Jump in a leaf pile
2. What's your pick for a hot summer's day?
   a. Water balloon fight
   b. Taking photos
   c. Planning an indoor fun house
   d. Chilling inside watching *I Love Lucy* or an Eddie Murphy marathon
   e. Exploring a new trail—hoping to stumble upon a waterfall
3. What are/were you like in school?
   a. Class clown
   b. Artistic
   c. Daydreamer
   d. Athletic
   e. Leader of all things
4. Of the following, which of these do you prefer most?
   a. Trampoline
   b. Costume set
   c. Colored pencils
   d. Car collection
   e. Xbox
5. Which of these apps do you use most often?
   a. BuzzFeed or Reddit
   b. Airbnb or Outdoorsy
   c. Minecraft or ProCreate
   d. Words with Friends or GamePigeon
   e. eBay or Etsy
6. If you could go on an adventure, which would you choose?
   a. BMX biking

   - **b.** Going to a carnival
   - **c.** Go camping cross country
   - **d.** Competing in *The Amazing Race*
   - **e.** Getting stamps from all the national parks
7. What do you enjoy most about sports?
   - **a.** Winning
   - **b.** Playing
   - **c.** Coaching
   - **d.** The write-up in tomorrow's paper
   - **e.** None of these
8. What is your favorite type of movie?
   - **a.** Adventure
   - **b.** Animated
   - **c.** Drama
   - **d.** Comedy
   - **e.** Documentary
9. If you could learn something new, it would be _____.
   - **a.** Party or wedding planning
   - **b.** Painting, pottery, or carpentry
   - **c.** Boxing, surfing, or yoga
   - **d.** Geocaching
   - **e.** Cinematic design
10. Which of the following would you enjoy?
    - **a.** Playing jokes on friends/family
    - **b.** Adding to your collection of cherished items
    - **c.** Exploring local creeks in search of new play places
    - **d.** Organizing group games with friends
    - **e.** Field days, mud runs, or escape rooms
11. When you are procrastinating, you
    - **a.** Flip through your collection of comic books
    - **b.** Relieve the boredom by sending funny memes to friends
    - **c.** Imagine you're in a movie and act the part of the scholar
    - **d.** Get fidgety and do something active to relieve the wiggles
    - **e.** Organize the work, then delegate or tackle each item
12. Which of the following careers would you most enjoy?
    - **a.** Anthropologist exploring new lands
    - **b.** Graphic designer for your favorite magazine
    - **c.** Sales for a gaming company
    - **d.** Antiques dealer
    - **e.** A novelist or news journalist
13. In your social group, you
    - **a.** Find ways to make every situation a game
    - **b.** Encourage group trips together
    - **c.** All have a common collection—books, journals, coins, jewelry, art
    - **d.** Take lots of pictures to use for the group holiday cards
    - **e.** Make everyone laugh, always lightening the mood

Highlight your answers below:

	#1	#2	#3	#4	#5	#6	#7	#8	#9	#10	#11	#12	#13
Artist/Creator	a	b	b	c	c			b	b			b	
Joker		d	a		a	b		d		a	b		e
Kinesthete	e	a	d	a		a	b		c		d		
Explorer		e	c		b	c		a		c		a	b
Competitor	b			e	d	d	a			e		c	a
Director	c	c	e				c	b	a	d	e		
Collector				d	e	e			d	b	a	d	c
Storyteller	d			b			d	c	e		c	e	d

*In item 7, no category receives points for choice e.

****

- Which play personality did you choose the most?
- What's your second-highest? Third-highest?
- Do you think this represents who you are? Have a conversation with a friend about your results.

You Have Results, Now What?

The outcome of your play personality quiz is valuable information for moving forward in your playful life. Self-awareness is a necessary starting point as we reflect and make plans for the future; before we can begin to fully embrace playful living, we really must take a deep look into ourselves.

There are play-based books in the world that give you a formula for *having fun*. We've read them. They teach the way to being a fun person is to plan it—every day, every week, every month, and every year. What a great idea . . . for a director. But how overwhelming and potentially disastrous would this be for the joker or the storyteller who doesn't find joy in the planning? They might feel like a short dog in tall grass and shut down from frustration, deciding they have no ability to play or be playful. We can't think of a worse outcome.

Honestly, I bet we've all tried to jump in with both feet for the wrong idea before. One year, against my (Jed) better judgment, I played Little League baseball. Basically it was an attempt to appease my stepfather and convince him of my "manhood" as I started middle school. The reality was this: I hated everything about sports. I was an artist, musician, singer, etc. But the stereotypes of boys coupled with pressure to please my stepdad led me to sign up for the team. WHAT A MISTAKE! It was so awful, y'all. I hated everything about it. I cried a lot. I wasn't any good. The only way I got on base was to get hit by the ball. I had a permanent bruise on my left love handle for the entirety of the season because I kept "taking one for the team." Thankfully after that horrid season was over, my family realized sports weren't my thing, and the band consumed me. I thrived there. It was my space, my people. The only good thing about my time in baseball was that it gave me a good story for this part of the book.

Learning more about our play preferences can help increase our understanding of playful memories. After taking our nonscientific quiz, many of our mutual friends have realized more about their play personality and play preferences. Some results were expected, and some were momentarily surprising but served to clarify what was previously ambiguous. This quiz has been slightly updated from its original version in our book *The Playful Classroom*. We originally created it so teachers could better understand their own play type as well as the play types of their students. How often were they including learning experiences that spoke to each learner? The same is true for you. In your own life, are you including experiences that speak to your definition of joy? In your work and interaction with others, how often do you consider the play personality of others? Knowing your play preferences will allow you to identify areas of your life that could benefit from a renewed focus. Knowing about others' play personalities will surely strengthen your interactions. It won't be an overnight transformation, and it won't flood every area of your life. But the smallest of rocks still causes ripples in a pond.

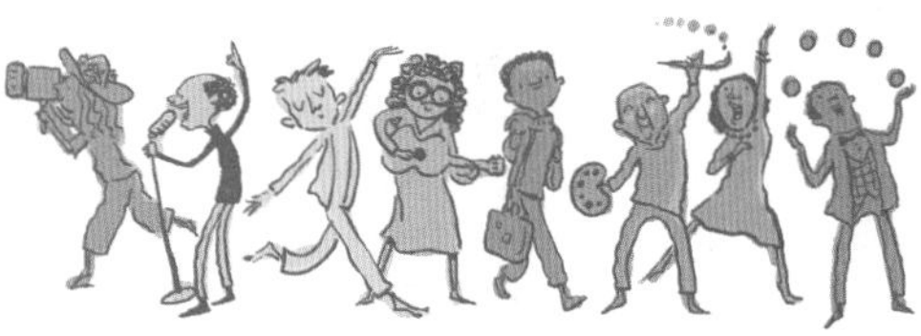

Play & Ponder

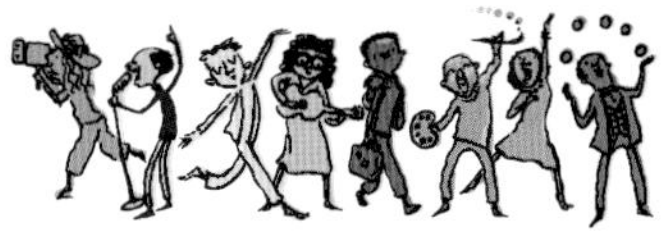

- What is your play history?

  Instead of writing down a list of all the ways you used to play, why not grab a ball (preferably one that will bounce) and play catch with a friend while you talk about all the fun things you used to do as a kid? No friend nearby? No problem, a wall will work just fine as long as the ball will bounce back to you.

  Catch isn't your thing? Maybe take a walk around the block and look for things in nature that prompt your memories of past play experiences. You see a rock and are reminded of skipping stones with Grandpa. You see a tree and are reminded of climbing with your cousins. You see leaves and remember trying to catch them as they fell while playing with a friend in a park.
- What did you learn from playing as a kid?

  This will be fun. Hang out with a friend and try this!

  Step 1: Gather 10 random objects from your house that remind you of childhood.

  Step 2: Ask your friend to do the same.

  Step 3: Combine all the items in a bag and take turns removing items one at a time.

  Step 4: As each item is revealed, talk about anything you can remember regarding your first interaction with said item as a kid. The lessons it taught you will spring forth as your chat! Julie and I did this and giggles were as plentiful as pigeons at a popcorn party.

Another option? Does your mama have any old home movies? Pull out those VHS tapes and have a giggle at your kid-self. You can even make it a movie night with friends, gathering all the old home movies y'all can pull together. What habits do you still have today? What has clearly changed?

- How accurate were the results of your play personality quiz?

So you got explorer, did you? Go out in the back yard and search for something you have never seen before. Think about how that made you feel!

You are a kinesthete? *Yes!* Try hula hooping without a hoop and then start to work on a task you have been putting off. We bet you'll feel better doing it after the hoopless hooping!

We love a director! Plan a popup party for your housemates. The purpose? Discovering the play personalities of the people you live with and providing them with an evening focused on playing their way!

SECTION 3

Mind

Our brains are tired. Does yours ever get tired, too? Lately the world has seemed so heavy it just gets more tired every time we try to make it more untired. We confess that sometimes we are so tired that we don't feel much like playing. It takes a lot for us to get ourselves going some days. But this we know . . . 99.99% of the time when we finally do get ourselves together and take the first step, the second, third, and fourth get a bit easier. If we will just read the first page of the book or open our journal to a clean doodle page, or put on our shoes and walk outside, the stress of the world begins to release. No, no, no . . . it doesn't all go away. And honestly, it never will. 'Tis the world we live in. But what does happen is that we forget about it for a bit. When we are reading about characters and their lives, our minds take a break from the ills of our own. When we doodle, we are bringing something new to life that has never existed before. When we go for a walk, we are able to peek into the lives of birds, and frogs, and squirrels, and beetles, and, yes . . . even the neighbors as they prune their bushes or play in the plastic pool in their driveway down the street. We know full well that these moments cannot happen all day

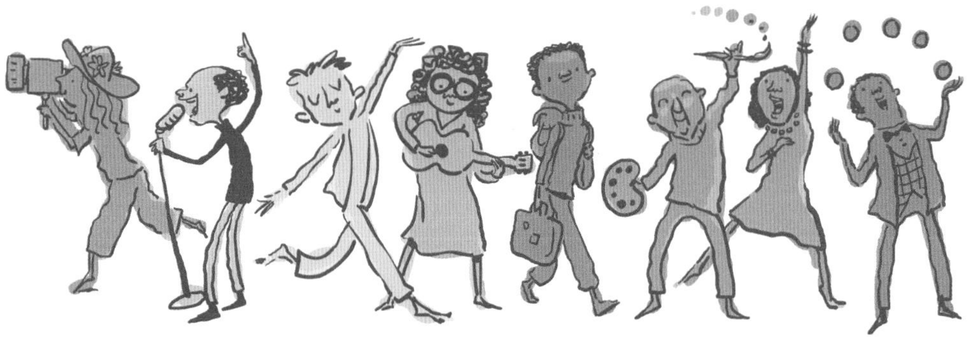

everyday. Even for those who are gozillionaires, life has problems that even their money can't solve. However, once we fully realize the way our bodies are wired to crave the moments of books, doodles, walks, or whatever tickles our fancy, then we can intentionally plan to bring those moments into our lives. Yep . . . we are wired for it. You read that right. Our whole existence as a species has brought us to this point of humanity where we are because of moments of brevity, moments of peace, moments of play.

CHAPTER 11

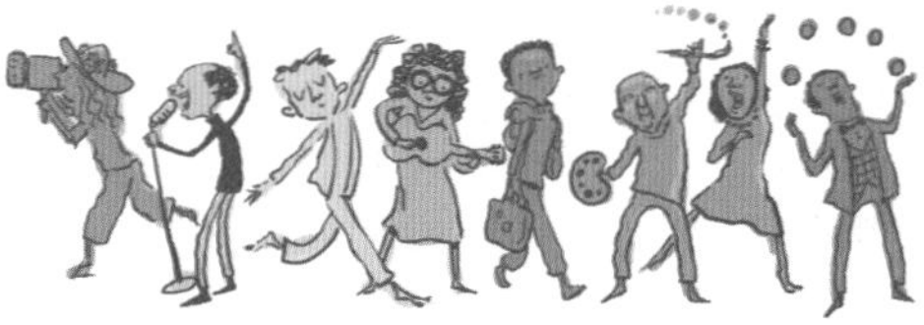

Biological Predilection

You read the story of Isabel Behncke (2015) and the bonobos apes. Well, let us tell you a story about Stuart Brown, one of our favorite play researchers, who is known for his work on the play histories of murderers, serial killers, and Nobel laureates. Brown has also studied play in animals—he recently shared with Jed and me about his friendship with Jane Goodall. Just imagine the conversations, y'all! Our (now) buddy Stuart uses his understanding of play in animals and compares it to his work with humans—arguing that to truly understand what play does for us people, we need to look at it in the context of biology and evolution. In one section of his book *Play: How It Shapes the Brain, Opens the Imagination, and Invigorates the Soul* (2009), Stuart tells the story of his conversation with Bob Fagen, another prominent play researcher. In all our conversations with Stuart, we've known him to be a curious individual. I've taken artistic liberty with imagining how this curiosity conversation might have taken place between Fagen and Brown, then a young whippersnapper. Picture it: two men standing at a safe distance from two bears playing. The scene takes place in Juneau, Alaska—in my mental picture, there is snow on the ground, and the two men are bundled up with toboggans (this is our Southern word for a knit beanie cap that you might wear in the snow) pulled low to keep them pseudo-comfortable in the biting wind. If it was me, my hands would be either stuffed in my pockets or in gloves (or both!). This is how I see Stuart standing. Bob, who in this tale is older, might be a bit more hardened to the climate. In my imagination, he's not wearing gloves. He sports a plaid flannel shirt and has a field notebook (you know, the kind with spirals at the top) poking out of his shirt pocket. There might have even been one of those short pencils tucked in the spirals, clearly sharpened with a knife. Young Stuart, being new to the field, was trying to learn all he could from Fagen.

Now, Stuart explains this conversation in his book, but I've rewritten it for you here as if they are characters in this mental play we're building. You might recognize this play from our first book, *The Playful Classroom*. I've added some stage directions to this one. Lights, camera, action!

Brown (looking at bears): Bob, why do those bears play?

Fagen (aloof): Because it's fun.

Brown (brow furrowed, turns to Fagen): No, Bob, I mean from a scientific point of view, why do they play?

Fagen (slight smile): Why do they play? Why do birds sing, people dance? For the *pleasure* of it.

Brown (stepping back, gestures with emphasis): Bob, you have degrees from Harvard and MIT, and an in-depth knowledge of bears. You're a student of evolution, you've written *the* definitive work on all mammals at play—I know you have more opinions about this. Tell me, why do animals play?
(Long, tolerant silence)

Fagen: In a world continuously presenting unique challenges of ambiguity, play prepares these bears for an evolving planet.

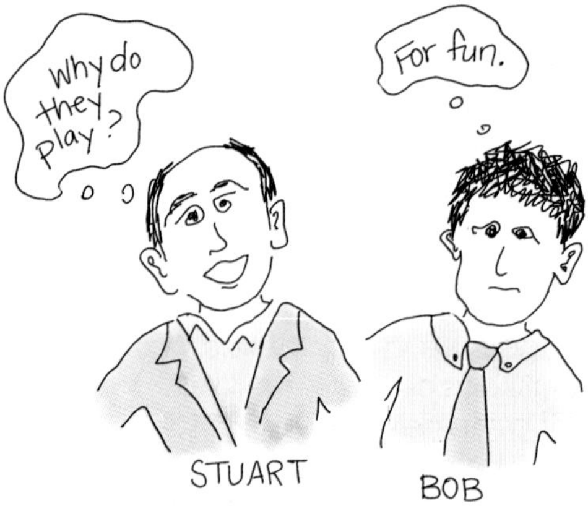

Can you sense the sarcasm in Fagen's response? I imagine it's there. Not condescending, but rather in a *bless-his-heart* kind of way. Why do we continually analyze concepts of beauty? Play exists—we all do it in some form or fashion. We all enjoy it. We all need it. Remember when Jed shared the story of his mama helping him create his play history? She knew intuitively that this experience was needed. Like the apes, bears, and cats (that story is coming), all studies point to the fact that play may be biologically wired in us all.

Let it be, sings Paul. But, alas, if that were so, you might not have purchased this book. Whether you are an evolutionary play theorist or not, play is pervasive across the animal kingdom. Not just in mammals, but down the evolutionary ladder or tree (pick your metaphor of choice), scientists have found play behaviors. Even the octopus has been observed engaging in "relaxed, idiosyncratic manipulations of objects," and ants are believed to engage in play-fighting (E.O. Wilson, cited in S. Brown, 2009).

Speaking of octopuses (yep we googled the plural to make sure we had it right. We may have giggled as we typed it, and we hope you giggle as you read it), have y'all seen the documentary *My Octopus Teacher?* In the story, the filmmaker becomes fascinated by an octopus living in a South African kelp forest. He visits daily, thus creating a unique friendship between the two. Once this bond is formed, the octopus and the human play together. One time, the octopus latches on to the human (as if holding hands), and they swim together. Y'all. This is a must-watch. More than once, the trust built between the two because of their playfulness helped to protect the octopus. One time, a shark attack was averted. The octopus knew it needed an ally. We wonder if this was its purpose for play. The documentary surely left us with all the feels.

Like the octopus, Brown (2009) explains that one purpose of play in animals is believed to be the learning process for making sound judgments. Play-fighting among bears teaches them when they can trust another bear, and when they need to defend themselves or escape. Biscuit and Bear, Jed's dogs, have multiple romps of frolic and fun daily. Here, play becomes a rehearsal for challenges they may face.

How about human lifeforms? So, I told this story in *The Playful Classroom*, but it's worth repeating here. When my brother and I (Julie) were younger, we often played together. Well . . . not always together, but I was certainly there when he played. He was often outside among the neighborhood kids practicing his breakdancing moves on a large piece of remnant, rolled-out linoleum. I wanted to be part of his group so badly. I was that little sister who wouldn't go away. Sometimes, they let me join them, but most times I'm sure he was ready to be rid of me. I remember clearly one particular afternoon ending with his size 10 Vans hurtling at me followed by a game of chase all around the house. He was quick, and my first-grade self wasn't as fast. I did what any sweet 6-year-old would do: I bit my arm and screamed bloody murder. Mama came a-runnin', and Jeff was grounded for weeks. We fussed and fussed. I'm not sure how that plate of spaghetti ended up all over his bedroom door later. It certainly wasn't because this innocent princess had had enough of his complaining. You're probably reading this and thinking, That's not playful. That's fussing and fighting. Nah—it was play. We loved each other. We still do. Even though he lives half a country away, we still look forward to our weekly phone calls to connect with the little stories of life. Do you see what play taught me?

It taught me how to defend myself.
It taught me how to strategize.
It taught me how to keep my head up even though the giants were all around.

Yes, biting myself and lying about it was wrong. (We're not condoning the sharing of false information. Although it does seem to be rampant these days.) However, it was the only skill I had in my junior plastic toolbox. I've gathered many more laudable tools since. We're sure many of you can relate to this story. Anyone with a sibling has had a fuss . . . has had a moment like this. Reflect. Didn't you also learn? Just like the biological predilection of the animal play behaviors we have shared here, play for humans is innate.

Learning is key to our survival—the learning that occurs through play is essential for us to continue on a forward path. Take for example the cult sensation *Survivor*. Yes, we know it's a TV show, but don't you think it mimics life in so many ways? The contestants must learn and adapt to be the last one standing; in this show, the learning happens through varied challenges, but also in the downtime between challenges. Intentional play and free play—alive for us all on the screen.

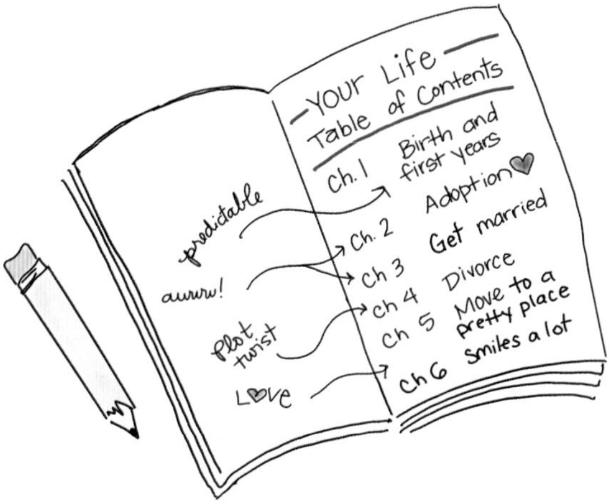

We hope you all played as kids. But to talk about play in the past tense alone makes us sad. Our lives aren't finished. As adults, we are gathering experiences on the daily. Chris M. Golde (2019) reminds us that "careers go in chapters." Pete Seeger sings, "There is a season. Turn, turn, turn." We're singing along. The thought of our lives as a book made up of many chapters is a powerful metaphor for connecting the many and varied experiences we have. Some of us have more chapters in our life books than others, and sometimes the book may change to a whole new story altogether.

Wired to Play

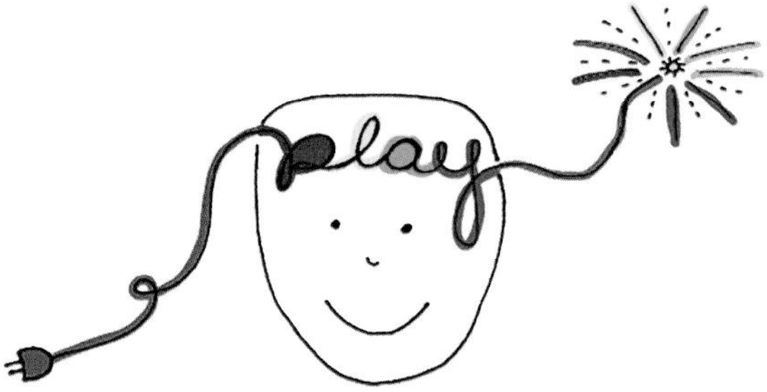

The jump from animal play to human play might be quite a leap for many of you. It shouldn't be, though; we humans are in fact mammals just like the dogs and bears previously mentioned, and the cats that are coming soon. We hope you take some time to watch some animals (ants, birds, squirrels, fish) when you have the chance. The next little tidbit we have for you isn't quite as big a jump for our understanding. The concept of play is also present in early human cultures. When we consider the notion that humans are biologically wired to play, some of y'all might be thinking, "Well, aren't we all wired differently?" Well, yes . . . we are, but there are some characteristics we all have in common, and the predisposition to enjoy play, or be playful, is one of them.

The traits of enjoying play and being playful present themselves differently in each individual, but there is a biological desire within us all to play. We know this through ethnographic studies of cultural groups across time and place. Hunter-gatherer societies, whether in Africa, Asia, or South America, all have common characteristics. They have common social structures, similar values, and like ways of raising children (Gray, 2013). The following are two of these similarities:

- **Autonomy** (personal freedom, sharing, and equality) is a common core social value, not unlike our modern democratic culture. Hunter-gatherer cultures take the concept of autonomy far beyond our common emphasis. Each person, the child included, is free to make independent choices daily—free from opinion, free from advice, free from interference.

- **Sharing** is expected, but a "thank-you note tradition" does not exist. (Here in the South we write thank-you notes thanking you for a thank-you note. It's a vicious circle of knowing when to stop thanking for thanking.) Instead of being a kindness, sharing is considered a duty; failing to share invites ridicule and disdain.

Connecting Dots

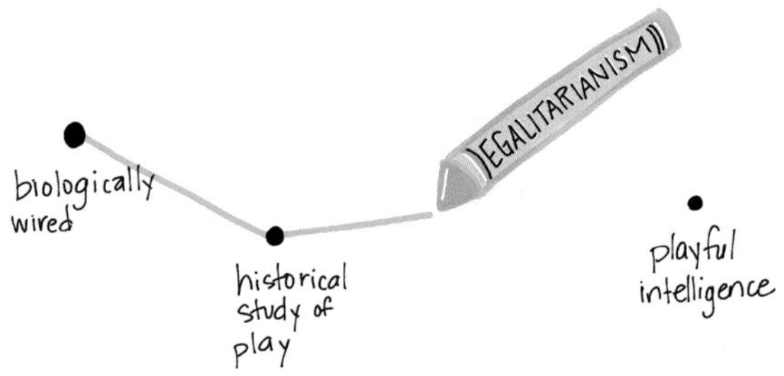

Moving forward with the understanding that we are biologically wired to play, we begin to see the similarity between the historical study of play and more current research on the topic. Sharing and autonomy are concepts intertwined in the larger idea of egalitarianism: everyone's needs are equally important. We see this concept manifest in DeBenedet's discussion of playful sociability (2018). Those with high levels of this quality focus on *we*, rejecting a *them-versus-us* mentality. Many hunter-gatherer cultures generally have no one person in a leadership role. There is no chief or "big man" who makes decisions for the group. Instead, those concerns are addressed through group discussions, treating women, men, and children with equal voice.

Speaking of children, you might be surprised to learn of **the high level of trust placed on the decisions of the child**. Children in these cultures are allowed to follow their own will; the reasoning here is that when trusted with their own decisions, when allowed to play and explore freely, children will develop the skills needed to contribute to the group's economy. Children are allowed to play with adult tools, even those we might consider dangerous, because they believe that only through playing with these tools will children become skilled at using them.

You can read more about these types of hunter-gatherer cultures in Peter Gray's work, *Free to Learn* (2013).

You may be thinking right now, okay that's nice (plastic smile on your face), but it's time for me to run. Good seein' you! (Internal script: What in tarnation do hunter-gatherer cultures have to do with having a more playful life in our culture?)

No worries, my friend. We get it—what we need to play and create memories is far different from what is needed in hunter-gatherer cultures. Yes, the cultures differ greatly. Yes, the conversation shifts. But you'll see the connection soon. It's like our friend and *New York Times* best-selling author Peter H. Reynolds said once at his bookshop in Dedham, Massachusetts, "The universe is constantly connecting dots. We just have to pay attention." Eventually, we hope to connect the dots for you and show you the ways that these cultures are sufficient for today's life. It's coming, but before that, let's look at a little more research.

A Story about Cats

Brown acknowledges preparation for the future self as a major theory of play literature. But even more interesting for our point here is his story about cats. Turns out, cats that are deprived of play-fighting turn out to be just dandy hunters. So, if the play-fighting wasn't preparing them for a future of hunting, what's it for? Listen meow. Hahahahaha. Too much? (*definitely too much!*) Okay, moving on.

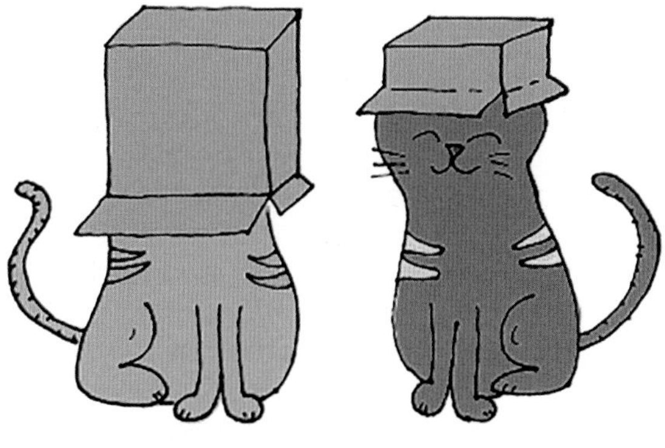

Cats that are deprived of play-fighting in youth actually lack another skill—the ability to socialize successfully. According to Brown (2009), these cats lack the ability to discern friend from foe, do not catch another cat's social signals, and choose to either act aggressively or retreat—both actions out of the norm for a cat's social graces. Talk about white paws after Labor Day! It's this play-fighting and mock combat that provide our feline friends with emotional intelligence—the ability to perceive another's emotional state and act accordingly.

In your world, there is likely a person who stands too close, talks a bit too loud, is unable to *read the room*, and always seems to say the most awkward thing. These characteristics served to make *Seinfeld* such a popular sitcom. We all know these folks. These are the cats we're referring to. We need play in our developmental years and throughout life to help us develop the social skills needed to participate in society. As we know, the norms of society are always evolving. Being playful helps us to stay with the times and change accordingly. Otherwise, we may be the ones saying and doing the awkward things.

CHAPTER 12

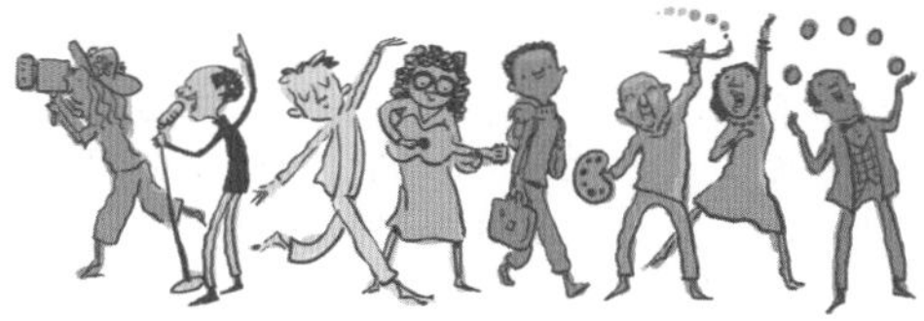

This Is Your Brain. This Is Your Brain on Play

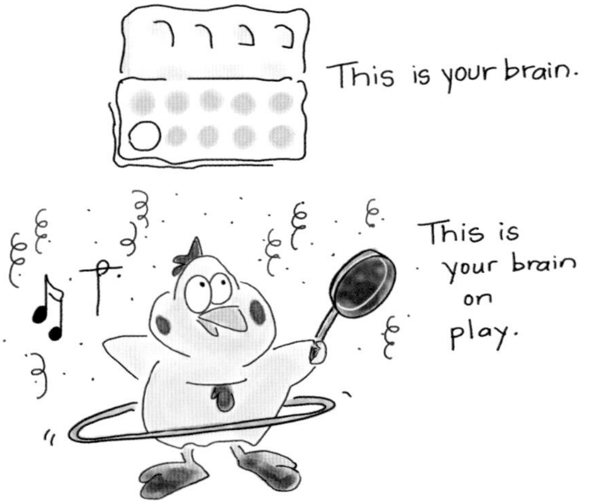

We aren't writing this book just so all of us can just play all willy-nilly-whenever-we-want-to-just-because. Although that would be okay with us, the bosses, the spouses, and the type A friends might need a bit more justification for inviting more playfulness into our lives. Understanding how play affects the brain is needed information for all of us who desire a more playful life. As you just read, play is in our DNA and the numerous benefits of inviting playful living into our daily routine are downright astronomical when you fully understand it. Our goal here is to help you wrap your brain around it all just a bit more. While this section might seem a teensy bit heavy, bear down and get through it so that you can better see what is happening inside your mind when you play.

Julie: "Bear down and get through it?" Really? This is among the best parts!

Jed: I said *bear down* because not everyone reading this is like you, Julie. Some of us are just regular folk. It's me. I am regular folk. Brain science is important, but also reading about it can be as difficult as being a rodeo clown with no barrel to hide in. It's a tad intimidating.

Julie (cuts eyes at Jed, but understands the assignment)

Let's start here with a bit of neuroscience we can ease into. What is playful is also memorable. Think back on the times you experienced playfulness with your family, your classmates, your coworkers. In Section One, we identified those times as your play history. These memories are easily recalled because the moment stuck in your brain. The playfulness of the experience is what did that. You may be thinking, "But how does one make a memory?" Now, Jed and I are not brain scientists, but after working in education for as many years as we have, we're well versed in how thinking happens, especially how learning happens. You could say it cranks our tractors! (Jed cuts eyes at Julie because it doesn't really crank his. In fact, he doesn't even want to own a tractor . . . but a nice man to drive a tractor for him sounds just right!)

As you've read this work, we hope you've had many thoughts. Maybe those were all about what kind of snack you want this afternoon or why you decided to wear these particular socks (today, mine are no-show and white, hiding in my sneakers). Maybe you've wondered why I just shared my sock details. Either way, you're thinking, so, what happens in our brains when thinkin' and wonderin' occur? It's pretty cool. Let's have an experience together, shall we?

Y'all do this:

- Hold your two hands out in front of you like you're pushing off a wall, fingers spread apart, middle fingers almost touching each other. These are brain cells. Your palms are the cell body. Your fingers are the dendrites.
- Okay, now. Think of a cow. Wiggle your fingers. See them getting all excited? Your dendrites are firing because you just had a thought. Imagine silly-string-like-spider-man magic coming out of one finger and connecting to a finger on the other hand.

- Are you brave? Now, moo out loud. Keep mooing until someone looks at you. Now you are having an emotional response. You're either giggly or you're super-embarrassed. Either way, your brain is now connecting cows with an emotion.

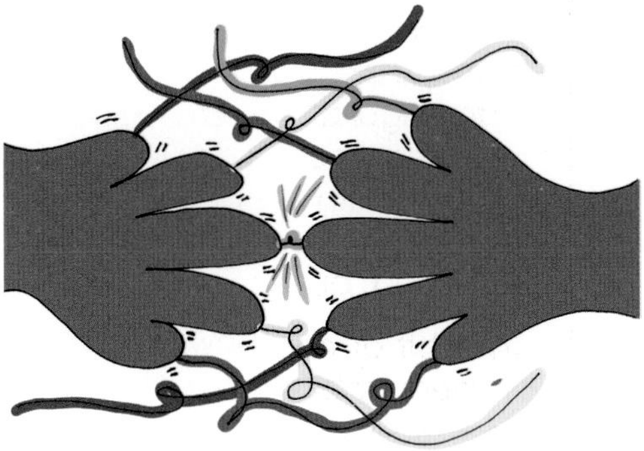

If you do this over and over, you continually build the connection between the emotional parts of your brain (the back and the bottom) and the part of the brain where that cognition is occurring. As you have repeated positive experiences with this concept (cows today . . . mules eating pickles tomorrow?), you build up your myelin sheath (my-a-Lin-she-th), the fatty tissue around these neural connections. You want this fat, y'all. It protects us from distractions or interference (so we can get in the flow—more on that in Chapter 13).

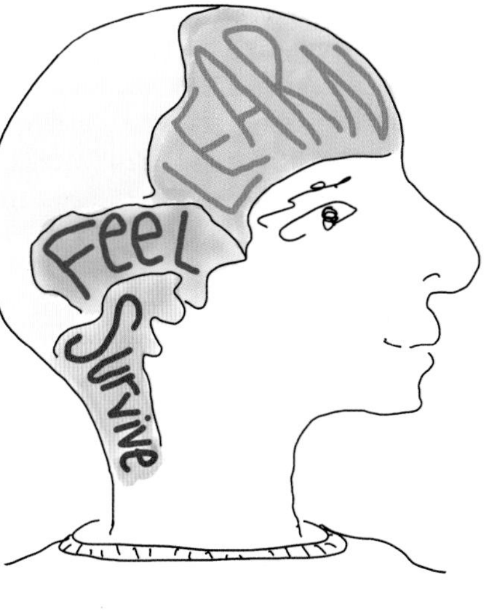

When we are in a state of play, part of our frontal lobe (that judgy executive functioning bit) seemingly gets unhooked, and connections are firing everywhere—imagine a *Fantasia* symphony experience in your noggin. Y'all saw that Disney masterpiece, right? Mickey is waving his wand and the colors are blasting, the instruments are playing, and everything is poppin' to the beat. As we play, in that process, we are creating new neural connections—new mental maps—and when emotions get involved (hello serotonin), we feel good, too.

Y'all. Play is learning. Learning is play. Yet, society has generally compartmentalized learning and play as two separate categories in our day. We learn/work, then we eat, then we play. Unfortunately, way too many of us still think this. Thus, the need for the book you are holding. But scientists now know this compartmentalized view of our experience is antiquated. We don't live in a compartmentalized world; now more than ever before, we live an integrated life. Consider how technology has changed humanity. Back before computers and phones, the workday consisted of an office, a classroom, a specific space where our daily tasks of employment or school had to take place. Then, after we were finished with that task, we moved on to home, or to our friend group, or to the gym. It was all segmented into parts. But now, we can all literally be in class, while working our job and exercising at a friend's house. And the reality is that we don't see our world going back to the days of boxes. The way life changed for everyone in 2020 is an example of this shift. It proved that the way "things have always been done" no longer had to be done the same way. The proverbial box we don't want to think in has quite literally been destroyed.

Living and learning (playing) happens within what Jensen (2005) calls the integrated paradigm. Cognition (learning/thinking/puzzling), emotions (joy, embarrassment, confusion, anger), and movement (whether physical or mental) are not separate. Instead, they are one heaping, happy spaghetti noodle tangle.

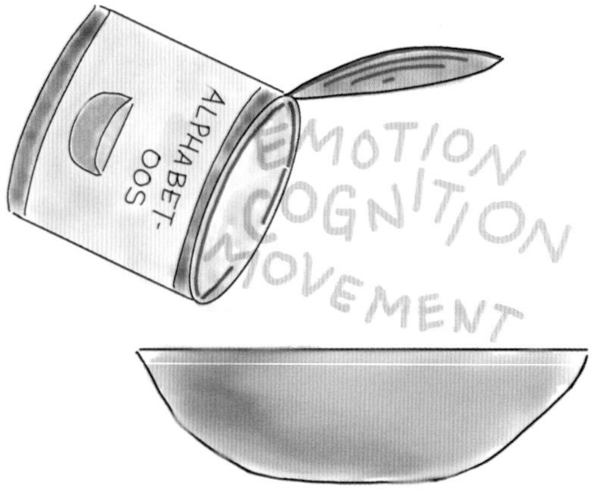

By adding more play to our days, here's what happens in the brain:

- Stimulated neural growth in the cortex and hippocampus (those are parts of the brain that teachers are super excited about—they contribute to learning, memory, logic, and language).
- Opportunities for developing social senses. When we move together, we read body language to successfully navigate our social group. This practice can reinforce friendships, and it also grows our confidence in adulting.
- When we play physically, our bodies are happy. Endorphins and adrenaline promote feelings of joy. Hello emotional connections. And don't forget about serotonin and the poop factor! Yes, we said it again because happy people are people who poop.

How to Create Experiences with the Integrated Paradigm

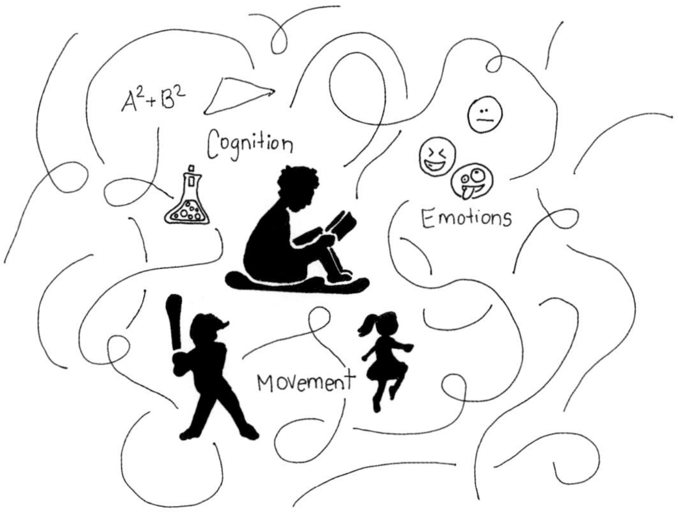

INTEGRATED PARADIGM

We get it: life is crazy. There is so much going on all the time that we need a reminder to set a reminder to look at the day's reminders. Life really is like that bowl of spaghetti. How in the world do we add play to the mix? My plate is full of noodles already. I don't even have room for a side salad. Instead, think of play/playfulness not as an addition to the plate, but as the plate itself. Go grab a plate and some scrap paper. Write all the busy-ness of your life on individual slips of paper. Work. Errands. Rest. Appointments. Family. Friends. Now put those papers on the plate. Play isn't one more thing. It should be what carries all the things.

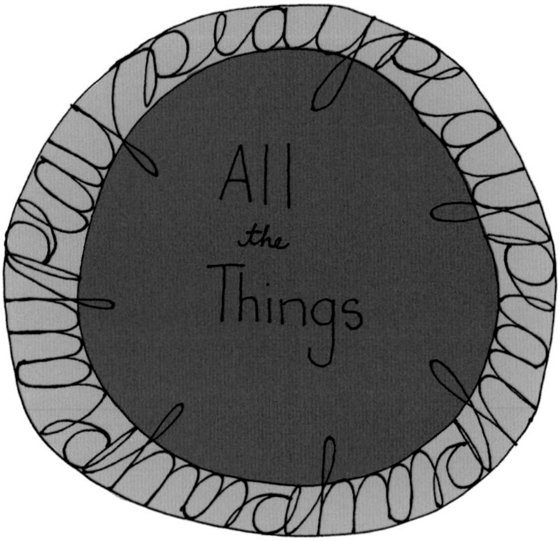

This sounds great, right? But, how do we do that?

Tip 1: Start where you are. Think about the results from the play personality assessment in Section One. Don't try to be someone you're not. A friend of ours who was not very artsy tried too much too fast to become an *artist*, and it was almost a disaster for him. Be true to *you*.

Tip 2: Start small. Don't rewrite your life's schedule. Decide which area of life needs a boost. Find a smidgen of time in your schedule that needs a bit more "oomph." You eat the elephant little by little, not all at once. (Now, you're imagining an elephant and a cow—you're welcome.)

Tip 3: Start with a friend. Plan a playful moment with someone in the next cubicle, a neighbor down the street, someone from your house of worship. Two heads are most times better than one, and it feels a little less scary to try something new when you are not going it alone. Having a friend to be a safety net makes it a lot easier to take the leap, and that courage spreads like kudzu.

Tip 4: Start simple. Too many materials, too many movements, too much too fast will likely exhaust you, and maybe even your bank account. Sometimes playful newbies buy things to make the fun happen. Dig deep in your brain and find the simplest route.

Let's dig deep into these four tips. Let me set you up with a scenario. Right now, I know I'll leave this coffee shop writing with Jed and go home to catch up on the work I've missed while we were writing. I adore my job. I absolutely adore it. But, I cannot stand email. Those people who would rather that meetings become emails? That's not me. Give me a productive meeting in which we work as a team to move forward *any day* over an email. My opinion of the email doesn't make the wretched things go away, though. It's like blaming the cow when the milk goes sour. (Mooo, what is it with us and cows?) For now, I need to change my way of thinking. Let me show you how I'm trying.

Tips	**Real-Life Application**
Start where you are.	My play personality is very much a joker/creator/explorer. As I tackle my emails, I look for funny word phrases or unexpected alliteration, and I jot them down in my journal. Sometimes, ideas for picture books about bunnies come from words in a work-related email.
Start small.	Do I do this with every email, every time? Goodness, no. (Thank you, Pete the Cat). But I do lean into it.
Start with a friend.	Email is such a lonely task. Sometimes, I send a silly text to a friend during the task. Jed and I often send knock-knock jokes and ridiculousness to each other throughout the day. We honor play breaks so much that now they come without us thinking about them.
Start simple.	I have 72 emails in my inbox right now. There is no way I can get to all of them. Each time I answer a few emails, I reward myself with a variety of treats—it could be chocolate, it could be playing the sound of an audience clapping. What if you created a fun little sticker chart for yourself like the one your first-grade teacher had? After you answer three emails, you get a sticker. Five stickers and you get to watch five minutes of cats jumping from cucumbers to relax your brain for a moment. The rewards can vary—you do you. Fun techy side note here: thankfully, Google has a feature called "snooze." I can read an email and snooze it until I need to see it again. I can also "schedule send" my responses. Snoozing an email takes it visually out of my inbox and removes the clutter. Scheduling emails means I'm not bothering colleagues with my reply at 8 p.m., and I avoid the reply, reply, reply that can add to my inbox, keeping me sitting in front of this screen forever. Starting simple can mean reading a few emails in a sitting before taking a break. It can also mean using the tools I have to simplify my process. Sometimes, I do both.

CHAPTER 13

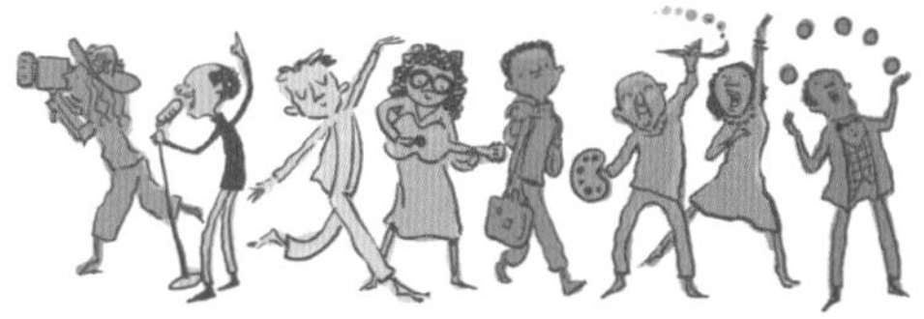

The Default Mode Network and Flow

Today is a cloudy day. The Northeast is about to get blasted with another snowstorm, and our sunshine in South Carolina is hiding. Jed and I have moods and temperaments today that honestly reflect the weather. We're scattered. Each time we get into explaining something to you, we go down a rabbit hole of googlin'. So far we've looked up the etymology of a word, the weather forecast in Chicago, cats and cucumbers on YouTube, and the new Book of the Month picks. You might see this as unproductive, but honestly we've accomplished A Whole Lot today. Why is this so?

Default Mode Network

When we check out mentally, our resting brains automatically switch to a default mode network (DMN). Located in the brain's midline, the DMN consists of a set of interconnected brain regions supporting autobiographical memory, our concept of the self, and our internal monologue (C. Brown, 2017). When the DMN is activated, we stop focusing on external tasks. What was being expressed outward now shifts inward. Say we couldn't think of the name of a particular actor . . . we puzzle over it a bit, but then move on with what we were doing. Y'all, the brain is still puzzling even though we're not cognitively aware of it. Later that day, the name of the actor suddenly pops in our brain and we text whoever we were talking to.

"Billy Porter! That's the actor!"

This is our default mode network in action. Fun fact: the DMNs of playful, creative people differ from those of the average person (Pang, 2016). Okay, great. So what? Okay, we hear you (sits up straight and adjusts glasses as we deliver scientific-speak): The complexity of the default mode shapes our capacity for self-awareness, empathy, moral judgment, and the ability to see from another's point of view. When we play, we build imagination, which is necessary for empathy. Exercising your imagination through daydreaming increases your capacity for empathy (DeBenedet, 2018; Frank, 1978).

DMN and Flow

I (Jed) have watched my niece Sophie really excel at soccer over the years. As she plays, she is totally zoned in on her role on the field. She makes it appear so seamless as she moves. She zips, she zags, she leans in, she backs up, she kicks a little bit, she kicks a lot. It looks like she's hardly having to think. I know she is, but the appearance to spectators is that her movements are as natural as breathing. She is definitely in the flow throughout the game. As soon as the game is over and the family is driving home, the reflection and self-analysis begin. "I should've zigged when I zagged" or "Next time, I'll do this instead of that" are common phrases she will speak about her performance. This is when her DMN is kicking in. During the game, she had no time to be critical of her skills or reflect on what she should have done. It was only after the game was finished that she could shift her brain's focus into internal thinking. Is this work vital to her success on the team? You bet it is. It's how she makes corrections, tweaks, adjustments to her footwork, running speed, and mental stamina for the sake of the team. Imagine if this part of her brain was in overdrive during the actual match. There'd be no way to focus and make the quick decisions needed as the ball comes hurtling at her face or foot. During the game, she is totally in the flow. Her self-criticism has to diminish so she can (1) protect herself from injury and (2) get the ball down the field and score a goal.

Our brains, even while we sleep, are always at work. But its various parts take the stage as the star at different times, thus allowing the other parts to take a quick dash behind the curtain before returning to the show. Of course while it is back there, it is getting

The Timeline of Flow

- Harvard philosopher Wililam James was one of the first to really explore what we call the flow state. He figured out that the brain can severely alter consciousness and improve performance.
- James's student, Walter Bradford Cannon, is who gives us an understanding of the fight-or-flight response. Ahhh—it's biology.
- Later, Maslow picks up on this thread of thinking, discovering that flow is a common feature for successful people.
- 1960s and 1970s, enter the famed Mihaly Csikszentmihalyi, who expanded Maslow's work from successful people to everyone. He asked as many people as he could about the times in their life when they felt their best. This is one of the world largest psychological studies.
- Mihaly Csikszentmihalyi writes the book on flow.

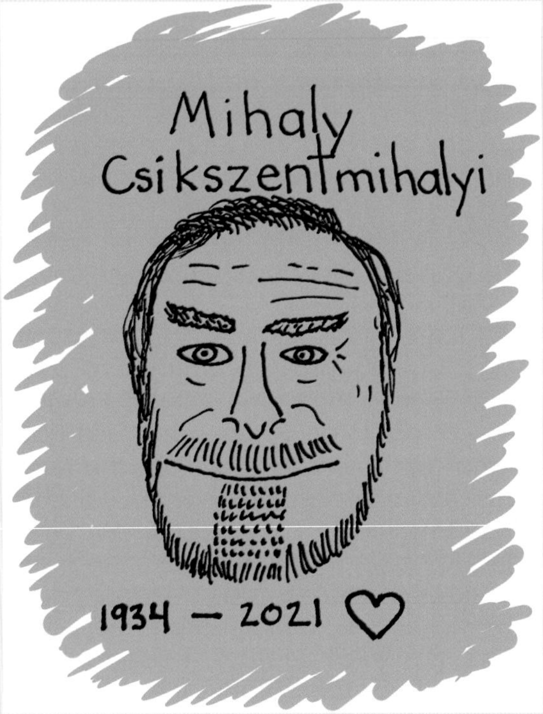

ready for the next act. In essence, our brain goes through a series of seeming "on" and "off." It doesn't cease to work, but works in unique ways depending on our needs at the time. When we play, the part of the brain that reflects and offers criticism is off-stage. Oh, it's there . . . taking notes.

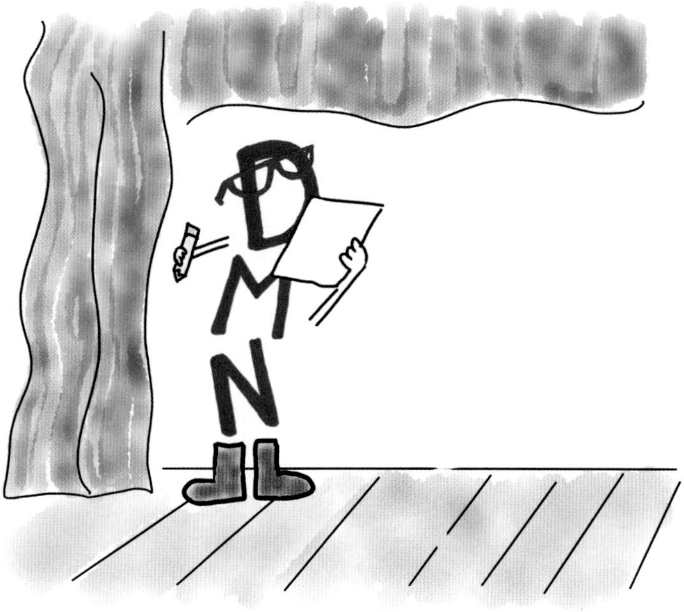

Think about Sophie on the soccer field during the game. Her DMN is backstage watching the performance, and when the game is over, it will appear from behind the curtain to remind her of all it saw as she engaged in play. But when we're in the zone, we are in a state of flow, we are "in it"—we are ON. Flow is Sophie as she makes her way up and down the field—it's a technical term for when we are so attentive that time seems to disappear. When Sophie gets in the car to ride home, her DMN is at the forefront considering her play-past and planning for her play-future. She's remembering, analyzing, editing for the "what if." In this example, Sophie is physically resting as her DMN is at work, but it doesn't have to be so. Our DMNs might take over when we're physically active too.

I (Julie) love to swim laps. On a good swim, I have conversations with others in my head, plan amazing classroom experiences, and wonder about the meanings of various song lyrics. You could be out for a jog, working on a different task, or running an errand. When our default mode network is active, our brains are essentially processing all we've internalized so we can use it later. This is why so many great ideas come in the shower. It often feels like a new thought, idea, or recollection comes from out of the blue. It's almost like our brain said, "SIKE! I have been working on your problem all this time and here is the answer." Our brain seemed to be at rest, but oh hunny—it has been working harder than a mule in May.

Both Flow and the DMN Are Essential for the Magic to Happen

Significant progress in the arts and major scientific breakthroughs are a result of what happens when creative folk play—when they're in the zone, in flow. Pattern recognition, future prediction, and other fundamental neural processes are amplified by flow. The default mode network plays a role in these creations as well. When we can see the connections between disparate ideas, when we can imagine something that's not yet so—that's what happens when we dig deep (flow) and when ideas simmer (DMN). Amor Towles, author of *A Gentleman in Moscow*, *Rules of Civility*, and *Lincoln Highway*, harnesses the power of flow and his DMN to cultivate creative work. He carries notebooks around with him and writes ideas as they come. A story might percolate over several years—he grabs that notebook each time and allows the adventure to grow. His process is not linear. He explores character and potential plots in the notebooks, and only writes the novel in a linear fashion when he knows the magic is ready.

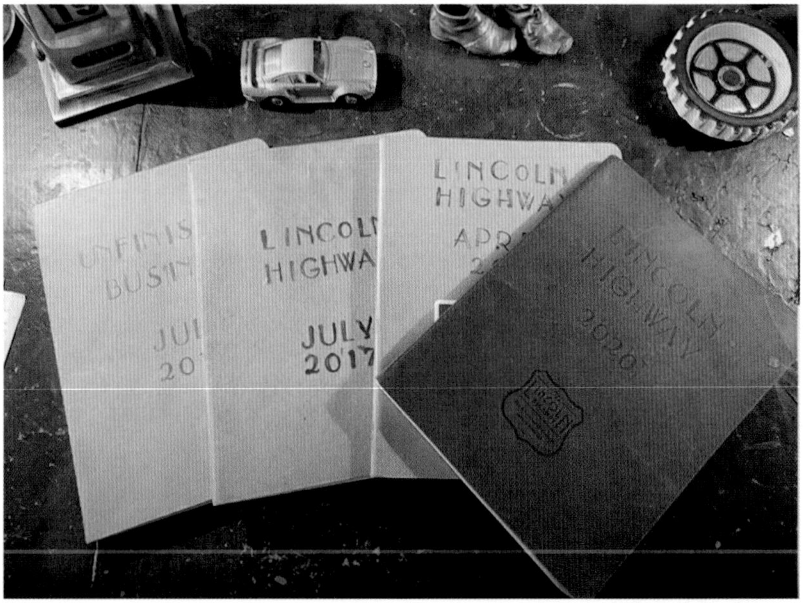

Consider how you handle your spurts of inspiration. Do you intentionally plan for blocks of play during which flow and activation of the DMN can occur? Why not try starting the day with a moment of fun? That could be a morning workout. It could be reading in your favorite chair. Think back to your play personality and before the craziness of the day starts, or right smack dab in the middle of the hectic schedule, drop a playful moment into the madness.

People Who Have the Most Flow in Their Lives Are the Happiest (Csikszentmihalyi, 1990)

Michael Pollan, who you likely know for his reporting on what we should all be eating, talked about the role of the DMN in a recent interview for his book, *How to Change Your Mind*. He described the DMN as the hub of the brain, like Grand Central Station: connections cross its territory all the time—but it's also a regulator (Pollan, 2018). It's where our brains go when we worry, it helps us plan for the future and consider the past. This is the part that's responsible for self-reflection and self-criticism. When we're in a state of flow, our DMN goes quiet, and we experience a dissolution of the self. In other words, our ego stops getting in the way. When we stop being so dad-gummed critical, when our walls are down, we begin to reconnect—with nature, with ourselves, with each other—and eventually we break out of the stories we have told ourselves. Our reflecting ability expands, and we can "change our minds."

When we're in a state of flow:

- We stop telling ourselves we can't.
- We stop saying we're not good enough.
- We release ourselves from the self-critical ego and allow ourselves to grow.

Let's give that inner critic the "what to and how for." If you are like us, you have daily, if not hourly, battles with the inner voice telling you, "you can't." Exhausting, isn't it? During a state of flow, the nagging inner critic is turned off. When we don't pay attention to this voice, we open up possibilities for play that were previously impossible. Creativity, risk taking, and performance all see increases. Many times during the writing of this book, which isn't always playful for us, we take moments to laugh, be silly, doodle, take a walk, etc. Because we are reflective writers, considering each word and phrase as it's put to paper, our DMN is often the dominant force—with a loud inner critic. Inviting moments of playfulness during our process, especially a trip to Hub City Bookshop—the smell of the pages, all the titles, our friends who work there—allows us to get lost for a moment. In a fraction of a second, we are lost in time, perusing the aisles. We can honestly say that the moments after a playful experience are often our most productive. Something we saw, said, or did while lost in the flow is almost guaranteed to inspire our work. That part about Amor Towles? I watched an interview with him while taking 10 minutes out for my at-home rowing machine.

The Neuroscience of Flow Impacts Both Skill and Memory

Flow is considered the source of intrinsic motivation and increases our memory recall for events. Previously, we mentioned what the brain experiences during flow, as five major neurotransmitters (norepinephrine, dopamine, anandamide, endorphins, and serotonin) rush the brain at once, creating a "creative high" not experienced naturally at any other time. Let's dig a bit more into this scrumptious cocktail.

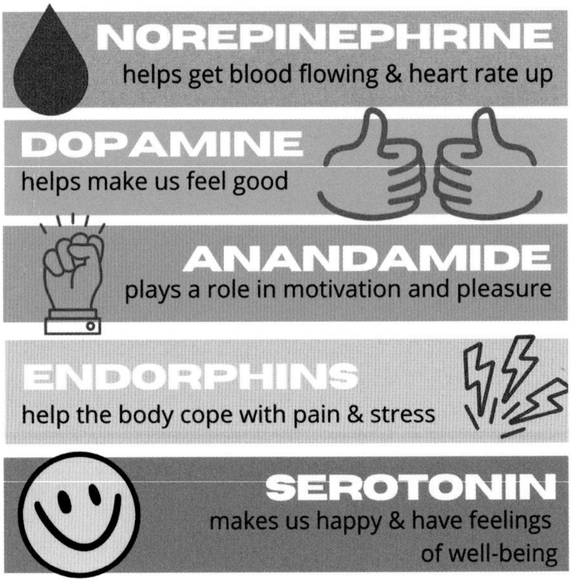

Some theorists believe that being in the state of flow actually trains the brain to be more playful. What does this mean for humans? The more these natural chemicals are present as we make memories, the greater the likelihood of us remembering the event. You've likely heard of Malcolm Gladwell's book *Outliers*—in this work, he explains that it takes roughly 10,000 hours to master a skill. He cites the Beatles and other playful folk as evidence for this claim (Gladwell, 2008). Imagine what flow could do for that 10,000-hour rule—talk about weedin' a pretty wide row!

CHAPTER 14

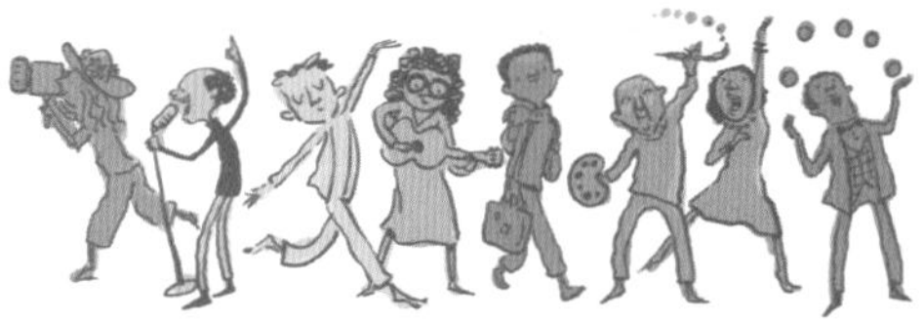

Playful Habits

How Habits Are Formed

Julie here. In 2015, my kiddos were in elementary school. I was at least six years past due on using baby weight as an excuse for my clothes not fitting quite right. In reflection, I discovered that much of this slow decline had to do with the sedentary lifestyle of academia—writing academically requires a lot of sitting. I wanted more activity in my life. I knew I didn't enjoy how I felt when I was sweaty, so I brainstormed movement opportunities that didn't include becoming overheated. Enter—swimming. My girls are swimmers. This sport was already a part of my life. I knew and understood the pool life—the rules of the lanes and the locations where the locker rooms were nice. One afternoon, I left work early and joined the local YMCA. Now I needed to figure out when I would work this new component in my day.

Here are some little-known facts about Julie:

- I'm a snooze-button repeat offender.
- I don't like eating breakfast first thing in the morning, instead preferring to sip coffee until ready for more.
- I also like a slow morning—one without stress of expectations and rules.

In academia, we often find ourselves teaching late into the evening. At the small, private university I teach at, we offer many courses at the 4 p.m. and 5:45 p.m. time slots. That can mean I'm not walking to my car until 8:30 some nights. So I was continually rising early and getting full-on ready for the day before

I took the girls to school. Where did that leave time for me to chill? Where was my time for movement? When was I letting myself decompress? Honestly, I wasn't. And I could feel it taking a toll. One day while driving home, listening only to the sounds of the road, it occurred to me that I was not using my morning hours well. I began to get up and throw on an outfit with a knit dress and slides. Now, with my hair pulled back and bag packed for the day, I have the time to chat with my oldest while she gets ready. I have time to help my youngest run around and ensure she has everything she needs for her day (lunch, charged computer, signed forms). Arriving at the Y, I can throw my bag in the locker, grab my cap and goggles, and get 30 meditative minutes of breaststroke before hopping out to shower and head to campus. Women, too often in our society, try to do all the things. I still try to do all the things. But by shifting my own expectations and my morning routine, I now have a habit of movement I look forward to daily.

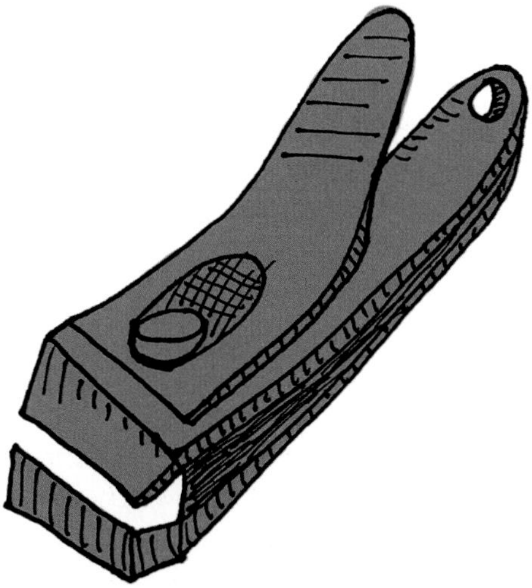

When I (Jed) was about 16 years old, I had a terrible habit of biting my fingernails. Anxiousness led to me constantly chewing on my fingertips. I often bit the nails way too far down and they would bleed and hurt for days at a time. My grandma used to fuss at me all the time about it. Not only was it painful, but it is a very nasty habit. One day, she got fed up with fussing and gave me a pair of fingernail clippers. "Keep these in your pocket, and it'll fix that for good," she said. At the time of this writing I am 43 years old, and to this day there has been and always will be a pair of clippers in my pocket. Ask any of my friends. They will confirm this is true. I don't leave home without them. I just showed Julie my current pair as I typed this. And just in case I accidentally leave them behind as I rush out the door, I have a backup pair in my bag, in my car, and have even been known to stop by the drugstore for a few extra pairs just in case one goes missing. Some would say it is a bit obsessive, but for me, it's a habit. It is a repeated action I do over and over, almost without even thinking about it. And what do I get out of this habit? No pain from hangnails and my fingernails are never bitten too short. I also have a handy device at the ready for snipping little strings and opening packages. For some 25+ years, this has just become my way of life. And thankfully, it squashed the bad habit of nail biting.

Charles Duhigg (2014) has done a lot of studying on habits. He even wrote a book about it, called *The Power of Habit: Why We Do What We Do in Life and Business*. In this work, he builds off hundreds of academic studies and over 300 interviews with scientists and executives. Our habits boil down to: (1) cue, (2) routine, and (3) reward. The cue is the trigger that alerts our noggins to go into automatic mode in which a habit follows. Once alerted, we have routines, both physical and mental ones. Finally, the reward stage helps our brains determine if this habit—this loop—is worth remembering for future experiences. When a habit develops, our brains essentially stop working as hard, now able to divert attention to other tasks. So, Duhigg writes, "unless you deliberately *fight* a habit—unless you find new routines—the pattern will unfold automatically" (p. 20).

Well, that's just hunky-dory, right? My brain can decide to do whatever I *cue it* to do. Nice (sips overpriced latte). How do I stop drinking this coffee then? How do I get myself up early to do all those things I lament not having done when I'm lying in bed late at night? That guy I see running in the rain—how does he get to that point? It has everything to do with cravings.

Did you know that brushing our teeth regularly wasn't a *thing* in the early 1900s? It wasn't until a Pepsodent campaign designed by Claude Hopkins spread the idea of toothpaste as the key to getting rid of that "cloudy film" on our teeth that the teeth-brushing habit took off. Pepsodent advertisers capitalized on the message that not removing this "cloudy film" would make our teeth be *off color* and *invite decay*. Who wouldn't want to be more beautiful? Who wouldn't want a shiny white smile? Who wouldn't brush with Pepsodent?

Cue (cloudy film feeling and desire for beauty) → **Routine** (brushing) → **Reward** (no film/sparkly clean teeth)

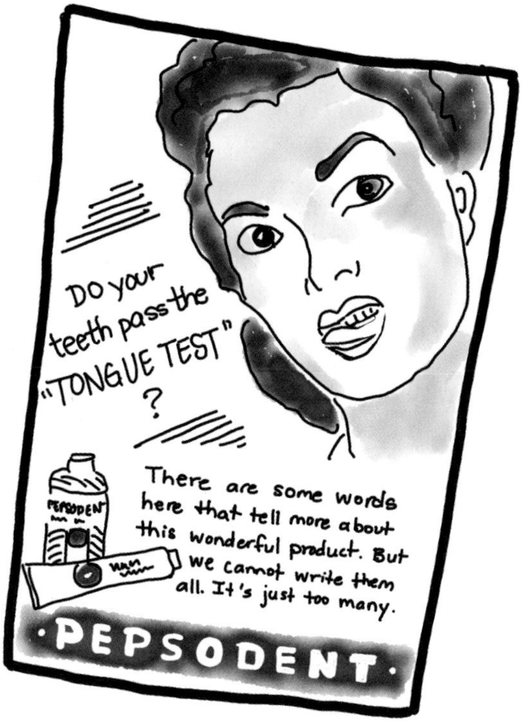

In the 1980s, a group of scientists began to pay more attention to brain activity in monkeys, curious about what parts of the brain were responsible for learning new skills or tasks. During an experiment, Wolfram Shultz, a neuroscientist at the University of Cambridge, saw a pattern emerge in the brain of an eight-pound macaque with hazel eyes, named Julio. Over time, as Julio received his reward (here, juice), his little brain began to anticipate the juice. In the brain, the activity began to occur *before* the juice arrived. If the juice was late or didn't come, Julio would get irritated, even angry. Why? Cravings. So these scientists did what scientists do. They applied this experiment to other monkeys—juice deprivation. They implemented distraction to see its effects. For the monkeys that had not developed a habit, that had no neurological activity showing anticipation of the juice, the distraction worked. But those monkeys that had formed a habit? Nothing worked. These are not cravings in the general sense of the word—these are neurological cravings, or, as we know them, an indicator of *habit* formation.

We know that cues and rewards alone do not create a lasting habit. Lawsy, if it did, we'd all look like superheroes and achieve every goal we threw into the ether. No. It's when our brains *expect* the reward—when our noggins crave the endorphins or atta-boy! that comes from a behavior that change occurs.

You Can't Teach an Old Dog . . .

So, I would bet that most of us reading these words are grown-ups. We have had years of life experiences creating our current reality. Creating new habits from scratch seems a bit much for those of us stuck in our ways. So then, how do we change an old habit? Tony Dungy, former head coach of the Tampa Bay Buccaneers, says the solution for changing habits in training NFL players came down to this process:

1. Keep the **old cue**,
2. Change the **routine**,
3. Deliver the **old reward**.

When we recognize the cues and rewards in our life that create such routines, we can use them to begin shifting our routines. Whereas Pepsodent created a new craving, many of us need to focus on adjusting old cravings. We can do this by analyzing the cue and the reward in our behaviors, looking for opportunities to shift routines.

Let's revisit Jed and his fingernails. Lots of people are nail-biters. But some are so extreme in their habits that they cause damage to their hands—scabs and bleeding fingers. Some so much so that they keep their hands in their pockets, hopeful of keeping others from seeing the results of this bad habit. By simply keeping clippers in his pocket, Jed inserted the opportunity for a new routine in his life. Running his hands along his nails in search of hangnails or a rough edge is a cue that continues to this day. The new routine of reaching for his clippers creates the same satisfaction of a smooth result—now, though, without the injury or drama of continuous biting.

For those of you who need a visual:

Jed's clippers

Old **cue**:	New **routine**:	Old **reward**:
Anxiety	Reaching for the ever-accessible clippers	Smooth edges and no pain

What about Julie's swimming habit?

Old **cue**:	New **routine**:	Old **reward**:
Need to be ready for the day when everyone else is ready	Less prep in the morning that includes swimming daily	Get to work on time without struggle

No, this cue-routine-reward (CRR) formula isn't a Charlie-chocolate-factory-golden-ticket. Habits are tricky and everyone's are different. What keeps us going? What will keep us coming back to the attempt at new routines? Belief. Belief that what we're doing will create the outcome we desire. Belief that you can keep going. When taking large leaps, this belief is best achieved in group settings. Our probability of success increases dramatically when we take on challenges as a group.

Want to be more positive? Surround yourself with positive people.
What to be a runner? Join a running club.
What to read more? Make friends with readers—join a book club!

Creating Playful Habits

Our days are full of opportunities to invite playful habits into our living. If we start with our everyday, ordinary experiences, these small shifts in thinking can create a habit that spills over into all the nooks and crannies of our lives. As you read the examples that follow, look at how each one responds to the cue-routine-reward rule, while also incorporating thinking, movement, and emotion.

Once we create new routines, honoring the integrated paradigm for learning will only reinforce our new behaviors. You don't need all three in each situation. Remember, it's a paradigm—a model, a way of thinking, not a direct path from A to B that must be followed step by step to achieve desired results. It ebbs. It evolves. Mix it up. Play with it.

To change a habit, we need an old cue, a new routine, and a previously consistent reward.

The reward of being more playful is multifaceted: when we play, there is a physical response in the body (the release of neurotransmitters), which leads to a positive emotional reaction (feelings of happiness, joy, less stress), thus increasing productivity and overall well-being (because you feel better, you do better).

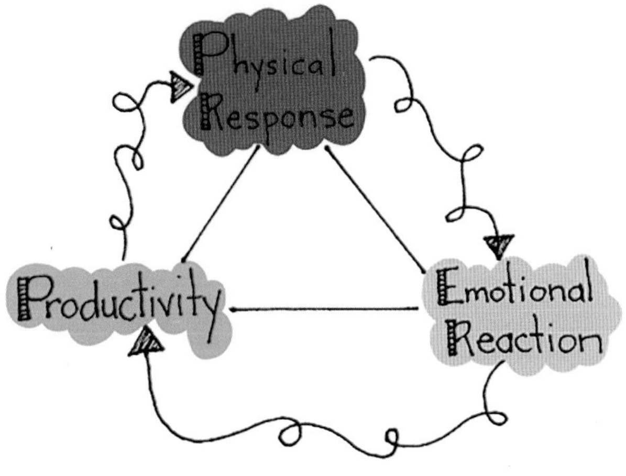

The following is a chart we created of some of life's mundane tasks that many of us have to face on a regular basis. These tasks have created many habits for most of us, whether we realize it or not. We are confident that all of you have a certain way that you fold laundry and wash dishes and you most certainly have a favorite radio station, playlist, or podcast that is your go-to when you're stuck in traffic. These habits have developed as you continue to complete the same task over and over. We don't give you cues and rewards here because those are different for everyone. What we do give you is a window into what could be a new routine . . . thus a new *playful* habit. Many of these actions have the potential to create stress or momentary unpleasantness. It is these types of experiences that need a playful pivot most.

Situation	**"Needs More Play" Me**	**"Playful" Me**
Need to fold laundry	"Ugh. . . this mountain never ends!"	I put the tunes on shuffle and fold with the mood of the music—quite theatrical.
Washing dishes	I get a bit salty, in my brain fussing at all the people in this house who dared to drink out of more than one glass.	I will look for pareidolia while I wash. Suds and bubbles often make for great surprise faces.
Need to share information to my team	I'll make a bulleted list and from that prepare my usual slide presentation.	I am bringing markers and Play-Doh and we will sketch and sculpt all the new information.
Shopping for a gift	If I have to go into a store, I may scream. I will just order something from Amazon.	I will pretend I am working with James Bond on a covert mission to retrieve a special antidote inside my friend's favorite local store.
Planning a party for a friend	I love my friend so much, but I wish I had let someone else plan this.	What does my friend love? How can I bring all the things they love together for a playful evening?
Completing a school assignment	I CANNOT STAND HOMEWORK! I ain't doing it. (Begrudgingly begins worksheet.)	I still think homework is ridiculous, but until the system changes I have to complete it. I will do that by giving myself a tiny snack or 30-second dance party for every five math problems I solve.
Organizing the junk drawer	I open the drawer. I see a mess. I close the drawer. I walk away.	I take items from the drawer and talk to each one as I begin to sort them on the counter. Each item has a personality and a voice. I ask what each is thinking and answer in the voice of that object.

Situation	"Needs More Play" Me	"Playful" Me
Extended time in a waiting room	I look around to choose a seat far away from others. I open social media and scroll until my name is called.	I sit in view of the whole room, and I imagine the backstory of each person. What do they drive? Why are they here? What's their mama's name? What are they eating for dinner? I create my own daytime drama while being careful not to stare too hard.
On hold with customer service	I talk back to the little phone voice using *not nice* words and dare it to put that awful music on again. "I want to speak to a real person please."	I challenge myself to a private dance party. Each time the voice comes on to thank me for holding, I freeze. Unfreeze when the music plays again.
Stuck in traffic	I will change lanes as much as possible, all the while cussin' those who refuse to let me over.	I will breathe deep breaths and listen to my favorite meditation podcast, album, or app.

You may read this and think, okay. Sounds good, but how do I begin this shift of thinking? Where do these playful ideas come from? First and foremost, they come from practice, practice, practice. It takes time to develop the habit because we have been so conditioned to seeing playfulness as a lack of productivity. The practice of play isn't just developing a new skill, but in many ways it is rewiring your brain's thinking. Leveling up is how we began to develop our own practice.

Level Up

Julie and I don't consider ourselves old just yet, but we do remember the world before cell phones and the internet. We had a great discussion as we typed this about how those of us born in the late 1970s/early 1980s are the last generation that will understand what it means to

- Call collect
- Check movie times by calling the automated hotline
- Pull an encyclopedia off the shelf at your house
- Pull the game out, blow in it, reinsert
- The thrill of the sound of AOL connecting your computer to the world

We also remember when the very first Nintendo introduced us to the world of *Super Mario*. I can still remember the first time

I saw him on the screen of my 13-inch black-and-white TV in my childhood bedroom. Again, I am not that old, but the TV in my room was. I digress. As Mario came to life I was immediately drawn into his universe. Walking mushrooms with eyeballs, hopping turtles with wings, and my ever-favorite, a magical flower that gave him fire-shooting power. You were almost invincible thanks to the ability to launch a fireball at the infamous Hammer Brothers. Of course tiny Mario could just run under them, but with firepower he earned extra points for taking the brothers out, and he didn't have to worry as much about timing his run to get past the boogers.

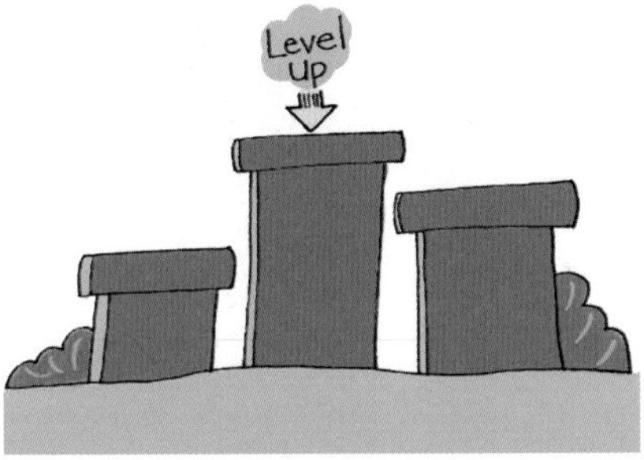

I spent hours and hours trying to beat the game and take down Bowser and save Princess Peach. The more I had the ability to hurl a flaming ball, the easier it was to do that. Could tiny Mario beat the whole game? Sure he could. But one little touch from an evil creature or its weapon and down he went. It made the game a bit easier when he would *level up*. The flower wasn't his only way to do that. There was the mushroom that made him large, and the star that made him momentarily invincible. These level-ups weren't always readily available. Sometimes he had to hunt for them hidden in bricks, behind bushes, or down drainpipes. But when he did have access to their help, it made his ability to conquer life in his world a bit better. Like we said, he could've done it without them, but man, how much more difficult it was.

As our understanding of play continues to develop—the benefits it brings, and the overall well-being it can provide to our lives—we mustn't forget the story of our tiny plumber friend and his *level-ups*. We certainly know that we can have a decent life without inviting all the aspects of play into our world. But don't we all want the best life possible? We want to strive for less anger, more happiness. Less stress, more calm. Less turmoil, more peace. Cultivating a playful life will not ever eliminate all of the anger, stress, and turmoil we experience, but, just like Mario with all of his *level-ups* while fighting the Koopas and Goombas, it will definitely make it easier to survive in the universe in which we live. Let's examine a bit more what a level-up looks like for us humans, unless of course you know where we can find a magical flower that gives fire-shooting power.

We've created some level-up steps for ya. We love a good acronym because it helps us remember them easier.

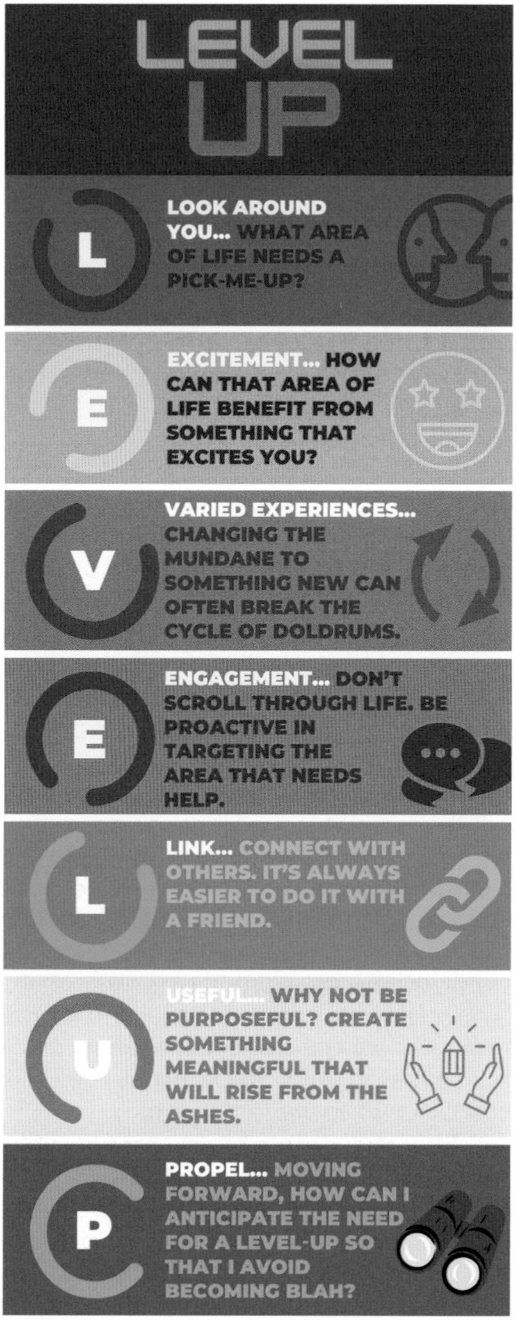

1. **Look** around you . . . What area of life needs a pick-me-up?

   Reflecting, I do spend a lot of time in my office. I need to get up and get out a bit more.
2. **Excitement** . . . How can that area of life benefit from something that excites you?

   I know that moving and doing will create more energy and will make me more productive. I love the feeling I get from a walk around the block. I'm awake, I've had time to think, I've moved my body. I like it.
3. **Varied** experiences . . . Changing the mundane to something new can often break the cycle of doldrums.

   There are a lot of ways I can add more activity in my life. Yes, I can take a walk. I can also play Just Dance with my kiddos. I can skip to the local coffee shop. I can get in a boat and paddle the lake. I can cut grass while jamming out to my favorite tunes. I can plant flowers and name them like pets (or new friends).
4. **Engagement** . . . Don't scroll through life. Be proactive in targeting the area that needs help.

   I went to a meeting once, full of people who speak in a heavy Southern drawl. It was all I could do to sit on the bench with a straight face. Y'all. It was thick (and that is saying something because both of us are very Southern)! Anyway, a woman in flowy clothes and wild (*wild*) hair stood up and invited all the "ladies" to her house for coffee on Monday mornings. She said, "Life is a contact sport. You gotta show up and play." Her words perfectly explain why I need to get moving. I want to be out there more. I want to participate and *engage* in my own life. It's time for me to get moving.
5. **Link**: Connect with others. It's always easier to do it with a friend.

   Hey, Jed. Whatcha doing on Tuesday morning?
6. **Useful** . . . Why not be purposeful? Create something meaningful that will rise from the ashes.

   You know how we meet to write and always spend the first 30 minutes shooting the bull before getting down to business? Let's start with a walk on the trail. We can get all our chattin' out while we're moving.
7. **Propel** . . . Moving forward, how can I anticipate the need for a level-up so that I avoid becoming blah?

   In my reading of therapy and play for healing, I know more about listening to my body and paying attention to my emotional reactions. I'm gonna do more of that.

CHAPTER 15

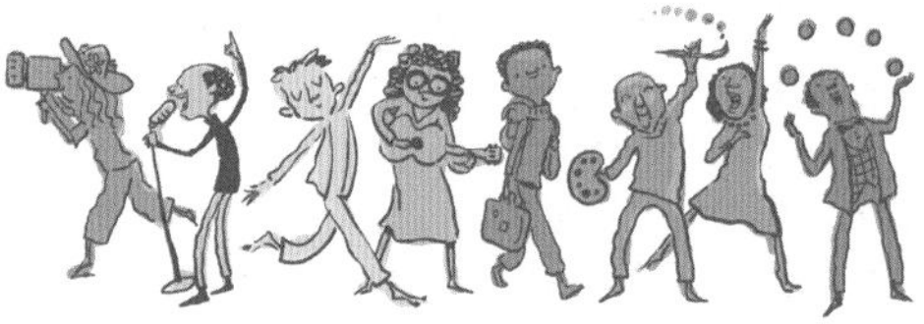

Play as Healing

We hope that, as we approach this point in the reading, you have already begun to identify areas of your life that are playful. Dance parties while cleaning the house, singing to the top of your lungs on the morning commute, doodling, crossword puzzles, or game night with friends are all forms of play. Maybe you have discovered some of your unique habits are also a form of play. Creating puppets with the socks as you sort the laundry, tapping your feet to the beat of the coffeeshop music, and humming *Happy Birthday* to time your hand-washing are also great playful experiences that can have a great positive impact on your day. These moments, even the briefest of ones, aid in decreasing stress levels. Who doesn't need less stress, right? Less stress helps us to sleep better, lowers our blood pressure, and improves digestion. (There it is again . . . *poop*!)

Play for Emotional Healing

Stress in our lives is directly related to experience—both present and past. Think about your physical reaction to certain songs that come on the radio. When I (Julie) hear *Killing Me Softly* by the Fugees, I have a bodily reaction—I tense up and immediately feel inferior. Play therapists call this implicit memory—a memory understood through physical reactions to a stimulus. This song creates an embodied memory from my college days of a Friday evening gone wrong. On the flip side, when I hear Tori Kelly sing *Hallelujah!*, I'm filled with hope and joy. I can see the end of the movie *Sing!*, as the elephant character Meena transitions the movie to its happy ending. My experiences with this movie always involve happy moments with my children. Recognizing the role of stress in our lives may begin with paying attention to our bodily reaction to events. Many times, our bodies tell us how we feel before our brains understand what's going on.

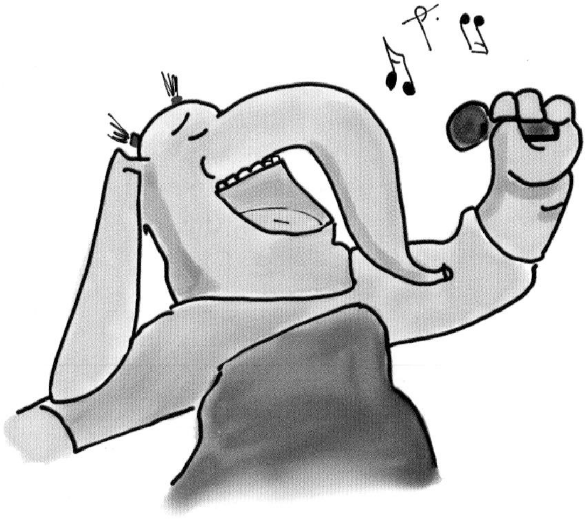

Decreasing the amount of stress in our lives is vital in regulating the amount of cortisol in our bodies. Cortisol is a hormone made by the adrenal glands located at the top of our kidneys. It is released at various times throughout the day. It helps us get out of bed in the morning or press through the daily workout that we are dreading. It helps regulate our blood pressure and reduces inflammation. Cortisol also helps us in those moments of fight or flight. Lots of therapists like to explain our body's need for it by asking clients to imagine being chased by a lion. We would need all the cortisol we could get at that moment. GET OUT OF THERE SO YOU SURVIVE! Personally, we have never been chased by a lion, but a herd of elk, yes, for me (Jed), once on the top of Donnelly Dome, a mountain in Alaska. Thankfully the cortisol was in full effect that afternoon!

You may be seeing all these benefits here and be wondering "why do I need to manage the level of this magical hormone?" Well, on the downside, too much or too little cortisol can have a very negative effect on the body. Like everything, we need it in moderation.

Symptoms of too much cortisol include (Healthdirect, n.d.):

- Weight gain, particularly around the abdomen and face
- Thin and fragile skin that is slow to heal

- Acne
- For women, facial hair and irregular menstrual periods

Symptoms of not enough cortisol include:

- Continual tiredness
- Nausea and vomiting
- Weight loss
- Muscle weakness
- Pain in the abdomen

My therapist and I (Jed) talk a lot about cortisol during therapy. Once she realized the amount of trauma that I had faced as a result of being a gay man, we had no choice. During my childhood, throughout high school and college, and even now as an adult, I was/am constantly facing one thing or another that forces my body into that flight-or-fight mode. To me, it almost seems like I exist more in that mode than any other. As a resident of the Southern United States, I am forced to advocate for my equality and safety on a regular basis. I face bullying in the public square, the workforce, and religious institutions. My guard is constantly up. I am always looking to my left and to my right awaiting, expecting, the next traumatic event connected to my existence to occur. It is no wonder my cortisol levels are through the roof. My brain has experienced this same type of trauma so repetitively that defensiveness is my go-to reaction for anything that seems slightly threatening to my well-being. I wasn't born to respond/react this way so often, but through years and years of trauma, my brain was rewired to respond in this manner. Honestly, it's exhausting to live like that, but it's likely what has kept me alive. Thus, the need for my therapist. I recognize the need for healing: physical, in that I want to rewire the previous rewire of my brain after all the years of trauma; emotional, because I recognize the need to have more peace and less stress so I can be more productive in meeting my goals. The good news is that it is *more* than possible to do that. Over time, I have made great progress thanks to the help of my therapist. One of the things we do that is most helpful during my sessions is laugh. Almost instantly as she closes the door to her office at the start of my session, we laugh about something. It might be because of Gracie, her tiny dog, or a joke my therapist tells me. Sometimes it's me who brings the moment of laughter as I tell a story about something funny a student said once. The laughter instantly puts me at ease, and opens my heart and mind to the work that needs to be done. It releases stress that I carried into the space and instantaneously my cortisol levels decrease. Just a brief moment of humor, which is most definitely a type of play, impacts my whole entire body and allows for me to confront the pain of the trauma.

Often, the hour of my therapy seems to go by in a blink because we both get lost in the work. I will never understand how 50 minutes can seem like five. We definitely are lost in the flow of the work. Don't get me wrong, it's difficult sometimes, and can include tears, but throughout the session, there is so much more than me retelling stressful moments and listening to her therapeutic advice. Not only is there laughter, but there is storytelling, a collecting of memories, art making, and sometimes even movement. My therapy, while not specifically play therapy, is full of playful experiences that are leading me to healing each week.

When I am in a state of flow talking with my therapist, the neurochemicals involved not only regulate my cortisol, but they significantly elevate my immune system, while also resetting the nervous system. Flow, as we play, does this for us all. The safe relationships experienced during play allow us to release a preconceived agenda, rewriting new scripts. These new scripts, or new understandings of relationships and community, overwrite and rewire neural circuitry, resulting in healing. Those implicit and embodied memories that so affected us before shift to explicit memories, and we become able to tell the narrative of our past without the significant emotional response.

This is not a quick fix. Healing takes time. For those of us who have deeper struggles, our window of tolerance for strong emotions may be narrow (Siegel, 2012). Small nudges over time as trust is built may be how we move toward healing in these cases. Allowing for play and our own state of flow regularly lets our brains form new neural nets—connections that are not associated with trauma or illness. The more we do this, the closer we can move to emotional (and, for some, physical) healing. The rewiring of the previous rewire is gradually happening with each session.

Play for Physical Healing

Play can also be a form of physical healing. While Jed's story of therapy is one of emotional healing, researcher Dr. Stuart Brown says that play can provide physical healing. "Even in a dementia ward, when you bring play into a dementia setting that is specified for the play type that that person once enjoyed, their need for medication and their level of agitation goes down as they get playful. So this is part of from birth to death there is a presence in our beings for playfulness" (Raz, 2015).

Physical therapists often bring playfulness into their practices as well. Playing catch with a friend, going for a walk, stretching, and water aerobics—all forms of play—can have significant impacts on the body's healing after accidents involving physical injuries.

We love these words by play therapist Dottie Ward-Wimmer (2003), "Physical motion invites release; creativity nurtures insight. Play and its therapeutic value reminds us of the old song 'Dem Bones,' which says 'the head bone's connected to the neck bones,' and so on. Play, whether with games, puppets, drums, clay, sports, motion, drawing, drama, dolls, sand, or whatever else is available, invites a cascade of positive effects."

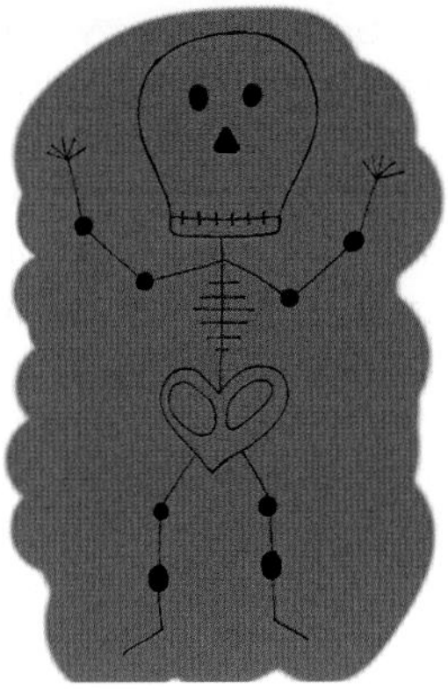

Let's break down some of these positive effects. When we play, we affect how our bodies (cells, tissue, organs, physiological systems) respond to exercise. When we upset our sedentary norms with short spurts of movement, we improve our health and fitness through physical activity.

How many of us have a sedentary lifestyle? How often throughout your day have you been sitting? Get ready: we're about to show you the weeds in your garden—but only because we see them in our own. A 2018 study from the American Cancer Society shows a link between long periods of leisure time sitting and a higher risk of death from all causes, including 14 of the 22 causes of death they studied. Y'all. This includes 8 of the 10 most common causes of death (Patel et al., 2018). Get up from reading this section right now!

Okay, glad you're back. Some scientists have even referred to sitting as the new cancer. Inactivity for long periods of time is linked to increased risk of health conditions, including hypertension, diabetes, cardiovascular problems, obesity, and early death (Suliga et al., 2018; Warburton et al., 2006). Thankfully, these health concerns can be addressed through lifestyle changes, including stress management, proper sleep, and regular physical activity. Wait a minute. Read that list again.

Stress management
Proper sleep
Regular physical activity

Play gives us all of that! When we play, we build our muscles, we improve systems, we release all the neurochemicals . . . and we can prevent disease and some disabilities. For example, strengthening the heart muscle through regular play reverses risk factors for heart disease and some risk factors for type II diabetes.

Pre-pandemic, we had the chance to attend a play workshop at the US Play Coalition's annual conference, led by Darryl Edwards, a former investment banking technologist turned movement coach. He is the founder of the Primal Play Method and writes regularly on physical activity, health, and play. He is also the author of the best-selling book *Animal Moves* (Edwards, 2018), which highlights why humans should move like the animals we are. Edwards's key point is that we need to be physical in our play. The learning experience we had in Darryl's workshop that day continues to be one of the most impactful classes we have experienced while researching the power of play and its effect on humans. It was also definitely the most humorous. The class was scheduled for the first day of the conference—you know, the day you show up looking all cute and clean. "Hey! Oh my goodness—so nice to see you!" etc., etc. Needless to say, neither of us were prepared for (read: dressed appropriately for) the amount of fun and play we experienced that day. Both of us had on restrictive pants (jeans, khakis) and there was definitely a pair of boots soon removed to allow for better movement. From the first moment of his presentation, Mr. Edwards had us moving up, down, and all around. To say that we laughed as we learned is an understatement: we downright guffawed, heehawed, and cried a comical amount of tears as we twisted and turned. The best part was that the room was full of "professionals" who, within the first five minutes, lost their inhibitions and soaked up the physical benefits of play. By the end of the session, we had learned to walk like a crab, hop like a kangaroo, build like a beaver, and strut like a rooster. Our heart rates were up, our lungs were strengthening with every breath, and minds were sharp as ever, all thanks to the animalistic movement we experienced as we played for three straight hours. It definitely set the stage for learning throughout the rest of the day. Our brains were primed from all the playful experiences. And on top of that, it was a total blast!

While we're on the topic of movement, we can't help but bring up location. As I write this in June 2022, the pandemic feels as if it's mostly behind us. Not that it's over, but the way we have started to live made available by the opportunity for vaccines feels very different now than it did in April of 2020. We are sure you remember the feeling of being trapped inside for fear of sickness or affecting our fellow humans. Some of us ventured out for walks through our neighborhoods, but many chose not to even leave their dwellings. This "staying inside" impacted the health of our world greatly, and not in a good way. Let us tell you about a study—conducted more than 10 years ago, well before the COVID-19 pandemic, a team of researchers conducted a series of five studies (Ryan et al., 2010). In the first study, they wanted to see if being outside was associated with vitality (surprise—it is). In the second study, they compared outdoor walks to indoor walks. In the third, they showed participants photos of nature or buildings. In the fourth and fifth studies, they looked at diaries of participants to determine if there were variations in where energy was derived—was it from being outside? You can likely guess that the answer is yes. They found positive effects across all studies—being outside is related to higher vitality, enhanced by as much as 40%. That's no shock to us—you either, we bet. What is very interesting here is that spending time indoors had the *opposite* effect (Taylor, 2022). Yeah, you read that right. The more we are inside, the more the sympathetic nervous system takes over. The primary job of this system is the fight-or-flight response to stressors. Conversely, the parasympathetic nervous system is induced by being outdoors (other things stimulate this system, too, but that's not our point). On an elementary level, the PNS basically undoes the work of the sympathetic system after a stressful situation. It heals. It lets us rest and restore. The lesson here? Get outside, y'all.

Our friend, Dr. Debbie Rhea, is currently working with her team to conduct research on cortisol levels of fourth-graders living in Texas. You may have read about her work in *The Playful Classroom*—she brought the ideas from Finland about the benefits of regular frequent recesses in schools and the impact on children's health and academics (Rhea et al., 2013). "Regular" here is 15 minutes for every hour—way more than American schools provide. These kids go outside at least four times a day for unstructured play breaks. Using hair samples, her team is measuring cortisol levels in fourth-graders in traditional versus LiiNK (Let's inspire innovation 'N Kids) schools. We won't spoil her big reveal of how much lower the cortisol levels are in schools allowing for play—that research will be released this summer. But, we can tell you that the levels in traditional schools (getting outside likely more than the average adult) was more than double what it should be. More than double, y'all. In 8-year-olds. How would you compare your outside time to that of children? More? Less? When is the last time you stepped barefoot in grass? Explored the feeling of a tree trunk as you stopped to rest? Watched a leaf be carried downstream? When have you simply taken time in a green space? The green part here is important. We've got another research story. Pull up a chair. This one examined the effect of houseplants on a group of 24 young male adults in their twenties (Lee et al., 2015). The group was randomly assigned to either a computer task or a plant-related task. With the plant task, the participants felt more comfortable, soothed, and natural than those with the computer task. As an added bonus, their diastolic blood pressure was also significantly lower after being with the plant.

Just a few weeks ago I (Jed) was pretty stressed out about some life happenings. The world seemed to be spinning out of control a bit, and I needed to just get away and "collect myself," as they say. My friends Nikki and Tony Smith sensed my emotional tremors, and sprang into action. They are avid hikers and know the outdoors very well. They are also craft beer experts. When outdoor enthusiasts and beer connoisseurs collide in one incredible couple, the time you spend with them is certainly gonna be fun. They took me to a place in Chimney Rock, North Carolina called Hickory Nut Brewery. It literally sits on the banks of the Broad River in Rutherford County about 30 minutes north of our home. On the path leading there, the trees are lush and green. There are occasional fields of colorful flowers, wild turkeys, and a deer if you're looking closely. Had we done nothing but drive the mountain roads, my soul would have benefited from the nature around me. I could feel my anxiety and stress falling away at just the passing of the earth around me. Once we arrived at Hickory Nut, it only got better. We grabbed a pint of IPA and headed to our outdoor seat just a few inches from the river. The temperature that day was perfect, about 73 degrees, and the water flowed by just quickly enough that it stirred a breeze in case you felt a tinge too much of warmth in the air. The first 10–15 minutes we all just sat there. No one spoke, but there was lots to hear—the splashes, the chirps, the rustles, the buzzes, the tweets. Gosh, it was just what I needed. We sat there for hours just taking it all in. After several IPAs we had a great discussion about where all the water was coming from. Needless to say the giggles ensued. After we finished up at the brewery, we had dinner across the street on the patio of Burntshirt Vineyards. The view while we ate was breathtaking. The official "Chimney Rock" bomed just overhead and the sun setting behind the Blue Ridge Mountains was the chef's kiss to a much-needed day outside. Like my student once said while on an outdoor field trip, "Today, I experienced the life of nature."

Green is good. Outside is even better. We've got to make changes, y'all. It simply must happen.

Play for Mindfulness

We all do so much. With our professional goals, work (or lack-of-work) stressors, our own mental health, our physical health, our relationships with friends and family . . . we could keep this list going all day. Meeting professional and social expectations is *tough*. Yet the pressures continue.

When we look at the impact of stress and trauma on our bodies, there's a deepening well of research to explore. Did you know the memory of helplessness is stored in the body as muscle tension (van der Kolk, 2015)? True. Take notice of how you are sitting. Lower your shoulders. Relax your jaw. Consciously relax the space where your nose meets your eyes. Why in the world were you tense? You're just sitting there reading these words, after all. Those who have experienced trauma and acute stress have memories that revolve around bracing for the unwanted—whether it's criticism, expectations, or a sensory experience. The autonomic nervous system is the brain's most elementary nervous system—using chemicals like adrenaline to fuel the body and brain for action. The parasympathetic nervous system uses acetylcholine to regulate bodily functions like digestion, healing of wounds, and sleep/dream cycles. At our peak, at our best, these systems work together to provide an optimal state of engagement—both with our world and with ourselves. We want these two systems to be in sync. This balance is measured by heart rate variability (HRV). Why is that important? I get it . . . we're going deep into the medical words here. Stay with us. (I am glad you said that, Julie, because I am gonna need a picture or an analogy soon.)

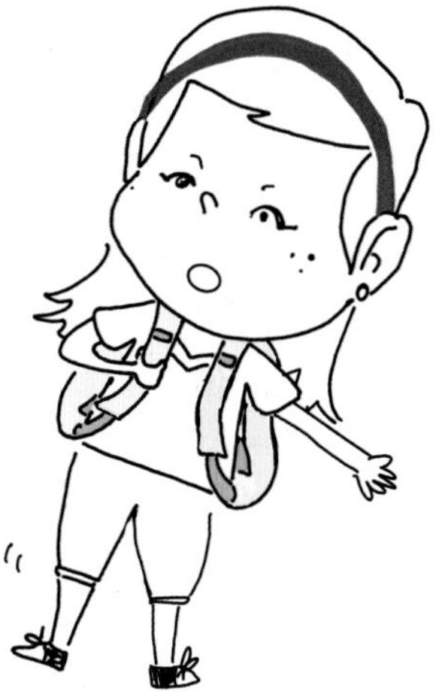

9 year old Julie off balance

When our autonomic nervous system is balanced, we have a good amount of control over our emotional reaction to frustrations and disappointments—letting us assess and respond calmly. If our autonomic nervous systems are off balance, so are we—mentally and physically. The autonomic nervous system organizes arousal in the body and the brain—measured by fluctuation in heart rate. A low HRV has a negative effect on how the body responds to stress. When we play, we engage in behaviors that improve HRV:

- Marathon running markedly increases HRV.
- Regular yoga practice improves HRV.

Which of those two is more accessible to you? I can tell you, I am not registered for the Boston Marathon. If you are, I am high-fiving you right now. However, I am a fan of yoga. During a yoga practice, the way one breathes can improve problems with anger, depression, and anxiety. Yoga has also demonstrated a positive impact on medical problems such as high blood pressure, elevated stress hormone secretion, asthma, and low back pain (Becker, 2008; Cuthbert et al., 1981; Khalsa, 2004; van der Kolk et al., 2014; Williams et al., 2005).

Almost all yoga programs include a combination of breath practices (pranayama), postures or poses (asanas), and meditation. With breath practice, there are variations in the speed and depth of breathing—using the mouth, nose, and throat with different results. The yogini grows to pay attention to the breath along the way. In the asana practice, rather than focusing on getting the posture "right," yoginis are led to pay attention to which muscles are active—creating a rhythm between tension and relaxation—with a goal of transferring this rhythm to daily life. Mindfulness, instead of being the focal point of a traditional practice, is touched by allowing the yogini to take note of what's happening in the body. Why do we feel completely relaxed and when do we feel physically safe? Here, we'd like to draw your attention to the world of mindfulness with a goal of combating toxic stress in our environments. Take a look:

Research shows that mindfulness practice...

- Can decrease stress and anxiety, and strengthen resilience and emotional regulation, and
- Can increase attention, improve interpersonal relationships, and strengthen compassion.

Reread those bullets again. Remind you of anything you have read lately? Sure sounds like play and mindfulness practice go hand in hand, if you ask us. Their impact on body and mind are essentially the same. In a world of overworked, stressed-out folks, with division aplenty we need mindful play more than ever.

Mindful Play

What brings you joy but also takes little effort? Consider rewarding experiences that allow you to lose yourself. These might include

- Cooking new foods
- Riding horses
- Visiting a new neighborhood
- Kissing
- Hiking
- Flying kites
- Playing a musical instrument
- Trying on fun clothes
- Browsing art books

As you play, let go of the need for control. Exist in the moment as time goes by. Focus on those around you. Take it all in, and enjoy yourself. Enjoy each other.

Imagine a world in which we all have compassion for each other. Do you see the link here between compassion and the life experience? The understanding that we come from all walks of life, have a variety of experiences, enjoy play with extravagance and without—that understanding combined with empathy is compassion. Our compassion helps us to be aware of and alert to all perspectives and allows for opportunities to validate them.

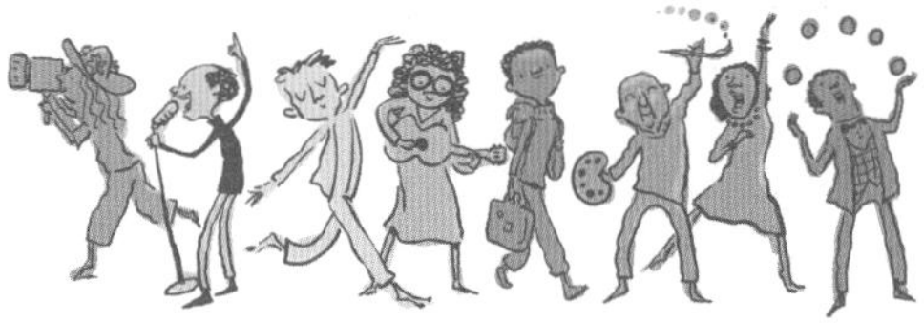

Play & Ponder

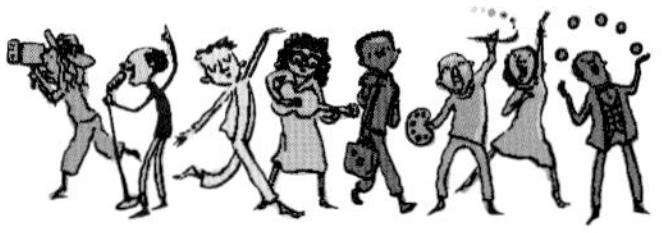

- Do you have some tinfoil nearby? Maybe you call it aluminum foil. Regardless of what you say, grab some and sculpt the best cat you can. It doesn't have to be perfect. Do the best you can. Put the finished product somewhere visible so that you will be reminded daily not to deprive yourself of play. Why the foil? Well, you have probably never made a cat from foil and we bet you will get lost in the process for a moment as you figure it out.
- Reread the chart in Chapter 14. Pick a situation from the list that you dislike the most. If possible, give one of our playful suggestions a try. Wanna make it really fun? Invite a friend to join you. Are there others that live with you? Get them in on the fun and see what happens.
- When was the last time you got "lost in the flow"? Was it when you went to the home and garden expo? Was it the day you reorganized your craft supplies? Maybe it was when you took a baking class or tailgated with friends before the big game. Take a moment to look at pics from that time. Let them take you back to the moment. Enjoy it, and make a plan to do it again soon.

SECTION 4

Mistakes

In a book about play, you may be wondering why we are talking about mistakes. There's no wrong way to play really, so how can we mess it up, right? It's not so much that you will mess it up, but there will be sidetracks, backtracks, and moments when you feel stuck in your tracks. You will have play goals. You will fall short. You will fail to meet your own expectations. How we respond is what matters. How do we know? We experience this on the daily. And you know what? We're in good company.

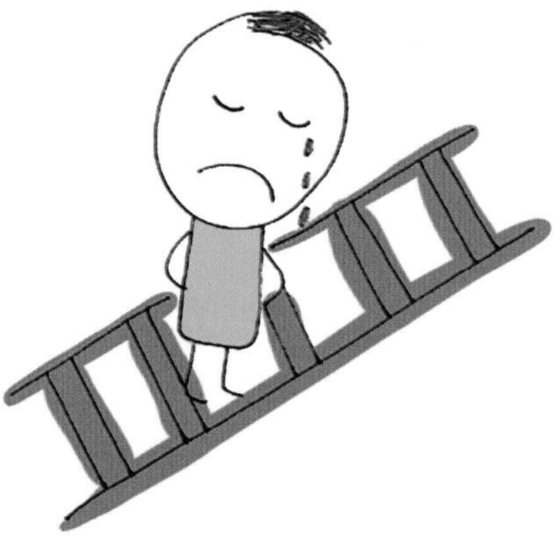

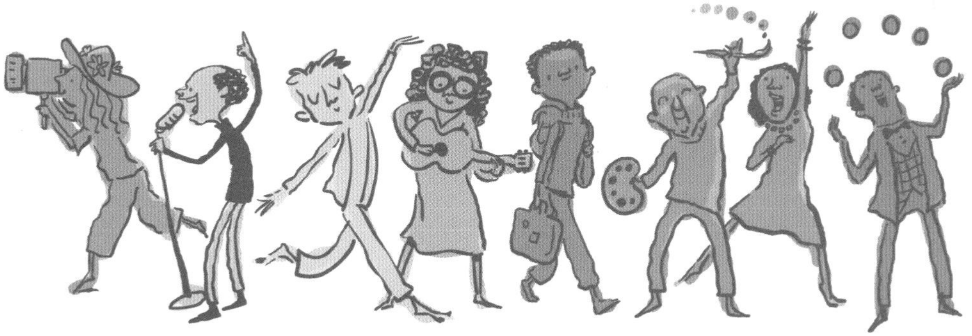

Walt Disney is a name almost everyone recognizes as someone who lived a playful life. He created so many characters, films, spaces, and places that millions of us enjoy. I cannot even fathom my childhood (or adulthood, for that matter) without Mickey Mouse and the gang. While his worlds of imagination, magic, and play are bedrock institutions in our society today, their beginnings were riddled with mistakes that almost kept them from existence. In 1955, when Disneyland first opened the gates, it was a catastrophe of epic proportions (The Grand Opening of Disneyland, n.d.). They were expecting about 15,000 people based on the invitations they sent out, but due to counterfeit tickets the crowd almost doubled in size. This led to long, miserable lines for the attractions and caused the park to completely run out of food. To make matters worse, many of the rides malfunctioned or didn't even open because they just weren't ready. No food and no rides—what else could go wrong, right? Well, more did go wrong when a tiger and a panther escaped from the circus, terrifying kids up and down the famous Main Street, USA. Speaking of Main Street, the asphalt was still so freshly poured that many shoe heels sank down into the path. The hits kept coming as the temperature soared above 100 degrees. And to top it off, there was a plumber's strike and many of the water fountains weren't working, thus unable to quench anyone's thirst. It was such a bad day that the employees named it "Black Sunday" (Klein, 2015). As the day's events unfolded, Walt was unaware of all the problems. It wasn't until the next day that he learned from the media about all the mistakes that were made. His reply? "If you do big things, you make big mistakes."

Imagine if Disney had given up right there in that moment—if he had thrown in the towel, dismissed the workers, and sold the entire venue to someone he thought would do better. We are thankful he didn't because we both have many memories at Walt Disney World—which, by the way, came in 1971, 16 years after the infamous opening of the first park in California. For Walt, mistakes were a part of life. He fully understood the concept that in order to create new things, mistakes would be made. Van Arsdale France, one of Disney's earliest employees, wrote in his autobiography *Window on Main Street: 35 Years of Creating Happiness at Disneyland Park* "I don't remember anyone getting fired for coming up with a dumb idea or making a mistake" (France, 1991, p. 68). By creating an environment that valued mistakes as part of the learning and growth process, Walt Disney afforded his workers and partners the freedom to dream big and not worry about the mistakes they made as they chased after the dreams. These are a few of our favorite Walt quotes that remind us to be courageous and pursue the playful lives we want in spite of mistakes.

"Everyone falls down. Getting back up again is how you learn to walk."

"We keep moving forward, opening new doors, and doing new things, because we're curious, and curiosity keeps leading us down new paths."

"I think it's important to have a good hard failure when you're young. I learned a lot out of that. Because it makes you kind of aware of what can happen to you."

"I dream, I test my dreams against my beliefs, I dare to take risks, and I execute my vision to make those dreams come true."

"All our dreams can come true, if we have the courage to pursue them."

CHAPTER 16

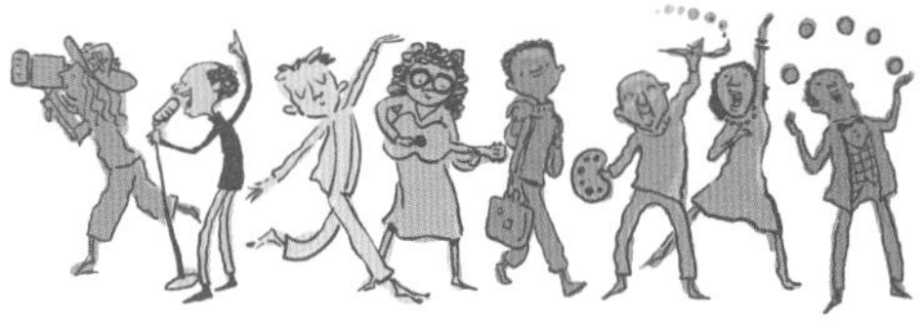

Low-Risk/High-Risk Play

Walt Disney fully understood the playful mindset as well as low-risk and high-risk play. His try, make mistakes, try again mindset led to new, meaningful results. In our quest to live playful lives, we too must embrace the reality that we will make many mistakes on this journey. But, like the dreamer himself, we must have the courage to pursue this goal even when we mess up.

We would have loved to have had the opportunity to interview Walt for this book so that we could ask him all about his process. What was his daily morning routine that invited playfulness into his space that led to his ideas? How did he take his ideas and move them into reality? When he was allowing others into his creative, playful circle, what qualities did he look for in those people?

We don't want you to misunderstand here . . . Disney is HUGE. Theme parks are such an undertaking for sure, and many of the ideas birthed by Disney were extremely risky and bold. Had he failed, it would have been on a grand scale. But at its core, Walt's idea started with a mouse. A mouse doodled in his journal. On one trip to Disney, I took a picture of this very drawing. It has been the wallpaper on my phone ever since—as motivation for me to keep going.

How did he do it? How did the doodled mouse even happen? How did Walt go from mouse to enterprise? We aren't suggesting that a playful life must always lead to enterprise development. Lord, that doesn't even sound fun to me. But the processes of playful creatives, and their learning and growth cycle, is reflective of playful living. It inspires us, and we hope it inspires you, to use their experiences as a guide for our own journey—inviting more play in our lives.

While we cannot identify Disney's exact thought processes, we can reflect about our own and how we are (or are not) inspired to think as we go through our days.

When was the last time a playful idea hit you? While watching *Hamilton*, and seeing all these impactful folk gathered together ("Raise a Glass"), I think—Oh, we should get a group of people together and. . . .

How did you respond to that moment? YES! I will call the group together and have them meet at . . .

Did you follow through? Yay! Everyone will be there by . . .

Did you write it down to revisit later? This was such a fun night, let's do it again on . . .

This is the basic thought process many of us go through when we are craving a playful moment in our lives. We think about it, we make it happen. There is not a lot of risk taking involved in hosting a game night. You want to play a board game, you invite the friends, and you play. We need both high- and low-risk play in our lives. Just as our moods ebb and flow, so does our predilection for taking a chance. And so much good can come from it! (Read about the health benefits of playing in Chapter 9.)

If you google "risky play" (OMG, Julie . . . you cannot tell people to google that. Lord knows what might come up), all sorts of information on how taking risks in playful behavior is so beneficial—especially for children. We know, we know . . . this is a book for grown-ups. We're grown-ups, too. We get it. Humor us a bit. Here are a few examples of childhood behaviors that are traditionally considered to be risky:

- Using things in ways that aren't intended (e.g., going up the slide)
- Rolling down hills
- Climbing seemingly treacherous terrain
- Playing at heights
- Running fast
- Walking in places that require balance

Every one of these situations involves taking a chance. Children are not often thinking about risks in the same way we adults do. They see an opportunity, and simply begin. Their gut gauges whether or not they feel safe, their focus on play allows them to take their time, and their perspective on learning (they don't even realize this!) encourages them to seek resources for assistance as needed.

How much of these behaviors parallel adults in play?

Do we know when we feel safe (both physically and emotionally)? Most of us as adults have developed a sense of what is physically dangerous (heights, traffic, wild animals . . .). Instead, adults are more concerned about what might hurt us emotionally or socially. We are not going to play in the road—we know that danger. Would we participate in a 5K on that same road even though we might not finish or we might be scoffed at for walking? Maybe not. We're afraid of the criticism.

Do we allow ourselves time to explore/focus on the present/be creative? Next to fear of ridicule, time is the enemy for most adults. Fun fact—Jed loves to bake. He wants to be good at it so bad. But the reality is he only tries to get better once every four to five months. The average time to mix the batter, bake the cake, and decorate it is about two hours, not counting cleanup. What if Jed gave two hours every other week to baking?

Are we comfortable enough with messing up that we try something or seek assistance to move forward? There are many times I've doodled in my journal and not shared my creations on social media. I have a canvas sitting in my home (two, in fact) that is incomplete. Why don't I schedule the time to play with paint and see what can happen? Again, judgment is my enemy. Instead of fear of others' thoughts, here I fear my own.

Now, there is nothing wrong with having fears. We all do. But when we live a playful life, we have to resist some of these fears because they keep us from enjoying new experiences. Simmer down. Now, don't go getting your fur up. We know you didn't buy this book so we could tell you to start rappelling off the side of a building. I (Julie) don't enjoy running. I likely won't ever sign up for a 5K. And that's okay. But some of the roadblocks to taking a chance described earlier are keeping us from living the playful life we could have. Some of us are ready to be all-in for playful living, and some of us like to go at it real slow (not Marvin Gaye slow, but a take-our-time kind of way). The approach we each take might be surprising.

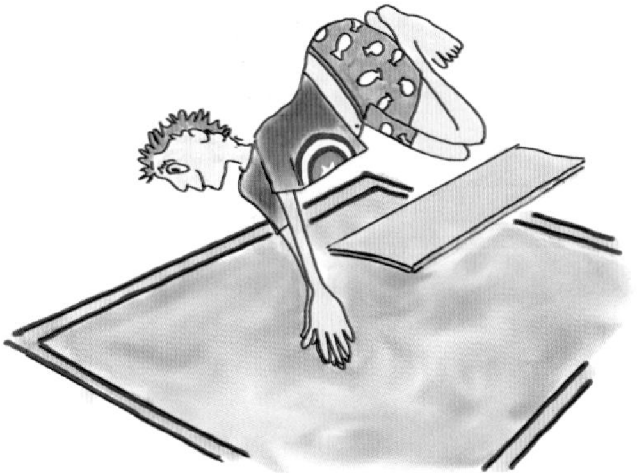

Funny story—Matt Matt, what I call my dear friend Matt Johnson, is one of those people who, when approaching a swimming pool, just jumps right in. I'm like, *what-in-the-world?! He didn't stick his toe in first? That water might be cold!* Jed and I are toe-first kind of people. We would be risk management folks if we worked in the business sector. Which is interesting because we are spontaneous in all other parts of our lives. Matt-Matt, in real life, is a quiet thinker. He does not jump in fast to any task. He weighs his options. Some of you might want to approach a playful life like Matt-Matt does a swimming pool. You're all-in with big ideas and risk taking. But some of you might want to stick your toe in first. We hear you. Play does not always have to be something big and loud. It can be quiet and still be playful. Low-risk play can be toe-in-first type behaviors. They are not overtly risky, but they are a start to a playful path. That start can be scary—these first steps may lead to something with a greater risk. What if Jed becomes a really good baker and suddenly his cakes are being ordered for weddings? Baking at home is low-risk. Baking for a wedding, a once-in-a-lifetime event, is much riskier.

Let's explore some more ideas for taking a chance in play that allows for both low-risk and high-risk action.

Personality	**Low-risk play (toe in first)**	**High-risk play (jump in deep)**
Joker 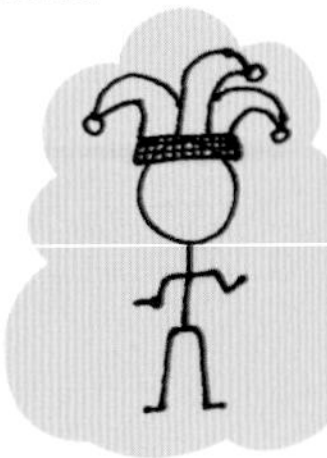	Reads joke book or memoir of a fav comedian	Signing up for open-mic night (move over, Amy Schumer)

Personality	**Low-risk play (toe in first)**	**High-risk play (jump in deep)**
Storyteller 	Animated retelling of a recent event for a friend	Auditioning for a role in the local community theater
Creator 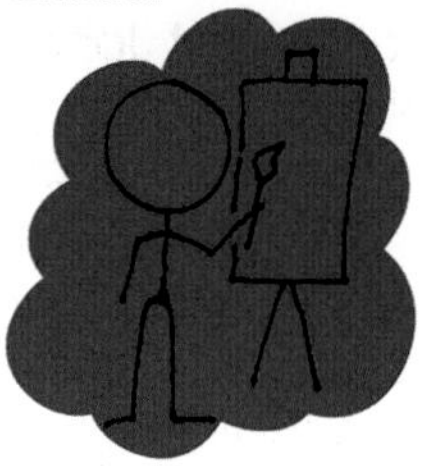	Doodling in your journal	Volunteering to teach a class on sketch-noting
Kinesthete 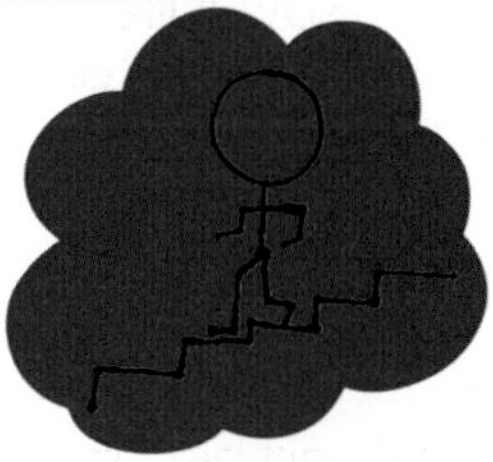	Taking a walk around your home. Try jogging some of it.	Signing up for a marathon
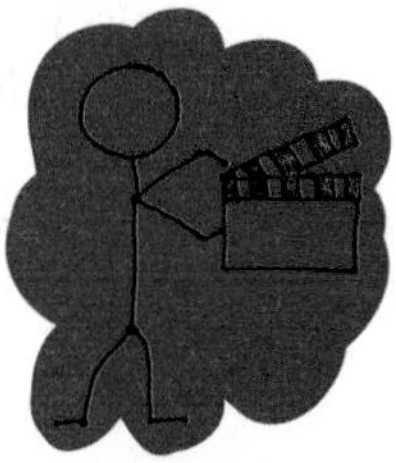 Director	Inviting your neighbor over for dinner	Organizing a charity fundraising event
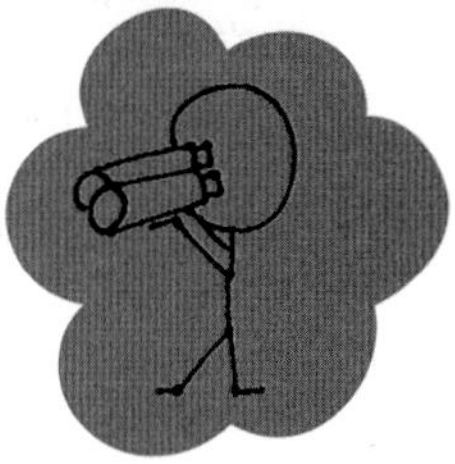 Explorer	Watching the Travel Channel. Dreaming.	Spontaneously purchasing a ticket to somewhere you want to go

Personality	Low-risk play (toe in first)	High-risk play (jump in deep)
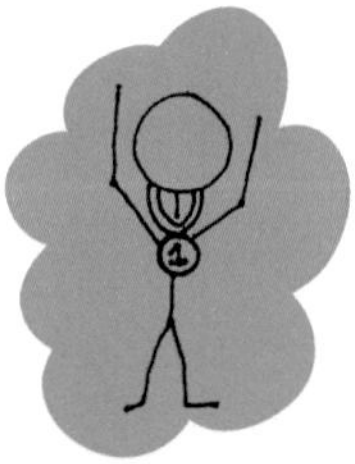 Competitor	Having a game night with your besties	Joining an adult sports league
Collector 	Arranging your pen collection by color	Creating a YouTube channel about your pen collection and revealing your obsession to the world
All 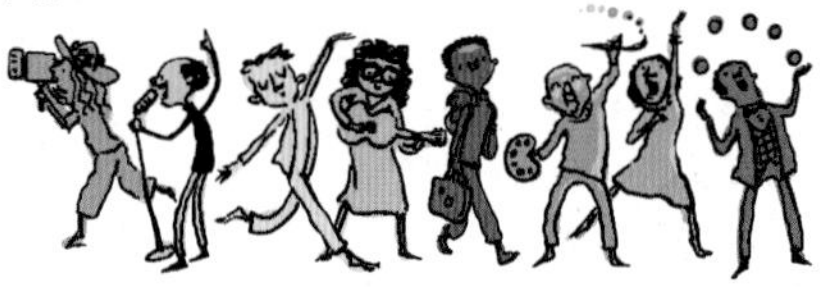	Listing goals in your journal	Publicly sharing your goals for the year on social media

CHAPTER 17

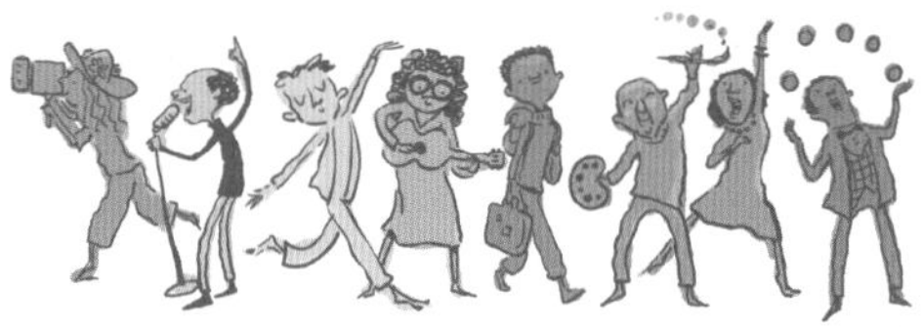

The Learning and Growth Process (RISK)

As you are likely thinking by now, some playful ideas may be a bit more involved. Auditioning for a role in the local theater or growing your own YouTube channel are definitely playful experiences but they may require a bit more of a learning and growth process. Mistakes are likely. Remember what Disney said about doing big things.

Here's a framework for how to cultivate thinking amidst the perceived chaos of our lives. Consider the following risk-taking process. Although the writing here makes it appear to be a linear model, it is more like a game of *Frogger*. If you have never played the game, it is basically moving up, down, left, right, back, forward, and repeat.

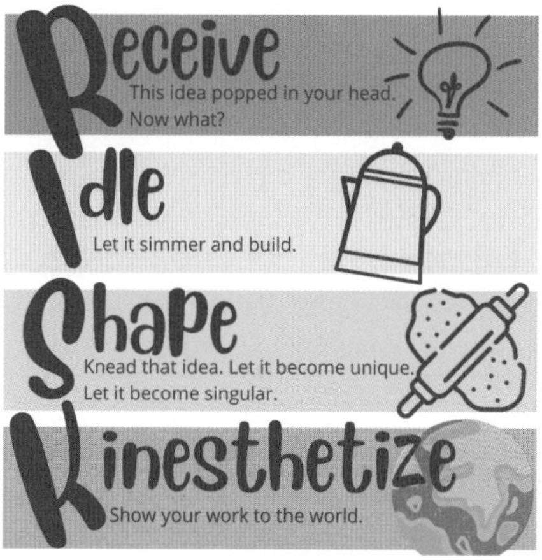

1. *Receive:* How does an idea happen? So you want to start your online video series about . . . Where did that concept come from? Were you

   Reading?
   Writing?
   Doodling?
   Chatting?
   Playing?
   Collaborating?

   Elizabeth Gilbert (2015) refers to ideation as *Big Magic*. The universe trusts us with ideas. If we don't act on them, they will travel to someone else until something is done about it. There are millions of online videos, but the world needs yours because the idea dropped into your mind. Now what?
2. *Idle:* According to the little box of quotes that we got at Target, actress Meryl Streep said, "Start by starting." Of course you could do this. You could turn on your camera and get to gettin'. But allowing ourselves the time and freedom to make an idea become our own often leads to an idea on top of an idea. Think of this like a car in idle. It is on, it is ready to go, but it isn't moving just yet. By letting an idea simmer and build in your default mode network, new thoughts can (and will) emerge. Creativity is an idea in motion. It's ideas doing something. This is what's happening when an idea leads to an idea, which leads to another idea and then a whole new idea. Howard Gardner, the John H. and Elisabeth A. Hobbs Research Professor of Cognition and Education at Harvard University, describes people in this phase as having a *Synthesizing Mind* (2020). In his book, Gardner writes about who he considers to be exemplary synthesizers—historian Richard Hofstadter, biologist Charles Darwin, and literary critic Edmund Wilson. Gardner goes further to emphasize how synthesizing minds are particularly valuable now as we process and propose ways to cultivate a unique human experience.
3. *Shape:* You have mulled it over. You have given it thought. Like a lump of clay, at this point you are pushing and pulling. You're kneading this concept. You're showing it to your inner circle and asking for their feedback. During the shaping process is when magic occurs. At some point, the work becomes unique. It becomes singular. You have something unlike everyone else's something. This may feel like innovation. This is extraordinary. This is an opportunity.
4. *Kinesthetize:* This is a made-up word. You won't find it in the dictionary, but our play mentor Dr. Stuart Brown once made

up a word to capture his thoughts, so we are following his lead. Basically, it means to get moving and reveal your idea to the world. Think kinesthetic, movement. Your idea has been gifted to you, you've thought it over, you've shaped it, and you are now ready to move this buggy forward. If the work has an audience of one (ourselves), nice. Srinivas Rao has an excellent book, actually titled *An Audience of One: Reclaiming Creativity for Its Own Sake* (Rao & Dellabough, 2018) on this very topic. You should get it. By focusing your creative work on pleasing yourself, you can increase your productivity, happiness, and (eventually, paradoxically) the size of your audience. But y'all . . . greatness is often meant to be shared. It is meant to inspire. It is meant to impact others. Is this the last step? No! It could be the first. In fact, it can be threaded throughout the process. But it is an essential element. Without it, we have no feedback. Without an audience for our work, how do we move forward?

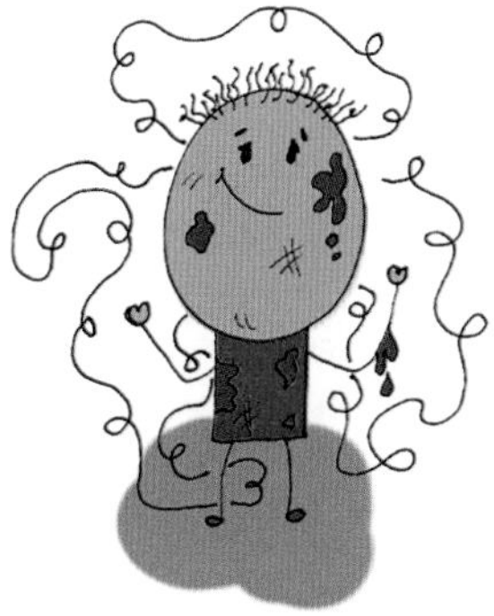

This looks like a linear process, but y'all—sometimes it's a muddy mess. We have to be brave enough to get dirty with it. (Jed here, Julie is laughing hysterically because her middle school mind cannot handle what she just typed. She coughed herself into a fit and is now getting herself together.) (I'm back.) Truth is, time is as much an element here as is the risk we take. We can't have an idea unless we honor the need to have time, space, and opportunity to play with concepts. It is through play that we can be creative. Anytime we have been creative, it feels like play. It feels good (hello, serotonin). We get lost in the moment. And none of this can authentically exist unless we play. But this whole process involves risk. Risk of failure, risk of success, risk of exposure, risk of difficult conversations, risk of judgment, risk of pleasure. Taking a risk is scary. And the reality is . . . we will most certainly make mistakes.

CHAPTER 18

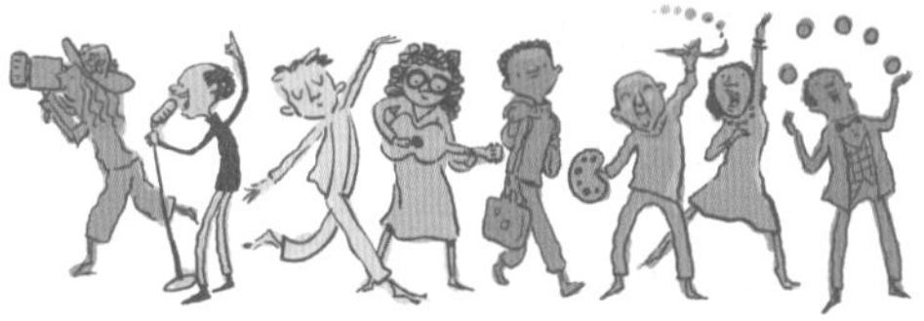

Mistakes and Fear

We fully realize that most of you reading this book don't have the luxuries that Walt Disney did that allowed him to make mistakes on such a grand scale. He had investors and lots of money that afforded him the time, space, and opportunity to function in and create an environment that embraced mistakes. In the normal world, where the majority of us live, it can be very scary to live like that. We get it. Fear is real, y'all. We know this from our own experience with writing. While we enjoyed the book publishing process and many aspects of it were very playful for us, when our first book launched it was downright terrifying. We felt like we were standing on Main Street, USA stuck in the asphalt, buck-naked while singing in front of thousands of people. Gosh, the day people started posting pics on social media as their preordered copy arrived in the mail made us have such emotions. You feel very exposed to have all your thoughts in print, readily available for anyone to read, dissect, critique, scoff at, judge, mock, review on Amazon/Good Reads, etc. Oh Law. . . We are getting nervous all over again just typing all that out because we know that when this book comes out those fears will all return. Oddly enough, here we are, doing it again. We are basically standing here with no pants on right now as you read this. Okay, okay, we are not actually in the coffee shop with our underpinning showing, but we want this metaphor to be strong due to the transparent nature of our writing. We want to be raw, authentic, "FRFR" as the young people might text. We want to communicate that we are in this game of life with you. That we struggle, we cry, we panic, we fall flat on our face . . . we fail too, a lot. Because of that—fear of the unknown, fear of repeating mistakes, fear of making new ones—we often feel paralyzed at the thought of taking a risk.

Being a grown-up who is playful is definitely risky. Even as we are writing this book, one of us was challenged professionally for being "playful" and not rigorous in our work by a superior at our job. No joke. A sit down, let's-have-a-conversation kind of conversation. Mind you, this person had never observed our work, read our books, or attended any event we hosted. They invited us in for a closed-door conversation based on the hearsay of us being known as a playful human. Seriously? It really shows what they know about the power of play. Bosses who don't get it are often life-sucking leeches that drain us and hinder our playful spirits. They are a reality we as adults must face, but hopefully those bosses are reading this book and change is a-comin'.

Play, and its effects on learning, living, and life, is in fact innately rigorous. Utilizing a playful approach to your work is beneficial for not only you, but those around you. Your increase in productivity benefits the company you work for as well. Bosses everywhere should want you to be more playful. You read in Section One all about the neurological benefits of play, so we won't go through all that again. But, be sure to give your boss, coworkers, spouse, friends, family, etc., a copy of this book so they can become more informed about how playing makes us all better humans. All that said, we realize that society has programmed us to:

Fall in line.
Stay in our lane.
Be the good responsible adults that we are supposed to be.
Keep our nose to the grindstone.
Work hard.
Pay our bills and taxes.

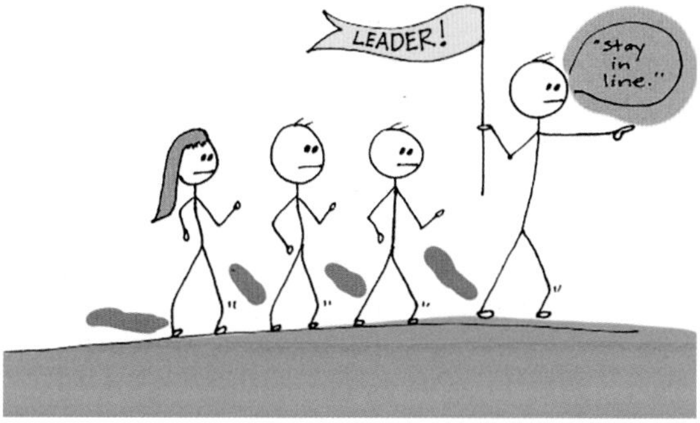

"Life isn't all about having fun" is an unfortunate mantra we have heard more than once. Sometimes it was from the adults of our youthful days, parents, teachers, preachers, etc., and as mentioned earlier we've even heard it recently. When all of this pressure of adult expectation piles up on us, it can certainly create a genuine fear of being seen as "too playful."

According to Merriam-Webster, fear is an unpleasant, often strong emotion, caused by anticipation or awareness of danger. We love that they used the word "unpleasant" in the definition. Southern folk tend to use that word when something is happening that they don't wanna talk about. It is unpleasant to talk about bowel problems, their cousin's most recent bad habit, or the surprise Susie Jane revealed at last year's Thanksgiving. We shake our heads and bless their hearts. But we don't talk about it.

Fear is in fact unpleasant, and the emotions that result from fear can be detrimental to our health. Some folks suffer from atelophobia, which is an obsessive fear of imperfection. They are literally terrified of making mistakes and often avoid situations in which they will not succeed. This condition isn't great for the body. In fact, too much fear of any kind can be very harmful. Just as being playful releases all the feel-good chemicals in the brain, the opposite happens when fear arrives. Remember, that's a good thing if a lion is chasing you and death by fangs and claws is nearby. It's not so good if you live in a constant state of worry and panic. The part of the brain that controls all of this is called the amygdala. It is a tiny almond-shaped blob found in the temporal lobe.

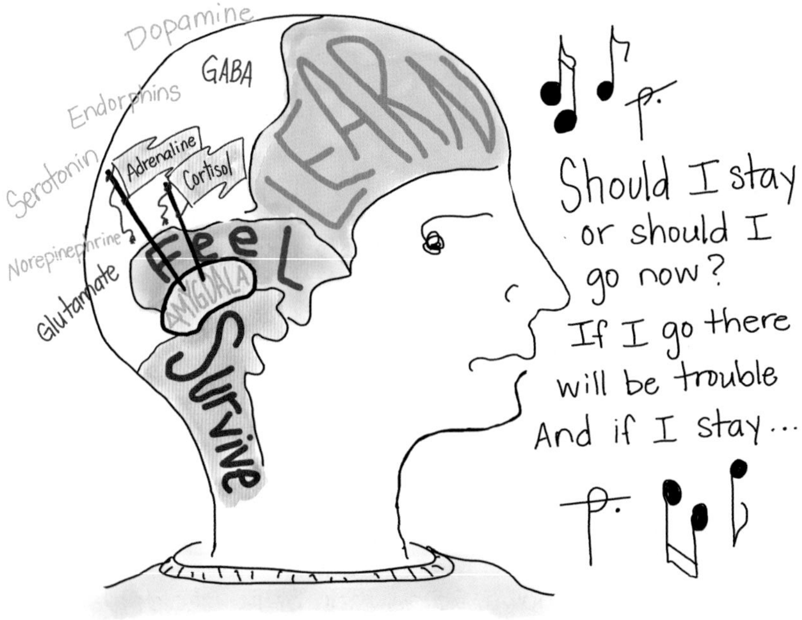

Most humans have two functioning ones from birth, but sometimes they can be damaged by stroke or other diseases. They can also be damaged by anxiety and depression. They play a role in a variety of emotions, but they are most closely associated with fear. They alert us when we are in danger and need safety. If we hear a bump in the night that could be a burglar, our amygdala becomes active. Increased heart rate, sweaty palms, stomach in knots, and the overall feeling of impending doom flood our body. Small doses of fear can be helpful. A Halloween haunted house, a scary moment in a horror flick, and someone shouting "boo" at just the right moment. All of these can be good for us—when programmed in our nervous system, fear keeps us safe from danger. However, fear can damage every part of our lives if we allow it to consume us. This is when fear becomes unhealthy and in many ways can squash the joy right out of life. Unchecked fear can damage our physical well-being, memory, brain processing, reactivity, and mental health (Delagran, n.d; Dubuc, n.d; van der Kolk, 2015).

When I (Jed) was on the cusp of adulthood known as high school graduation, I faced my first health issues because of unhealthy fear. I was absolutely terrified of graduating. Most seniors cannot wait to ditch the textbooks and embrace the "freedom" of being a grown-up that awaits in the college or career on the other side of high school. Not me. As much as I hated high school because of bullies and ignorance, at least it was my norm. My routine. I didn't want anything to break that. I had the marching band and a small group of friends that gave me safety and stability. I craved those relationships due to a tumultuous childhood caused by my parents' divorce and an abusive father. Band life and my tiny circle of friends gave me comfort. The impending doom of what lay ahead post-graduation was almost more than I could bear. I started having some pretty severe intestinal issues because of it. At the age of 18, I had no choice but to have an endoscopy and colonoscopy to make sure there was no damage inside. The results of those tests were conclusive. My issues stemmed from the stress I was placing on myself from the fear of the next step, and the concern of losing my life's consistency. This was not healthy fear. It was damaging to my body. It was damaging to my mental health. And most of all, it was damaging to my spirit. All the goodness that made me *me* was being suppressed and drowned out because of the fear that strangled me. I only wish I had had the understanding of the playful mindset and risk-taking at that age in my life. It seemed like so many of my peers embraced the idea of the unknown. Rather than being afraid, they were excited about dorm life, about the freedom from parents, about the lack of curfew. I often wonder what opportunities I missed out on because of that fear. One in particular I know that I missed was an opportunity to learn at Appalachian State University. I got accepted, went to orientation weekend, and even met my roommate. Those two days sent me over the edge of fear into full-on panic. I backed out and never went to App State. Instead I enrolled at a local university and stayed home. I eventually transferred to a college nearby and lived on campus, but it was only 30 minutes from home, and I could be with my mom and sister for dinner any night that I needed safety and stability. Don't get me wrong here. It is totally okay to want those things. It was totally okay for me to feel afraid at that time in my life. The unknown is scary. But, when it limits our lived experience and creates health concerns, there is a problem. A playful life can help us to overcome those fears.

As we seek out playfulness in our everyday lives, we have to limit the presence of fear. Think about it . . . if you want to bring more play into your life by. . .

Creating art . . . You are gonna have to put off the fear of "messing up."
Reading more . . . You are gonna have to put off the fear of "wasting time."
Dancing at work . . . You are gonna have to put off the fear of people laughing at you.
Singing in the car . . . You are gonna have to get over the fear that someone hears how bad you sound.
Playing cards . . . You are gonna have to get over the possibility of losing.
Taking a walk in the woods . . . You are gonna have to get over the fear of sweating and bug bites.
Writing letters to friends . . . You are gonna have to get over the fear of not getting a note back.
Build a shed . . . You are gonna have to get over the fear that it might leak or fall down.
Plant a garden . . . You are gonna have to get over the fear that the Brussels sprouts won't make.
Travel . . . That plane isn't going down. And if it does, well. . . .

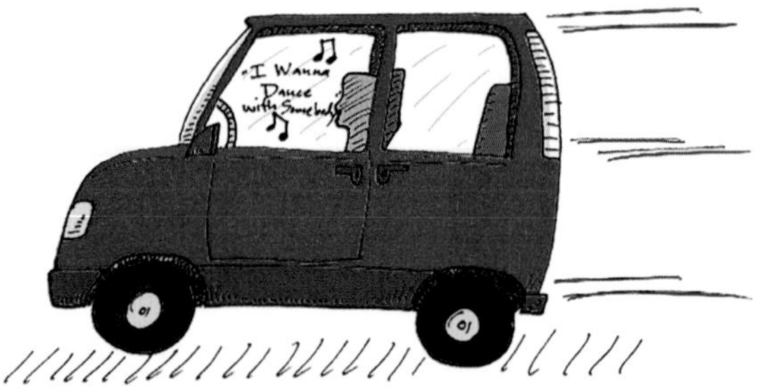

See what we are saying here? Fear keeps us from playing in so many ways. This is how fear can be associated with mistakes. We are afraid of the outcome of being playful so we don't even attempt it. There is a quote that we say often in our day-to-day lives as we come up with new ideas to bring play into our workspace. Remember Meryl said, "Start by starting." Don't wait 'til you are ready to start because you won't ever be. Don't wait 'til you know everything to start because you won't ever know it all. (Even though a lot of people think they do.) Don't wait 'til you have the money because if you are like us you may never have enough. Can you see how that Streep quote gets things moving? You will likely always experience fear as you are facing something new and unknown, but the less it controls you, the freer you are to experience the benefits of a playful life.

CHAPTER 19

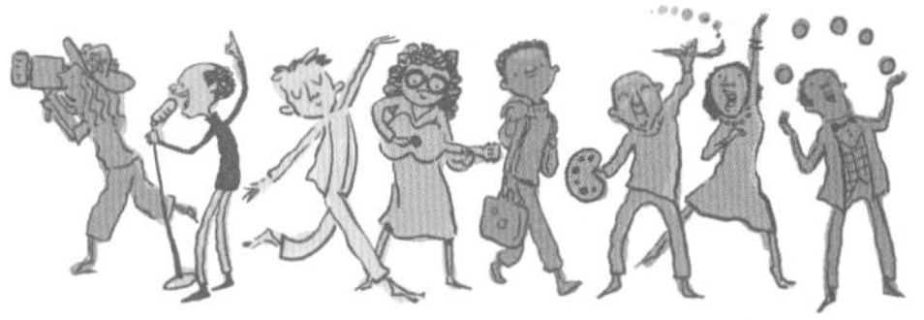

Excuses Are Mistakes

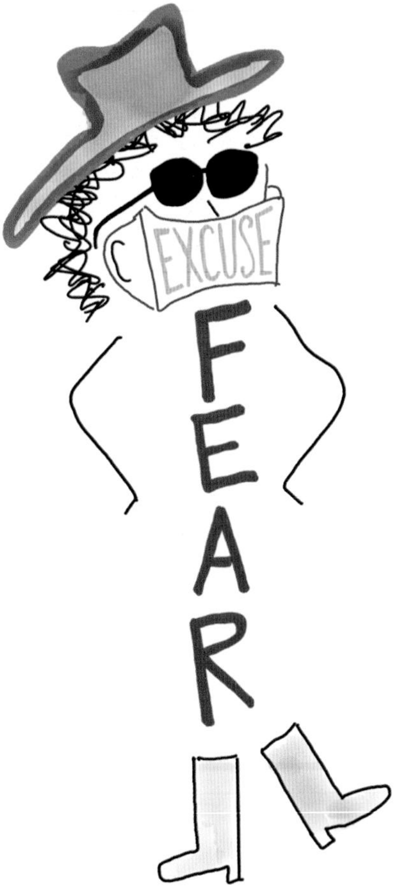

Sometimes fear masks itself as an excuse. It is a lot easier for us to come up with a reason that we cannot do something than it is to admit that we are afraid of doing it, or messing up while we attempt to do it. Mistakes are misguided errors. When we make excuses, we are misguiding ourselves. You know those moments just before exercising, going for a run, lifting weights, or *Sweatin' to the Oldies* with Richard Simmons? Those moments are the hardest part of the entire experience—making changes to our lives to bring more play into our spaces is easy to excuse away. Side note: If you don't know Richard Simmons, you aren't as old as us, and you must stop right now, open up a tab, and search for him! Tweet us when you do: @juliepjones and @mrdearybury.

Our brains love to come up with a million reasons why we don't want to work out. I am tired, I am hungry, I need to run that errand. Excuses are common deterrents we come up with to avoid discomfort. However, when exercise is complete, the excuses seem so silly in comparison to the brain and body benefits that fill us up thanks to the movement, weights, or dancing. *Why* do we do this to ourselves?

Overcoming our excuses to avoid change in our daily routines and real-life challenges is crucial to developing a playful life. Elimination of excuses is a must. Elizabeth Gilbert (2015) tells us that fear is one of the primary excuses that many of us have in pursuing our creative endeavors. We tend to agree that those same fears lead to excuses that limit our playful living. We bet some of your excuses sound like this.

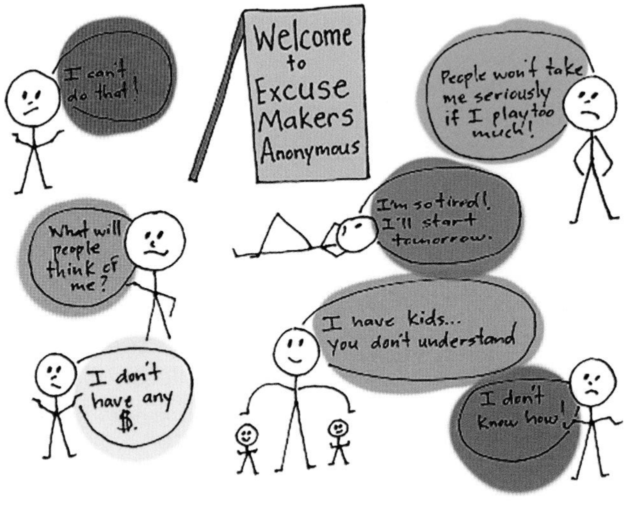

We know there are a lot more of them, but these are the ones we hear, and make for ourselves, most often.

Why Do We Make Excuses?

Before we unpack one of the top excuses that we have heard from others during our work, let's first take a moment to think about why we make excuses to tweak, change, reimagine, the daily practices that inhibit our playful living.

1. **Comfort Zone.**
   Change is hard and is rarely fun. Excuses allow us to stay snug and warm in what we know. Who wants to get out of bed when the covers are so warm and snuggly? It's cold out there. There are responsibilities waiting on me. I will have to commit to the day once my toe peeks out from under the blanket. Okay, okay, that analogy has worn out its welcome, but you get it. Leaving our comfort zone is difficult.
2. **Self-Doubt.** Many of us may feel incapable of making changes to the work we do, so excuses make the feelings of incompetence go away. Some psychologists categorize our behavior of making excuses as "self-handicapping." By hurting our own motivation, we distract ourselves from potential achievement. We remain in a safety net. Freud would say that our ego has a subconscious desire to protect us from anxiety or embarrassment (I hope you read that with your pinky out 'cause that's exactly how I said it when I typed it). Instead of taking the risk, our self-doubt fuels the construction of barriers—anything to keep us from putting ourselves out there. These barriers shift the focus away from ourselves and onto the external (really onto anything else).
   The teacher didn't like me. They wouldn't stop laughing. It was raining. She said it first.
3. **Status Quo.** How many times have you had an idea to do something differently, but know that your family, peers, coworkers, boss, etc., won't like it? So, rather than use your own idea, you join the excuse bandwagon of why "it just won't work." Look around. How many of your coworkers or friends are idea people? Are you the only one imagining a new way? Are you the only one who seeks a brave new world? (Okay, Julie. Enough with the literary puns).
4. **Fear.** Gilbert (2015) says perfectionism doesn't just stop people from completing their work, it often keeps them from beginning. She's talking about us . . . well, maybe not all of us, but perfectionism is common in many walks of life, and it can be a breeding ground for excuses. We fear the whole thing will be wrong, incorrect, a big ole pile of. . . . And we

never even start to try for fear of messing it up. For years, I had stacks and stacks of blank journals that sat on my shelf. Why didn't I write? I was fearful that I had nothing to say.

How many of these hit home for you? Likely more than one of them. We felt it too. Still do. Remember, the playful life isn't one to arrive at. This is not a book where you can do steps 1 through 10 and arrive at happiness. We have to work at it. Constantly. It's not easy. We're right there with you.

CHAPTER 20

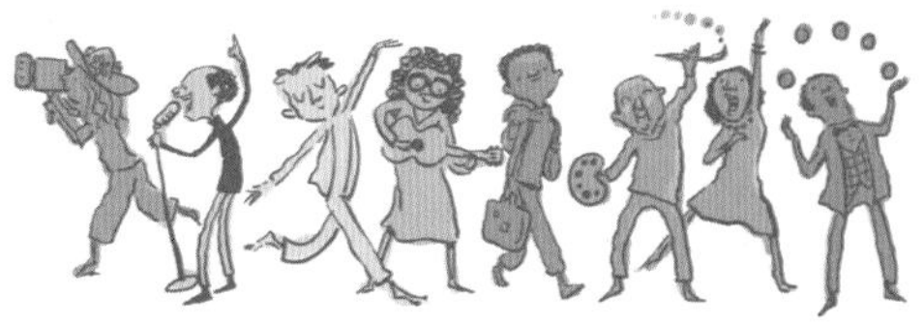

A Path to Eliminating Excuses

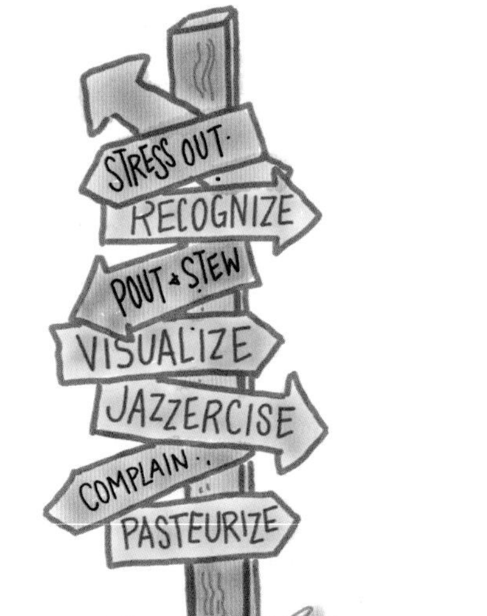

Ridding ourselves of excuses is vital for authentic playful living. Excuses often serve as roadblocks to any and all work we hope to do for the betterment of our lives. The following four steps will help us eliminate excuses and stay on the path toward meeting the goal of bringing more play into our lives. FYI, #3 is our favorite.

1. **Recognize.** We have to be able to admit when we are making excuses. While there are some valid hurdles we often face, many of the reasons we come up with to avoid change are based more on fears, lack of motivation, or worry regarding the opinions of others. We (both of us are included here, because we do this too) have to stop telling ourselves why change cannot happen. We must start telling ourselves how it can.

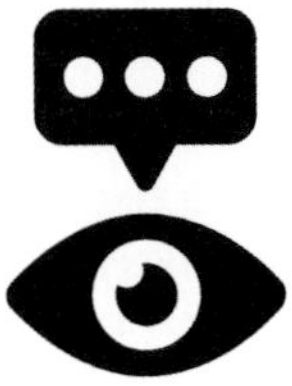
recognize

2. **Visualize.** Start dreaming. What does your ideal life look like? What playful experiences would occur? What moments for joy would develop? What resources do you need to make it uh-may-zing? The excitement of the new, the possible, the reimagined is powerful. The endorphins released just by daydreaming about the changes we want to make can often be a catalyst for eliminating excuses.

visualize

3. **Jazzercise.** Now get movin'! Go back to that visualized list, and create an action plan. The number-one factor prohibiting almost all of us isn't money, nor time—it is simply inaction. There are countless opportunities for play throughout our day. It is all a matter of prioritizing the need for play and inserting playful moments into any available space we have. This throwback to the jazzercise days is intentional—man, those people know how to move!

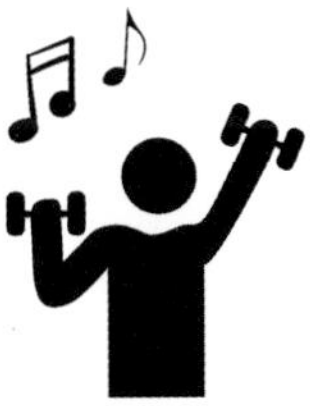
jazzercise

4. **Pasteurize.** Yes, like milk. The purpose of this process is to extend the shelf life of perishable goods. Once your excuse is debunked, don't get too comfy and think you're safe. Excuses creep their way back into the work often, no matter how deep we get into it. Even as we write this book, there are some other projects that we are both working on, and the excuse demon is trespassing in the midst. We must arm ourselves with the latest research to justify our decisions. Research is continually advancing—we can't let our forward movement become stagnant.

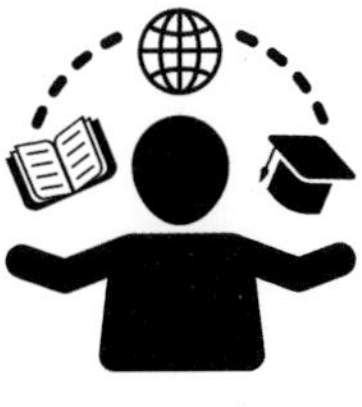
pasteurize

Let's Eliminate One Excuse Together

One excuse that we have used, and others often use, when considering playful living is **"I just don't have time."** We agree fully that the daily schedule for any of us is fuller than a tick on a dog's ear. We have so much to do. Time is definitely of the essence, and there are only so many hours in each day no matter which way we slice it. Meetings, soccer games, swim meets, paperwork, feedback, supper fixin', phone calls . . . on and on and on and on. But if we follow the steps of eliminating excuses explained earlier, there's a way to move this excuse right on out of the house to make room for something new and exciting.

Recognize: To recognize a misguided belief as an excuse, we must first acknowledge that we need to make time for things that matter. Our grannies used to say, "You make time for what matters." Aren't grannies always full of wisdom? Instead of leaning on the excuse, let's ask ourselves, "*How can I make time?*" or "*How can I restructure my day so the time showcases what matters to me?*" To do this, we suggest conducting a benefit analysis. This is simply a process by which organizations (our households/lives are like a mini organization) can analyze decisions, systems, or projects to determine a value for intangibles. The model is built by identifying the benefits of an action as well as the associated costs, and subtracting the costs from benefits.

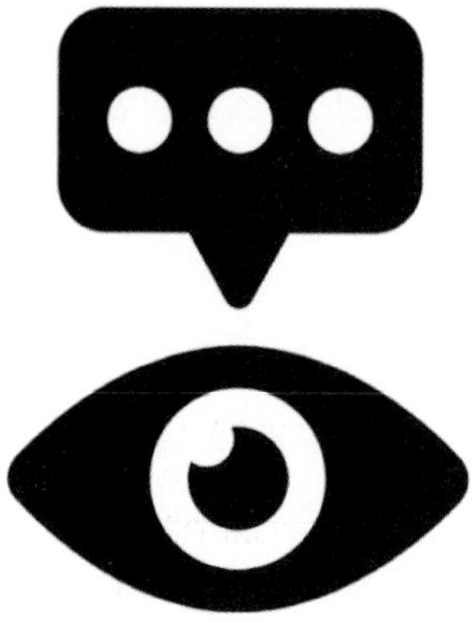

You might know it as ROI: your *return on investment*. Questions we often ask ourselves to help with this evaluation include:

- Does our current schedule give meaning and depth to the lives we want to lead?

- Does our current schedule maximize the time we have, or are we wasting it with things that don't help us achieve the playful life we long to live?
- Does our current schedule invite us and those we live and interact with to laugh, move, or create?

While these are not questions a traditional business would ask of its performance, for the purposes of our work, contemplating the answers to these questions helps us to see the areas of our schedule that may be soaking up our time, thus making us feel like *not having time* is a valid reason for inaction. Recognizing these thoughts, these excuses, as misguided errors will help us to move to the next step in this process.

Visualize: Once we recognize that "not having time" is an excuse, it is helpful to visualize how we want to fill the spaces of time that are revealed as a result of the benefits analysis. The visualization process is key to making the changes happen, but without caution, we may fill the spaces with other activities or events that use more time without keeping the goal of developing and leading a playful life as our focus. The following questions often help the visualization process yield the best results for us:

visualize

- Does the new use of time give meaning and depth to the life I want to lead?
- Does my new schedule maximize the time I have or am I still wasting it with things that don't help me achieve a playful life?
- Does the new use of time invite me, and those I live and interact with, to laugh, move, or create?

If the answer to these questions is no, then we continue to visualize a better use of the time until we answer yes to at least one. While we were writing this book, we often visualized, rather comically we might add, how we typed that serotonin makes us go poop. If you have missed that part then you have missed one of our favorite parts of this work. We hope y'all won't forget that! We regularly attempt to apply that fun bit of playful mindset and humor to our writing to help connect it to you, the reader. Think about it: lots of books, meetings, courses, etc., need some serotonin ASAP! In the words of Mr. Coach Klein, "Visualize and attack!"

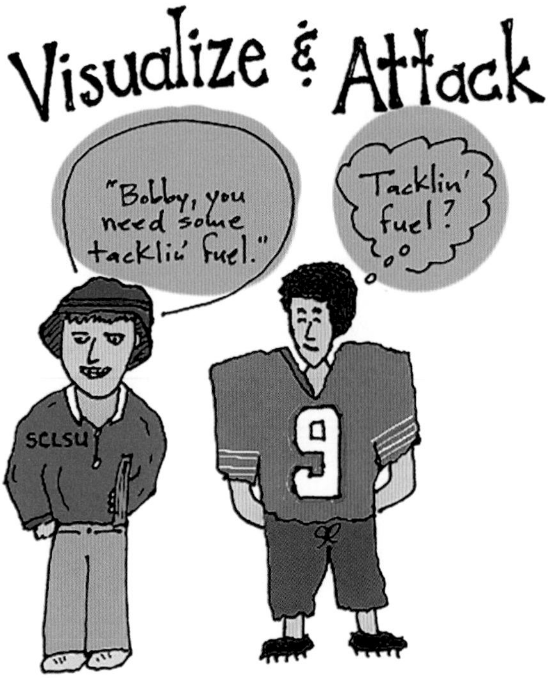

Jazzercise: If you don't get the preceding doodle, it is meant to represent a scene from a classic Adam Sandler movie *The Waterboy*. We confess that we never thought that we'd be quoting Mr. Coach Klein in a book about play, but, when the musket fires, that dog'll hunt! For those not familiar with the movie, Bobby Boucher (Sandler) becomes a college football star. From time to time, he needs a little help with his athleticism, and his coach, played by famed actor Henry Winkler, encourages him to visualize how he will attack his opponents. They call this his "tacklin' fuel." It's what gets him moving and it leads to huge gains for his team when he does. Ask yourself:

- What huge gains does my life need most?
- What fuel do I need to tackle the objective of living a more playful life?
- What can I do to motivate myself and others around me to live the playful life—like a coach motivates an athlete?

Regardless of how we answer these questions, we have two desired outcomes:

1. We need to get moving toward our goals.
2. We gotta get our families, friends, coworkers, etc., moving with us.

Do you see the need for our fun use of the word Jazzercise for this step of the path? We know many of you are aware of this 1980s (it was actually founded in 1969 by Judi Sheppard Missett) workout routine, but for those who haven't heard of it, it is a "pulse-pounding, beat-pumping, body-blasting fitness program that gets you results . . . fast. It's a high-intensity dance party that fuses cardio, strength, Pilates, Hip Hop, yoga and kickboxing" (About Jazzercise, n.d.).

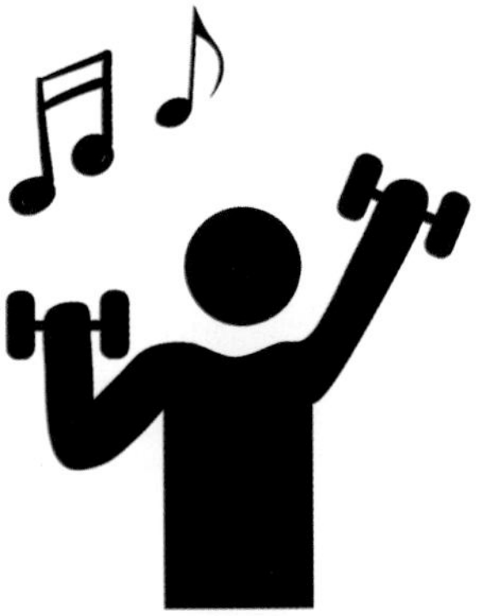

jazzercise

Imagine with us for a moment that every one of us lived a life that was described as a "pulse-pounding, beat-pumping, mind-blasting experience that got us fast results by utilizing music, visual arts, creativity, critical thinking, problem-solving, and playfulness to develop our brains, empathy, and compassion and strengthen our bodies and communities!" See now why we call this step Jazzercise? It fits, and the heading makes us want to get moving away from the excuse of "not having time" and closer to the reimagining of our schedules to make more time for meaningful, relevant, and fun lives filled with play.

Pasteurize. If you haven't figured this out yet, we like words, and we like to use them in unique ways that some folks aren't used to. Our Southernisms, for example, which are prevalent throughout our work, are there in order to capture who we are and to invite a playful spirit to the work. And at that . . . pasteurize enters stage left and all are a-wondrin' what in tarnation it has to do with the path to eliminating excuses. Read on.

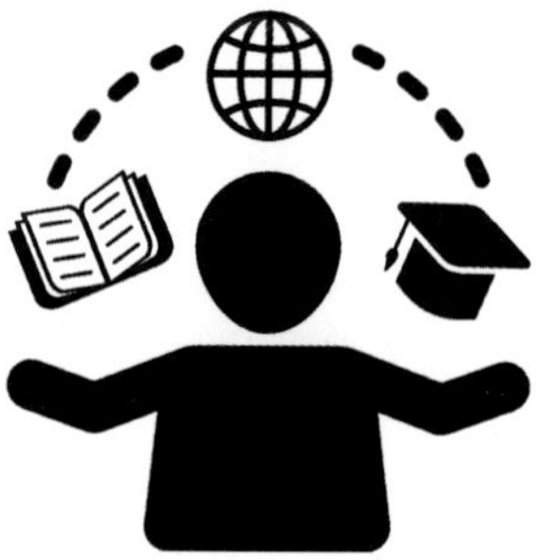

pasteurize

In the 1860s, scientist Louis Pasteur wanted to extend the life of products like wine and milk and other dairy items. To do that, he developed a process using heat that destroyed the harmful microorganisms that led to spoilage as well as reduced contaminants that led to human illness. Pasteurization, as it was named, revolutionized many food industries, and it is still used today.

If you don't see the connection yet, allow us to explain. When eliminating excuses (misguided errors known as mistakes), the process isn't full proof. Recognizing, visualizing, and Jazzercising are great, but unless we take the steps to prevent contaminants such as complacency, lack of motivation, and stagnancy from creeping back into our living space, new excuses may emerge and create hurdles that hinder the meaningful, relevant, and fun lives we long to live.

How then do we pasteurize our lives to eliminate the excuse of "I don't have time"? We do it by intentionally cultivating a circle of support. We are the average of the five people we hang around the most. Y'all. If your circle isn't cheering the loudest encouraging you on, you need to get a new circle.

We pasteurize by asking these questions.

- Does my circle of friends help me analyze my time and support my ideas for change?
- Is my circle playful? Do they encourage play and playful thinking or do they tend to squash my playful ideas?
- Is my circle dreaming with me—are they laughing, moving, or creating?

Learning and growing as a human is a never-ending path of discovering, trying, discovering more, and trying again. Because the process includes risk taking and failure, our circle of friends is vital to our success. We go down this path time and time again because it's what leads us to more playful experiences and greater social, emotional, physical, and academic gains.

Now What?

Having walked through the elimination of an excuse along with us, we encourage you to think about other excuses you may have, and consider how you can use this framework to eliminate them as well so that your playful mindset will grow faster than a milkweed in June. Trust us . . . those things'll grow!

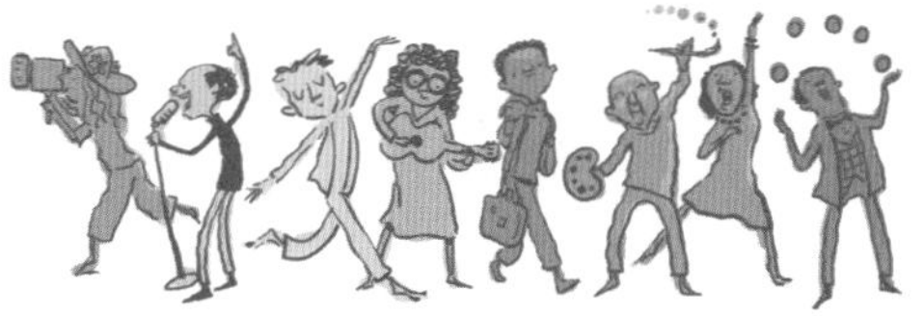

Play & Ponder

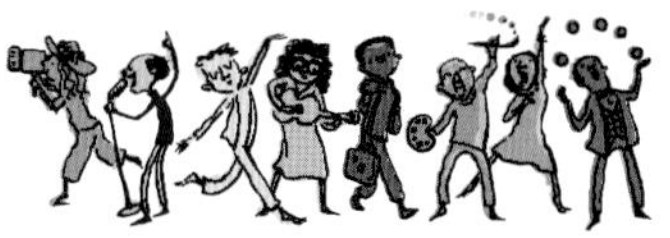

- Do you have an empty cereal box nearby? Maybe some cardboard that protected your last online order as it was shipped to your house? Grab that box. Destroy it. Yep, cut it up, rip it up, however you see fit. Just proceed with caution as you do. No time for paper cuts here. Once the box has been dismantled, use all the pieces to create something new. It doesn't matter what it is: a cat, a house, a flower, a re-creation of your favorite Lego masterpiece in cardboard form. We assure you, your creation will *not* be perfect. What it will be is a real-life model to remind you that nothing is perfect, including you. No matter how hard you try, there will be mistakes. Keep the sculpture you make as a visual reminder to keep you focused when you worry about messing up your playful life journey.
- Reexamine the high-risk portion of the chart earlier in this section. Make a list of what scares you most about each item. How many of those things you list are connected to mistakes, or your fear of them? Share the list with a trusted friend and have a conversation about your fears. Good friends can often help you see past the concerns you have and help you peer into a future where those fears are overcome.
- Journaling isn't what it used to be. You don't have to have an A5 dot-grid Leuchtturm1917 bullet journal like us. You might

have voice memos and notes on your phone. There are hundreds of apps that can help you. A friend of ours wrote a whole book on the back of receipts that he collected while working at a job that wouldn't allow him to journal while on the clock. (The book is *Bleak* by Ben Honeycutt, and it's fantastic.) Regardless of your method, capturing the thoughts, memories, ideas, lessons, melodies, etc., that are gifted to you by the universe is important to leading a playful life. When the moments of reprieve from the rat race come, these doodles, scribbles, words, *twiddles* and *drawzles* (words Jed made up) will help you to recall what brought you joy in the moment.

SECTION 5

Movement

No, this is not an exercise book. We promise. There are a gozillion ways to invite playfulness into your life other than running (there's a story comin') or visiting the gym.

Julie: Here . . . gazillion?
Jed: No, I said GOzillion for a reason. I am Southern, and that's how I talk.
Julie (raises hand): Umm ... South Carolina, right here.
Jed: But I am writing this section at the moment. Mind ya own beeswax.

Siblingish banter aside, playful living does in fact require some movement. Yes, you can absolutely play while being fully rooted to your couch or gaming chair, but even then your mind is moving. Let's say you are reading an exciting book, playing your "best-good" video game, or binging an intense thriller on your favorite streaming service. What's happening inside us at that moment? Our brains are actively engaged (moving) to the source of stimulation. Our hearts are racing. Our blood is pumping (moving). Our endorphins are releasing (more moving). See . . . all that movement is happening even while you're sitting still.

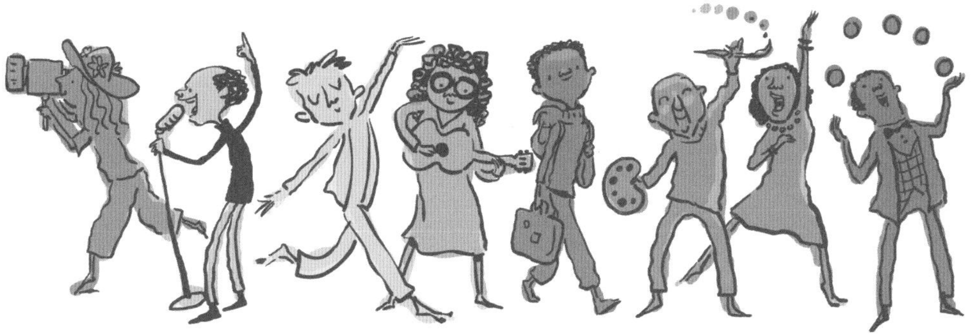

I had an experience like this as I read Margaret Atwood's *The Handmaid's Tale* several years ago, before it became a popular series on Hulu. I had a visceral reaction to it as I finished. I was frustrated as I neared the ending and my blood pressure was definitely up. It was like I was watching an intense boxing match or the last few moments of a championship game. As I read the last words, I was left hanging with so many unanswered questions. I was outraged at the religious zealots—the antagonists in the book. I was worried about the handmaids. I closed the final page, and I literally threw the book across the room. I then proceeded to text all of my friends who had read the book so I could debrief about the whole experience. You know what else was happening during all of that? I was enjoying Atwood's storytelling gift, and my mind wasn't on work 24/7. Because of her exceptional writing skills and creativity, I then connected with my friends on our shared experience.

In the coming chapters you'll read about play as *A Movement*—intentionally written with multiple meanings. It's physical, it's social, and it's mental. Leading a playful life is healthy. It's balance. In Chapter 21, you'll hear the story of wellness—how the status of Jed's blood and weight was directly related to his overworked brain. There were no moments of downtime. It was always work, work, work. He had no balance, and it took a negative toll on his health. In subsequent chapters, we show you how playful living should be *A Movement*. We have to be playful in our individual lives before we can be playful with others. In starting with ourselves, we begin *A Movement* of growth that we hope will spread *A Movement* in our communities.

We start small, where we all are. Gandhi is credited with saying, "If you want to change the world, start with yourself." So that's what we'll do. But we also know the work on ourselves is never really complete. At some point, we hope to feel ready to expand our movement to include friends and family. When we include others in our play, the benefits are exponential and the outcomes can be great. The tractor is cranked now. Once it begins rolling, you'll see the *movement* take shape and there can be a community influence.

Be the good, y'all. Be the good.

CHAPTER 21

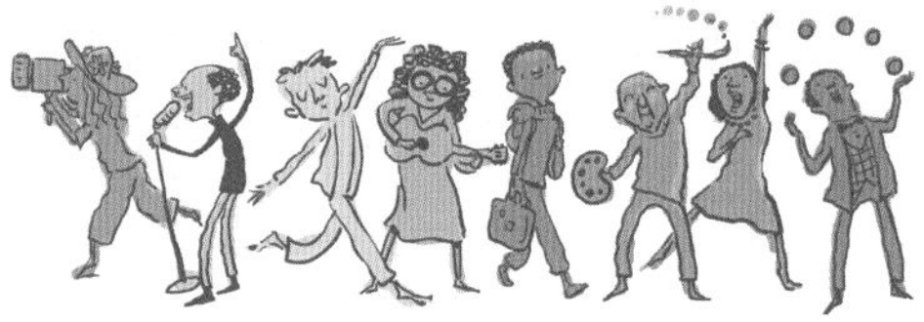

When Play Is Missing

In late September of 2009, the school where I (Jed) worked began partnering with a local organization that would conduct bloodwork testing for teachers at a discounted rate. I was 31 years old at the time, and having bloodwork done seemed so silly to me. That was what "old" people did, right? So I thought, anyway. I wasn't old yet, and that was something I didn't need to worry about 'til much later in life. I didn't have any major health issues that I was aware of. I wasn't morbidly obese—maybe a slight bit fluffy, but no worse than a lot of 31-year-olds. I chose not to sign up.

Little did I know, the school secretary was checking over that list more times than Santa checks his, and she noticed my name was missing from the sign-up sheet. She was like that, as secretaries often are—efficient and aware of what was happening in the building. She knew everything there was to know about our school.

She started talking to me about it one day while I rested in the rocking chair next to her desk. "Jed," she said, "You really should consider this. It will never be this affordable anywhere else, and you will learn things about your insides that you don't know."

I caved to the pressure, and maybe a bit of nagging by my coworkers, and signed up.

Weeks later, the results arrived. It was all there in numbers and percentages. Because this was my first time, I had zero clues about what I was reading. I took it to the secretary, who was also an all-knowing health guru for our staff and asked her to interpret it for me.

Almost immediately she looked concerned. Long story short, she said I needed to call my doctor and let him guide me through the numbers—they weren't good. Cholesterol was high, triglycerides were through the roof, and my liver enzymes were all whacked out.

"*Yikes!*" was my doctor's reply as I shared my numbers. Apparently the 50 pounds over my ideal weight had done more than just round me out. My insides were a mess.

Weight wasn't the main contributing factor here. It was a by-product of what was happening inside. We know lots of very thin people who also have things going on inside. Don't read all this as us saying anything negative about weight. This is just my personal story, and I am getting to the point.

After hearing the words *stroke, heart attack, heart disease,* etc., come out of my doctor's mouth, I was terrified. What did I do? I called my mama. In an instant, she activated her motherly role. We went straight to the grocery store. Why there, you ask? I was eating poorly. I worked a lot, but healthy eating was not on my priority list. For example,

- I'd swing by Hardee's and grab a biscuit for breakfast on the way to school.

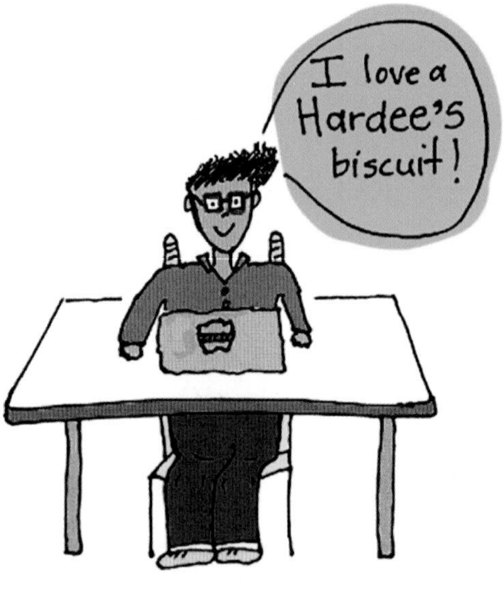

- The awesome cafeteria ladies LOVED filling my plate full of extra tater tots at lunch, and my good Southern upbringing required me to clean my plate so it didn't hurt their feelings. I couldn't be seen as rejecting their gift of bite-sized goodness. Like Blanche said on my favorite episode of *The Golden Girls*, "That would be . . . unsouthern."

- I usually worked at school 'til 6 or 7 p.m. and on the way home I would hit whatever drive-thru struck my fancy for dinner. I would scarf it down, finish up the lesson planning for the next day, then crash.

Exercise? Nope. I had no time for exercise either. I made time for work, but failed to prioritize myself. I realize the irony that I am now sitting here writing a book about playfulness and its benefits for all areas of life, but clearly, being aware of the benefits was not always the case with me.

Teaching, like many careers, can be all-consuming if we allow it. The day-to-day rat-race mentality often convinces us that if we take a pause, if we spend time indulging in activities/experiences that are not helping our work, we aren't successful. I am sure it's because many of us (in the United States) equate money with success, and the only way to make money is by working. The more we work, the more money we make, the more successful we are. But wait . . . I would venture to say that many of you reading this are salaried employees, and you don't make any more money the more you work. In fact, all of the teachers who worked in the building with me who left right at 3 p.m. every day made the same amount I did, even though I was there 'til 6 or 7 every night. They were out there living their best lives apart from work and still had the same amount of money as me. Talk about a letdown. I thought the way I was using my time made me more successful, but in reality I was destroying the vessel that was specifically designed to carry me through life. Rather than increasing the value of my life through walks in nature, reading books, creating art, and making memories with friends and family, I was shortening my life in servitude to a hierarchy that didn't value me for the extra I was giving. I am confident that many of you reading this right now will feel the same about your job. As we type these words, we are in the midst of what some call *The Great Resignation*. We found there is a way to work better, more efficiently, while also tending to ourselves.

Y'all see where this is going now? A playful life isn't just rainbows and glitter. It isn't just fluff that we are peddlin' here like some mystic guru living on the side of a mountain. It isn't just taking time away from work. The playful life is literally a matter of life and death for some of us. My bloodwork revealed that my overscheduled, overworked life was literally killing me. I was sacrificing myself for the sake of the job, for the sake of the dollar, for the sake of my own health. In reality,

I didn't want to eat junk.
I didn't want to avoid exercise and playful living.
I just didn't feel like I had much choice.

After my visit to the grocery with Mama, things began to change. It wasn't easy at first, but it quickly became a new way of life. How'd I do it? Well . . . I made it fun. Counting calories, buying new foods, making myself and my health a priority turned into a habit because I told myself it was a game. A game with awesome benefits for the winner, and quite honestly, possibly death if I lost.

About four months into the change, I had lost 40 pounds and had taken up running. At six months in, I ran my first-ever 5K on my 32nd birthday. Not long after that first race, I was *hooked* on running. I ran my first half-marathon, followed rather quickly by my first full marathon in March of 2011. By that time I had lost another 45 pounds, my bloodwork was exponentially better, and I had rediscovered the playful Jed I knew prior to being consumed by years and years of working too much.

CHAPTER 22

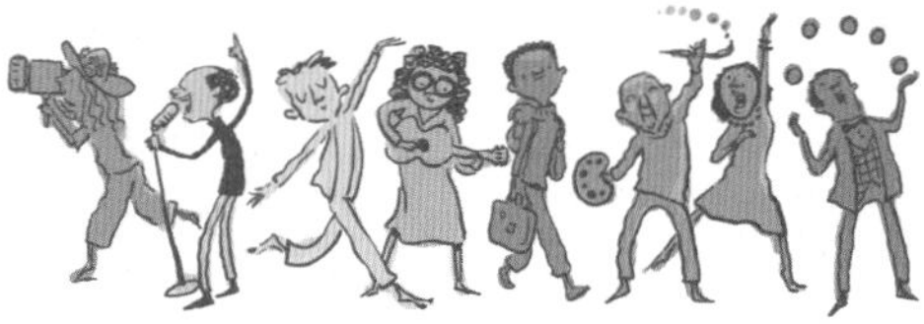

Start with Yourself

Playfulness is not a destination. We don't go there and come back—it's a way of living. It's taking the juice of our DNA—the way we were created as humans—and using it in our daily lives. Can we go to a spot and play? Yes. But the goal of this text is for us to shape a life where play and being playful exist as our intention. Full transparency here—some days we're just not playful. We're hitting snooze, pulling the covers over our heads, and wishing we could go into hibernation mode. And that's okay. Recognizing this need—and giving ourselves grace in times we crave rest—is a necessity. Sometimes the healthiest decision we can make is to let ourselves go offline for a bit. We recommend that you keep up with how often this happens. We often journal our days so we can find patterns more easily. Even more recently, I (Julie) have paid attention to my initial bodily reaction across situations. Certain people may enter the room, and I have a physical response—joy at their arrival, or a sense of dread and caution. As you read earlier, this past semester, one of us got a talkin' to about being perceived as "too playful" by our peers. Y'all, it was me. I was perceived as being too playful—as in, *not rigorous*. I politely fired back—come see me teach. Y'all know that didn't happen. Those people? Yep—bodily reaction when they enter the room. Shoot fire, there's a bodily reaction when an email pops in from them. Our bodies often know how we feel before our brains do. We have to be in touch with where we are emotionally to begin our personal movement forward. If you recognize a bodily reaction in a certain situation or around certain people, pay attention. Let's explore this a bit further.

Trauma is stored in our brains as isolated images, sounds, and feelings. Instead of recalling details in narrative form, such as beginning, middle, and end, we embody the memory. Interestingly enough, sounds and smells are stored separately in the brain from the story memory itself (van der Kolk, 2015). If you have ever smelled cinnamon during winter and suddenly had a flashback, you've experienced this phenomenon. It can also be negative, such as my relationship with the Fugees. Picture it, August 1997: party downtown. The DJ selects *Killing Me Softly*, and the end of my first serious relationship plays out before me on the dance floor. That was hard times, y'all. Every time I hear this song, I'm right back there. White T-shirt, acid-washed jeans, carefully coiffed hair dulled from the Southern summer heat, and a heaviness in my soul.

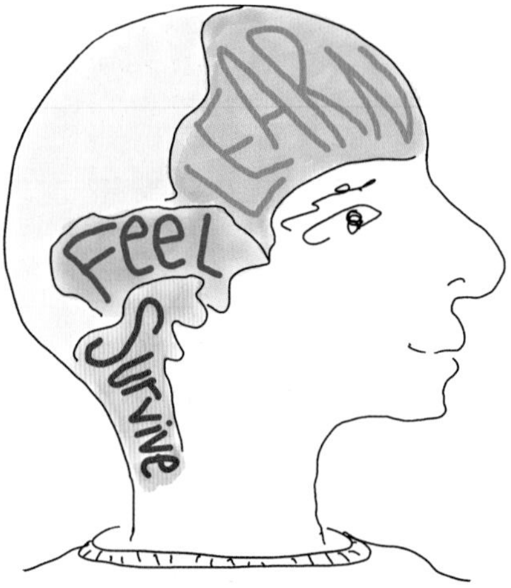

If our memories are positive, we'll have warm fuzzies. If they're negative, our bodies may respond as if the event were happening in the present. We might experience elevated blood pressure, heart rate, and oxygen intake. Why? You see, the most important job of the brain is to ensure our survival. Everything else is secondary (van der Kolk, 2015). When we feel loved and accepted, our brains can focus on exploration, play, and cooperation. When we feel unwanted or frightened, our brains focus on management of fear or abandonment. Let's think about it this way: as a growing child, we explore through movement and experience. We experiment with our surroundings—we play—we learn. These experiences shape the brain structures for emotion and memory. Each experience we have as we grow and develop modifies these structures—positively by a beautiful first love, or negatively by assault, bullying, or neglect (2015). Have you heard the phrase

"What fires together, wires together"? It's referring to our brain's beautiful capacity for healing and growth. The concept of neuroplasticity explains our brain's ability to modify, change, and adapt as we go through life. It is almost as if when the cosmos created us, it knew our brains would experience difficulties and need the ability to heal and move us forward. Remember when we were told that an IQ test defined our intelligence? Lies. Read Chapter 4 again. Read *The Playful Classroom* for a breakdown of that terrible tale. When our brain circuits fire repeatedly, those settings can become engrained, thus leading to a repeated pattern of behavior. Neuroplasticity shows that we have control over these settings—what great news! This means that no matter what we've experienced in life, we have the incredible ability to retrain our brains. While we explain this so simply, we need you to know this is NOT easy work. It may take a licensed therapist. It may take medicine. It may take a new friend group, a relocation, a career change, a walk in the woods every single day. The point here is that it's rarely easy, but our brain makes it doable, and it's always worth it.

I (Julie) have recently walked through a very difficult time in my life. I have been sad. So sad that the feeling began to encroach upon other areas of my life. When I realized I was focusing on the sadness and loss I'd experienced, I began to intentionally look for the good. It was no easy task for me. The hurt and pain sometimes came in moments where I least expected it. My journal became a place of solace. Sometimes I made lists of all of life's joys and the quirks about myself that I loved. Other times I doodled and sketched through my grief. I drew the parts of my life I wanted to remember. The view from my seat on the plane, watching my children talk to each other on the couch, a sketch of a sweet letter I got in the mail. While I am still on this journey through the dark valley, I find myself writing about rewiring and firing the brain to a new place. Ironic, huh? But this I know—my brain, and yours, is an extraordinary organ within our bodies that will lead me through this time.

According to the National Institute of Mental Health (2022), an estimated 17.3 million (7%) of adults in the United States had at least one major depressive episode in the past year. These statistics rank depression as one of the most common mental illnesses in the United States. Stuart Brown, play advocate and researcher, explains depression as the opposite of play. These two, play and depression, are incompatible. Where one exists, the other cannot. This state of mind, this depression, is one way trauma robs us of the feeling of being in charge. To recover, we have to reestablish ownership of our minds and bodies. Sometimes, we can shape these changes on our own. Sometimes, we need others to help us through. Thankfully, the conversations around mental health and the role of therapy for healing have increased and become more transparent in the past five years. Just yesterday, I saw a commercial for online therapy with Michael Phelps as the spokesperson.

Whether you have a therapist or not, let's explore some ways in which play and being playful can facilitate our personal movement toward healing.

Personality	**Playful Experience**	**The Science Behind It**
All play personalities 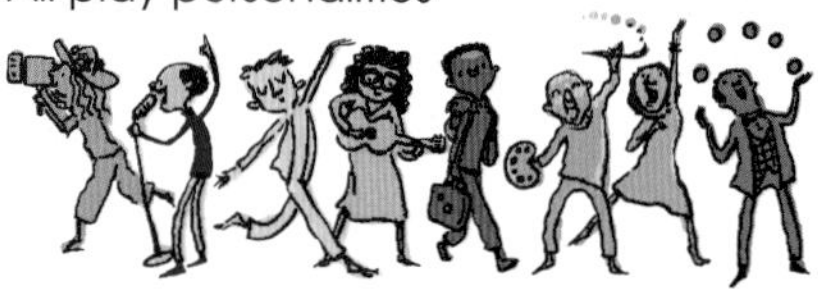	Get a therapeutic massage.	The most natural way we can calm down is through touch. Mindful touch and movement grounds people and allows us to discover tensions we might not have been aware of before (van der Kolk, 2015, p. 218).
All play personalities 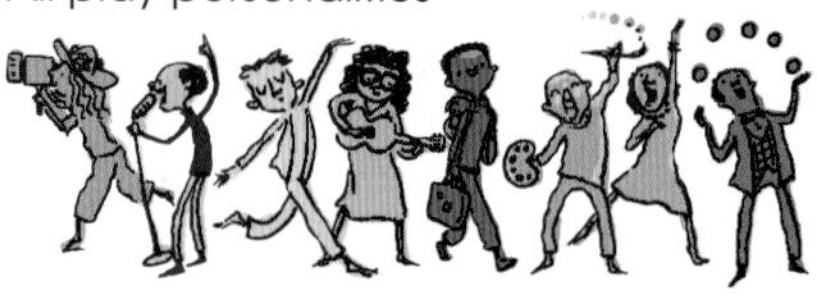	Meditate.	Meditation decreases glucocorticoid levels, sympathetic tone, and all the bad stuff that too much of either can cause (Lazar et al., 2000; Sapolsky, 2004).
Storyteller 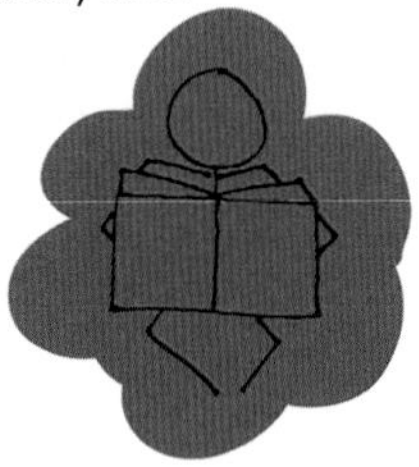	Write your story. As much as you want to tell.	Telling our story is important. We possess two forms of awareness: one that keeps track of the self over time, and another for the present self. Our narratives change as we tell them, and our perspective changes as we incorporate new ideas (Badenoch & Kestly, 2016).

Personality	Playful Experience	The Science Behind It
Artist/Creator 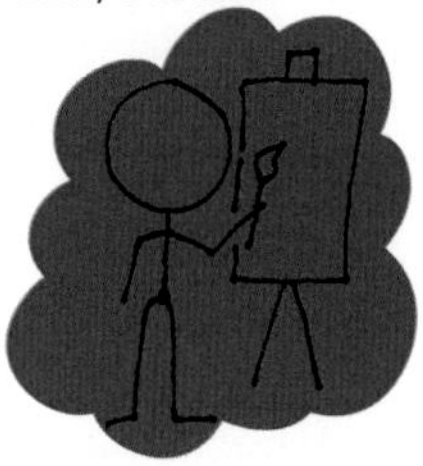	Paint a picture, write a song.	There are many ways to share your experiences. When we know ourselves, we put images and feelings in context. Without memory of the story, we cannot imagine how things can be different (van der Kolk, 2015).
Kinesthete 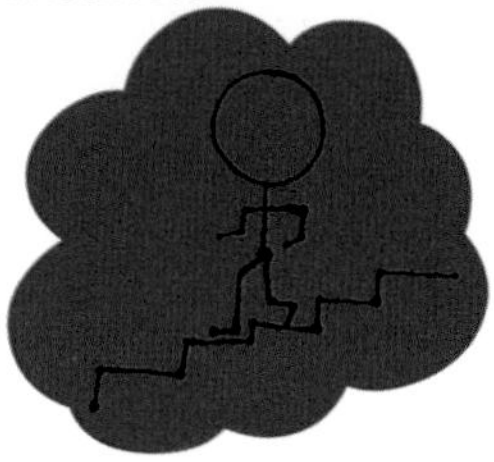	Practice yoga.	Memories of helplessness are stored in the body as muscle tension. Yoga practice will not only work out that muscle tension, but it also regulates our digestion, healing, sleep, and dream cycles. When our systems work together, we are primed for engagement with ourselves and others (Gulzhaina et al., 2018; van der Kolk, 2015).
Explorer 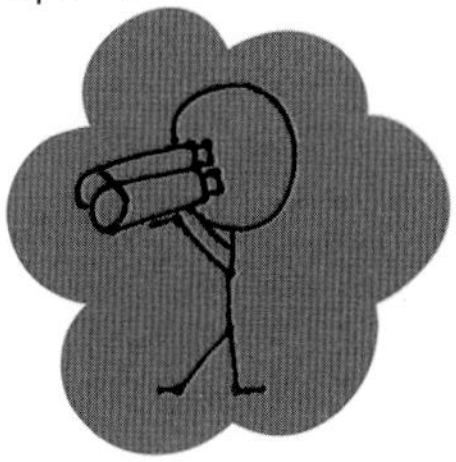	Look for new experiences in outdoor spaces.	A study in June of 2016 found that 10% of participants lowered their blood pressure if they spent just 30 minutes or more in a park each week. An earlier study in Japan found that people who spent 40 minutes walking in a cedar forest had lower levels of the stress hormone cortisol compared with when they spent 40 minutes walking in a clinical setting (Sifferlin, 2016).

Personality	**Playful Experience**	**The Science Behind It**
Collector 	Gather up what you love. Art? Books? Photos? Experi-ences? You name it.	Collecting, whether objects or experi-ences, is reinforced with anticipation. The collector's desire allows them to imagine any-thing they want to about the desired returns of the object (Mueller, 2009). Imagination, a quality of playful intelligence, is a precursor to empa-thy (DeBenedet, 2018).

CHAPTER 23

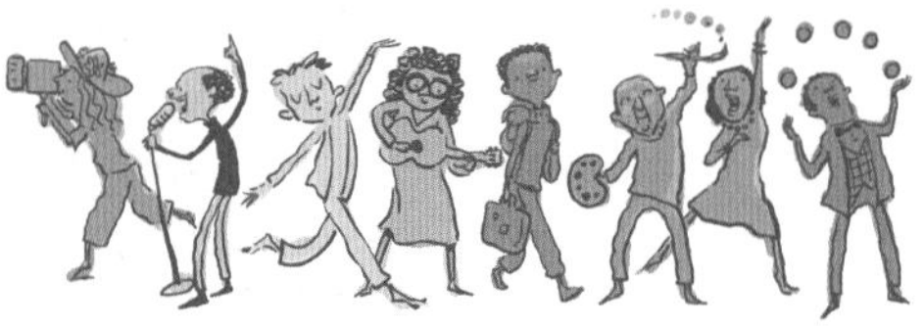

Grow and Play with Friends

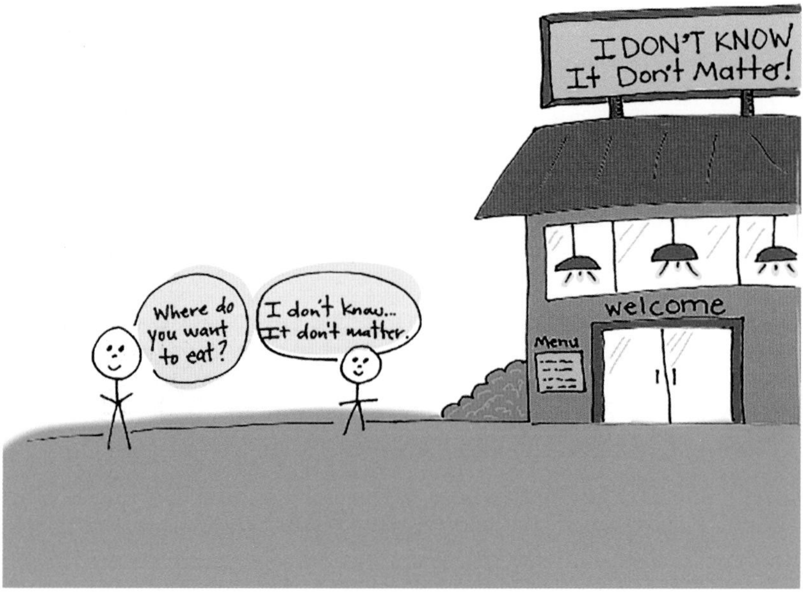

Sometimes I (Julie) am really indecisive. What game to play? What shoes to wear? Where to go for lunch? When I'm hesitant or indecisive, I often play this mind game: I let someone else decide. I know my preference by that feeling I get when someone else speaks their mind. If there are two dessert options on the menu,

I pretend there is only one of each left. I let Jed tell me which one he wants, and then I know. I know which treat I want based on how I feel. I'm either mad he got the last sweet potato pie or I'm happy the key lime is mine.

Jed interjects: Y'all, one time Julie and I went to a local restaurant for lunch. She played this exact game where she let the server decide our lunch choice because we weren't very decisive that day. I am not as adventurous with my food selection, but reluctantly agreed because Julie can convince you of anything (read that as peer pressure). Anyway, the server delivered a pastrami sandwich to our table and sat it in front of me. She said, "Thank me later." Admittedly, it was *not* something I would've ordered. In fact, at that moment, I don't recall ever having eaten pastrami . . . but since then . . . *Hunnnnnny* get back! That sandwich was the best thing I had ever tasted. I have eaten it countless times since that day. Gosh, I am glad I played Julie's game! Letting someone else decide our lunch was golden.

JULIE: You should listen to me more often.
JED: {bleeped out by the editors}

Julie takes back over. . . . We shared in Chapter 20 about how we are the average of the five people we hang around the most. By hanging around me, Jed is clearly affected by my food-ordering process and has secretly started playing it when I am not looking. I caught him last week. You may be wondering, how am I shaping his behavior? How do we explain this phenomenon? You're gonna love this. Let's dig in.

Have you ever noticed yourself sitting the same way as the person across the table? They cross their legs and before long, you've crossed yours? Maybe you have been sitting at a coffee shop and heard someone cough and then you yourself felt the need to cough. Do you relate? Yeah? Want to know why? Okay, but first, a story about monkeys. (Jed—*For the love of Pete, Julie.*)

Picture it—a research lab in Italy.

JULIE: In my mind's eye, these researchers are listening to Elton John sing "Can You Feel the Love Tonight?" You know . . . that's when the Lion King came out.
JED: Raises microphone. Sways with one hand in the air. "*Nants ingonyama bagithi baba!!*" Simba.
JULIE: Yes . . . okay, monkeys. . .

Purely by accident, in 1994, a group of Italian researchers discovered the existence of mirror neurons. These researchers had attached electrodes to a monkey's premotor area of the brain, then set up a computer to watch which neurons fired when the monkey picked up a banana or a peanut. At some point, maybe while imagining Rafiki lifting baby Simba, an experimenter was putting food bits in a box when he looked at the computer screen. Y'all. The neurons were a-firing, but the monkey wasn't eating or moving. What's cooler than that is that the neurons were firing in the exact location where the motor command neurons were located. He was watching the researcher, and his brain was vicariously mirroring the researcher's actions. Enter mirror neurons, stage right.

Scientists around the world followed up with studies of their own. Turns out, these mirror neurons explain all kinds of things we didn't have explanations for previously: empathy, imitation, and language development. Not only do we pick up on other people's movement (synchrony), but we pick up on their emotional state and intentions as well (van der Kolk, 2015). You've walked in a room where there was tension before, right? You can feel it. It's thick. And uncomfortable. Now you know why this superpower exists: mirror neurons.

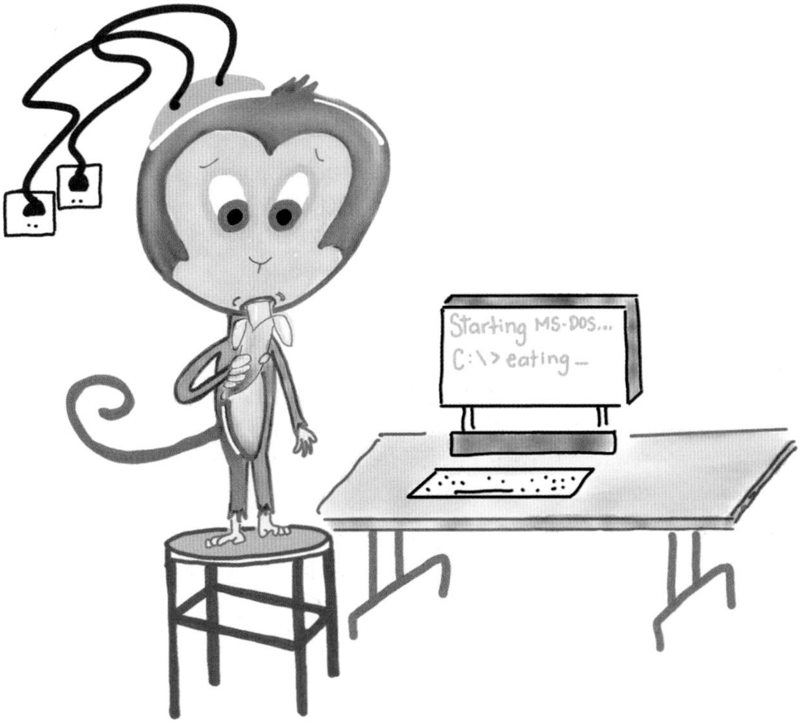

Empathy is housed in the frontal lobe of our noggins. Well-functioning frontal lobes are vital for healthy relationships with others. This area of the brain isn't actually fully formed until we are about 25 years old (Johnson, Blum, & Giedd, 2009). When we're young, we begin to understand that others have feelings and that those feelings are separate from our own feelings—this is the transition away from Piaget's theory of egocentrism. The understanding of the self and our role in a larger society continues to develop as we age. As we mature, if our frontal lobes aren't flexible and active, we risk becoming creatures of habit. Our relationships can grow stagnant, superficial, and routine. Without wonder, without discovery, without invention and innovation, our relationships are lacking. How can we keep wonder, discovery, innovation, and invention alive?

You got it. Play.

Playing with others and developing a network of playful friends is our greatest protection against emotional threat. The presence of familiar people, faces, voices, and physical contact offers comfort and safety. When we feel safe, we can play. When we can play, we can grow together. We are bonded; we are attached.

This word *attachment* is important here. A history lesson: When threat of war in the 1940s came to England, many families sent their children to live with friends or other family members in the countryside for protection against German bombing raids. Studies conducted afterward found that children who were sent away fared worse than those who remained with their parents and endured nights in bomb shelters and saw death (Newcombe & Lerner, 1982). Of course, we would both probably send our children out of harm's way from falling bombs, but it is interesting what the study highlights. Familiarity often provides emotional stability. Bonds from our network are powerful, whether our connections are with family or friends.

There are numerous examples of how playing with others can be beneficial. Let's take a gander at a few of them. Just for kicks and giggles, we aligned this research to several different play personality types. Such a director kind of move—we know.

Personality	**Playful Experience with Others**	**The Science Behind It**
All play personalities 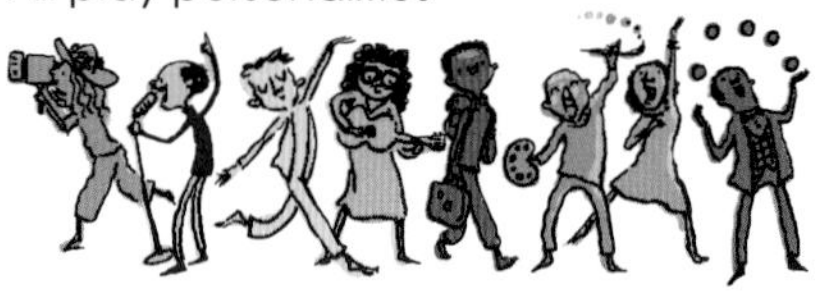	Play with others.	Study after study shows having a good support network is the most powerful protection against trauma. Safety and terror are incompatible (van der Kolk, 2015, p. 212).

Personality	Playful Experience with Others	The Science Behind It
Competitor 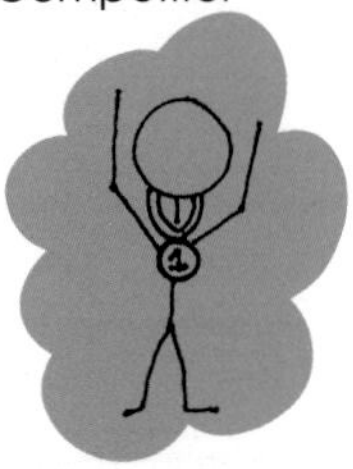	Challenge accepted.	Competing in a playful environment establishes trust and boundaries with others (DeBenedet, 2018).
Director 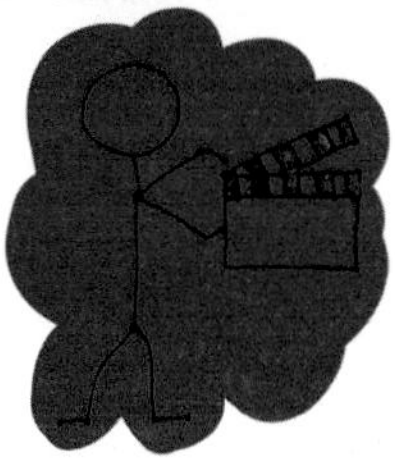	Organize a fundraiser or celebrate awareness for a cause near and dear to your heart.	Multiple studies have found a link between prosociality and well-being (Hui et al., 2020). "(Altruism, cooperation, trust, and compassion) are part of the shared culture of humankind," Hui said, "and our analysis shows that it also contributes to mental and physical health."
Joker 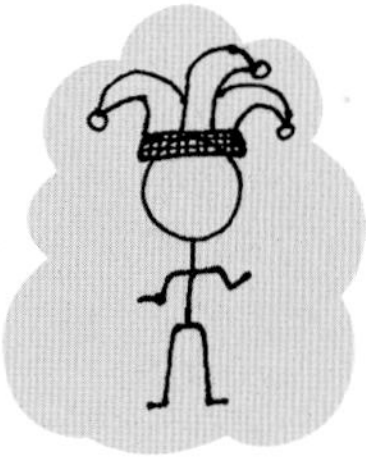	Tell knock-knock jokes.	A mutual creation of a synchronous synergy comes from telling jokes with others—human connection. Also, people high in self-monitoring (determining how the joke being told is received) are more likely to modify their behavior based on the social situation, and are more likely to take on leadership roles in social groups (Eby et al., 2003; Schmidt et al., 2014).

CHAPTER 24

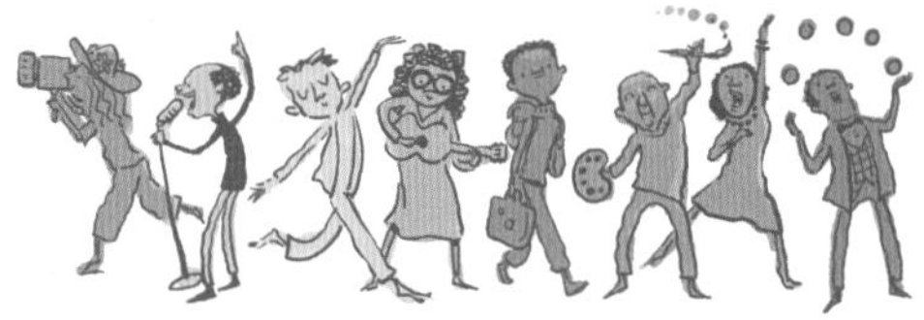

Play in Our Communities

As a result of my (Jed) marathon running mentioned in Chapter 21, and the revival of playful Jed, I began to pursue goals that I once would have never dreamed of. Completing the New York City Marathon was one such accomplishment I wanted to add to my list of running accolades. The thought of weaving my way through the five boroughs while on foot, being cheered on by thousands of city residents, was so exhilarating. I was fortunate enough to secure a spot for the experience upon my second time joining their participation lottery, and immediately began my training. The months of early morning runs passed quickly and it was finally time for the big event. It wasn't just a one-day happening. There was a whole weekend of festivities. We arrived in the city on a Friday. The race was scheduled for Sunday. I went immediately to the race expo, got my T-shirt, bib, and family photos with the official race step-and-repeat backdrop, then made my way to the Hampton Inn in Times Square. As I stood at the hotel counter chatting with the clerk while checking in, Mayor Michael Bloomberg appeared on the television near the desk and announced that the race would be canceled due to the impact of Hurricane Sandy on the region. While the worst of the storm had blown through days before, resources were stretched thin and many areas of the city were still reeling from the catastrophic blow of the storm. The entire lobby fell silent as he made the announcement. Everyone in the room was in town for the race and there was instant anger at the mayor. It wasn't pretty, y'all. People were big-mad. In hindsight, the race should've been called off well before runners arrived into the city so that all the extra visitors didn't add to the stress of the battered infrastructure. But alas, there I was, a runner with no race.

I was disappointed. Months of training for an event that was not happening seemed wasted at that moment. I am not gonna lie about it, I pouted that night, but the cancellation was exactly the right call. The city was definitely in distress because of the storm. Thankfully, I had family and friends with me to help move me quickly through the stages of grief I was experiencing. They, along with some frosty beverages at an Irish pub, helped do the trick.

The next morning I awoke with a new sense of purpose and meaning with my running. "Why not turn this into something good for others?" I thought. My idea? I would go home and complete a full marathon on the streets of my hometown, and ask the community to donate financially in support of my run to help those who had been negatively affected by the hurricane. Because I was an educator, I specifically asked that people donate to teachers whose classrooms and schools were damaged by Sandy through a website called Donors Choose, a nonprofit that allows the public to support the individual needs of teachers across the country. The organization helped me create a giving page filled with descriptions of projects written by educators who were directly impacted by the storm, and I began to share that on all my social media platforms. I contacted local media outlets and they added the good-news story to their nightly shows. Local businesses began to donate and sponsor food and beverages for the day of the event. Other runners began messaging that they wanted to join me in the run.

Looking back, it is incredible how quickly things got moving. I shared my plan on the day after Bloomberg canceled the race, and by the very next Saturday, one week's time, my own personal marathon through Spartanburg, South Carolina was happening. At the conclusion of the race, surrounded by over 150 of my closest friends, family, and fellow runners, I announced that we had raised over $13,000 for teachers and students in the Sandy-ravaged region. The news media came back and reported again about the outcome of the event, and money continued to come in. I honestly don't remember the final tally, but it was over $15,000. My mind was blown. In one week, y'all . . . all that money seemed to just appear!

I realize that in the big scheme of life and fundraising more money has been donated, raised, etc., but to be a part of what was named by the media "Dash for Donors" was an incredible experience for me. It showed me the power that one person with an idea could have on a community. At the heart of what we did that day was play. The runners were playing, the volunteers who worked our aid stations were playing, the folks who paced us as we ran on open streets played, the random strangers who lined streets and cheered when we passed by played, and the celebration at the finish line was most certainly playful.

The end of the race was not the end of its impact. About a year later, Donors Choose nominated me for *GQ* magazine's Male Leader of the Year Award.

I. Was. Shook!

I never in my wildest imagination thought that the run I basically threw together in a week's time would lead to being recognized by two national organizations. Talk about a playful experience! GQ flew my sister and me to an all-expense-paid weekend in New York City for the award ceremony. *The Gentleman's Ball*, they called it. The event was unlike anything this small-town boy had ever experienced. Cameras flashing, celebrities milling about on the red carpet, and food upon food upon food upon food. I will never ever forget it. There are pics out there. Give it a google.

CHAPTER 25

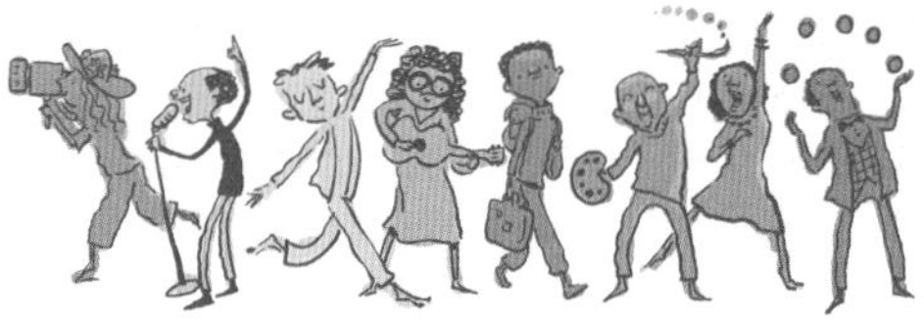

You Don't Have to Run a Marathon

As you read about Jed's story, maybe you thought that the point was to highlight that he was running and that we found running playful. Maybe you thought that we were wanting you to get moving and run. Remember, we promised this wasn't an exercise book. What we hope you took away from the entire pop-up marathon experience was that it created *A Movement* in our community.

Although running was a form of play for me (Jed), it led to something for the greater good. Digging deeper into your play personality can help you do that for your community, too. By no means does it have to be on a large scale like planning a race for hundreds of people. It can be something very simple like asking your friends to create holiday cards for a local nursing home. My sister and nieces do this every year. It randomly began one Christmas season when she was in a crafty mood. Her play personality type is definitely artist/creator. An afternoon of card making with her girls was a fun way for her to spend a cold December day. She and my nieces ended up crafting cards for several days and then delivered them to the senior living facility nearby. All the hearts—the seniors' and my family's—were filled with joy. Immediately my sister wished they had made more cards. The next year she did it again and included the rest of the family in the creativity. It has since become a tradition that she invites her friends on social media to join in. She has expanded the card delivery to local prisons as well. Our family has had loved ones incarcerated before (sometimes unjustly) and we want them to be a part of our holiday. My sister has a strong desire to share love and joy with others, and she uses her play personality to do that. Her approach to this work is so very admirable. Not in the "aww, look what she did" kind of way, but in a manner that speaks to the empathy and compassion she has for her fellow human. When play and a desire to do good begin to intertwine, the impact can be great. As of the writing of this book, over 1,000 cards have been made for those in our community thanks to my sister and her girls, and their social media friends.

We hope we have inspired you with a few stories about how play can lead to *A Movement*. Are your playful and giving spirits starting to mingle in your mind? We love to imagine that everyone reading this will create a playful movement in their home, in their school, in their workplace, in their community. But how does one even begin? Remember back to what Meryl said: you "start by starting." Be the good, y'all. Be the good.

Play for Community Healing

Play isn't just good for our personal health. Play and playfulness with others can positively impact the health of communities. It's time for another history lesson. (Stop rolling your eyes, Jed.) Did you know that play in the form of kicking a soccer ball around provided time for German and English soldiers in World War I to forget the harsh reality of battle for a while? It's true. When you have a moment, research "Christmas truce." This may even be the beginning of our modern-day games for promoting social good.

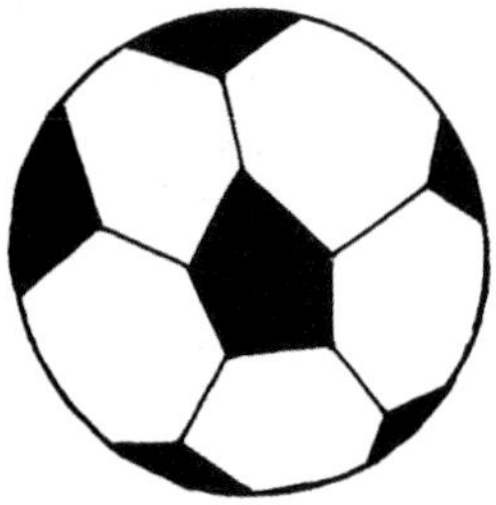

Nearly 100 years later, the London 2012 Olympics popularized using games and sports to impact communities, and spurred momentum for many organizations to build on the idea of play to affect social good. Team UNICEF's sport for development (S4D)

work uses play to bring lasting change to communities. In an interview with *The Guardian* (Anyangwe, 2015), Luke Dowdney describes how boxing became a vehicle for access in a rundown neighborhood in Rio de Janeiro. In the late 1990s, it was common to see young men, even 15 or 16 years old, walk the streets armed for war. Not that Brazil was at war with another country at the time—instead the community battled a skyrocketing homicide rate. Drug-related violence made every day feel as if the community was a war zone. *The Guardian* stated, "an estimated 15,000 young people (in Brazil) are armed and in drug factions." One day, Dowdney had a conversation with a young boy, which led to curiosities about boxing moves. The boy asked Dowdney to show him a few moves, and as this was transpiring, other children began to gather around. What became of that moment was transformative. Because of the relationship between boxer and coach—that discipline and respect—combined with the community experience of training together and supporting each other, Dowdney and his colleagues were able to establish and grow programs that led to peace and change. Instead of creating government programs that often miss whole groups of people, boxing provided access. "We put on boxing shows that traffickers leave their weapons behind and come to."

Play helps us reach people, and there are stories of play being a catalyst for community change all over the world.

- Dowdney's program, Fight For Peace, founded in 2000, offers young people an alternative to violence.
- A community-based program called Moving the Goalposts Kilifi (MTGK) uses soccer to help women and girls in Kenya get an education, learning the financial skills to establish their own businesses.
- AIR Sports Network, a government nonprofit in the UK, focuses on giving former offenders something constructive to do with their time. This group boasts a 65% success rate for helping young people refrain from reoffending. Sports insulate young people in the program from criminal influence (Gov.UK, 2016).
- The Gay Games, held every four years, exist to serve the needs of athletes, artists, and LGBTQ+ advocates. Their mission is to promote equality for all, and in particular for LGBTQ+ people throughout the world, and to provide a safe place in which to socialize and bond with other people with similar orientations.
- Adaptive sports are bringing health and happiness to people with disabilities now more than ever. Justin Laferrier led a 2015 study that found participation in wheelchair basketball and

other sporting events was a massive boon for disabled vets; the longer they participated and the more team-oriented their sports were, the more likely they were to be happy, healthy, and have better self-esteem (Neumann, 2015).

- PeacePlayers International works with children from conflicting backgrounds (Israeli and Palestinian, for example) to show that it is possible to have fun conflict, like opposing sides of a game, without violence. By bringing sports into these communities, their hope is to help children develop empathy through play—creating better, less war-torn futures.

But formal organizations and even play in the form of sports are not the only ways to impact communities. You know from Section Two that there are many forms of play, and all of these forms are valid for the player:

Reading.
Writing.
Planning an event.
Designing clothing.
Coding a new computer game.
Marketing a new toy.
Vacays.
Board games.
Art of any kind.
Solving mathematical puzzles.
Sitting on the shore for hours.

All of these are play.

Are board games impacting communities? Yes, honey! Take a look back at Section Two when we discussed how play improves social skills. What about reading? Of course. Our local Hub City bookshop hosts monthly book clubs, where the reading centers on a particular social issue. These events bring together people from all backgrounds to talk and build community. They don't have quantitative data on social change, but sometimes you can't quantify the qualities that make a lasting impact.

SDG 9: *Build resilient infrastructure, promote inclusive and sustainable industrialization, and foster innovation.*

SDG 17: *Strengthen the means of implementation and revitalize the global partnership for sustainable development.*

What about those techy friends in the crowd for whom computer coding is an escape? While it isn't necessarily playful for us, there are some who play for hours while designing code for the next "it" thing. Take a minute to search "Tech for Social Good" on your nearest device. One in particular, Github, supports the United Nations Sustainable Development Goals with open-source programming opportunities. In 2021, they had a high-volume impact on goals 9 and 17. Read more about their impact by scanning the code here.

Steps for Taking Our Play from Solo to Plural

1. **What do you love? What brings you joy?** Creating a playful movement—regardless of size—should never be more stress, work, or anxiety. Center this action around something that brings you joy. Maybe running and card making aren't your thing. So, what is?
   - Did you take the play personality quiz? No? Go back and take care of that, pretty please.
   - You could create a *map-a-doodle* (for more info on what this is, see Chapter 35) of all the things that bring you happiness.
   - You could create a Joy list of all those sparks of delight you experience throughout your day.

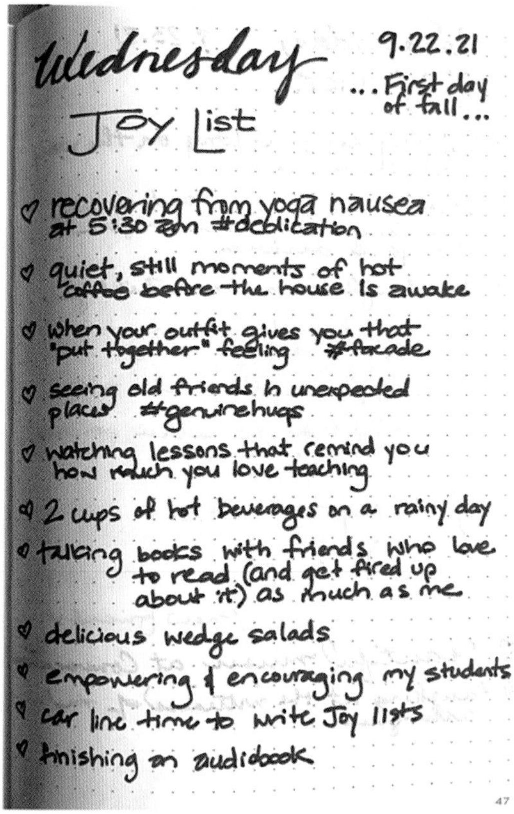

- You could ask your inner circle, "When do you see me at my peak? In my best moments?" Compare their response with your physical reaction to those ideas.

2. **How can you connect your love with the community?** Now that you've got your list, choose your path. Every community has its share of cat-loving, video-game-playing folx who are also **obsessed** with knitting. Or, those peeps who carry three books in their bag throughout the day because they want choices if they are ever in a moment of downtime. Or those humans who strum their guitars and make recordings on a private-no-link-shared YouTube channel planning for that one day they hope is coming. No matter what form your play takes, there's a group out there hoping to join in the fun with others. It doesn't have to be a big thing. We worry if you jump in too deep too quick, you'll wear yourself out and be a one-hit-wonder. Start small. Keep going. Let it grow. We can find our play-people by giving them an opportunity to join us in play. Remember, Jed's sister only made a few cards that first year.

3. **Level up—how can you partner with others for good in your community through play?**

   Do you ever find yourself doing your thing around town and come upon some event, some image that gives you pause? Your thought: *They should do something*, or *someone should do something*. There is no THEY. You are THEY. Many people will shake their heads and keep on going, but we challenge you to explore how your play-joy might make an impact.

   - Let your play be an action that cleans, builds, creates something new.
   - Bring the playful experience to those without the same access you have.
   - Use your knowledge to bring awareness to people, places, ideas that are often marginalized by the hegemony of the dominant culture—wherever you are.

What the world needs now, is love sweet love, and MORE PLAY!

CHAPTER 26

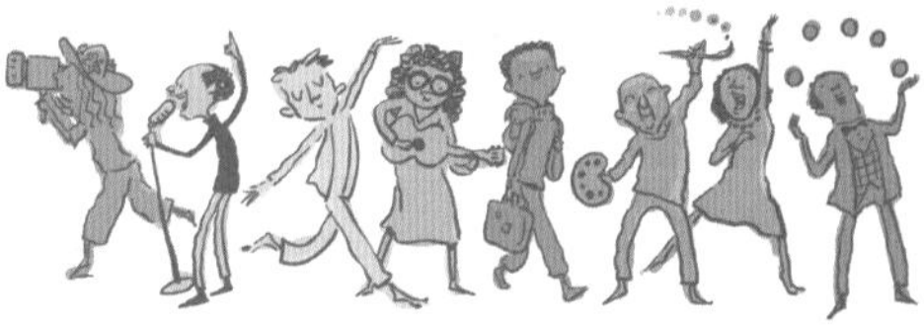

Advocating Through Play

Dr. Jemelleh Coes (@jemellehcoes), the 2014 Georgia State Teacher of the Year, Director of Teacher Leadership at Mount Holyoke College and Clinical Assistant Professor at the University of Georgia, is a fierce advocate for diversity, equity, and inclusion. Her accolades in the education world are plentiful, but it is her work to take education beyond the classroom that has impacted us most. A strong Black woman, she tackles racism and injustice at every turn. I (Jed) cannot tell you enough about the way she has inspired me as a gay man to fight for my own equality and civil rights. Just typing about her here makes me emotional as I am overwhelmed with gratitude for her influence and friendship in my life. When she and I first met, we used to text about our favorite music and books 'til very late at night. We would laugh hysterically about the ignorance of those who didn't like us, and we often shared comical memes that added to our laughter. When I examine my own play history, Dr. Coes is definitely high up on the list of people who I like to play with.

Recently, her playful life combined with educating the masses on the beauty of being Black, why representation matters, and the teaching of history in the most incredible of ways. Annoyed with a certain elf that arrived every year on her shelf, Dr. Coes wanted to create a daily experience for her child that was more than just wrapping the holiday tree in toilet paper. While nothing was inherently wrong with that, she wanted the daily elf play for her daughter to be meaningful and relevant, as well as fun. Of course her daughter was hearing about the elves from her peers at school and reporting them to the family at home, but the experiences seemed a bit less than desirable. Dr. Coes, wanting to give her daughter a similar experience while also seeing a need for her daughter and other children of color to be more represented, met that need for *all* with a playful movement and her own version of the elf.

She named their magical visitor Miss Georgia Roots. The family is very connected to the Peach State, as Dr. Coes is also a graduate of UGA as well as her title as Georgia Teacher of the Year, thus the name for the North Pole friend. When Miss Roots arrived for the first time, she came with a note that informed Gabby, the oldest Coes daughter, that as she slept each night her elf friend would be traveling to a different country on the African continent and deliver a report of her "roots" the following morning. Instantly, Gabby was hooked and the idea of daily acts of elfish comedy vanished from her mind and were replaced by playful learning moments about the heritage of her ancestors. Jemelleh shared the excitement and learning of Miss Georgia with her friends in the social media world, and we were equally intrigued. I couldn't wait to wake up each morning and learn where our new friend had traveled next. Angola, Congo, Nigeria, Kenya, Ivory Coast, The Gambia. In total, 20 countries were visited that holiday season. Each day was filled with the true history of the country and not a colonist interpretation. This is important to note because so much of the history learned here in the United States is told from a perspective of those in power. White people for the most part have controlled the way our history, and the history of other nations, has been taught. While this is not a book about the ills of systematic racism and its history here, this highlights the need for such an experience that Dr. Coes provided to her daughter. How beneficial this was for Gabby and for all of us who tuned in each day. And doing it in such a playful manner made the learning sink in deeply. Having lived in the West African nation of Senegal for a short period of time in 2001, I was transported back to my time there when the language of Wolof appeared in one of the daily reports from Miss Roots.

In the years since that first visit, Miss Georgia Roots has visited the island nations of the Caribbean and Latin America. The history and influence of African countries around the world weren't the only stops. Miss Georgia can also travel through time! One year she visited different eras of Black history: the civil rights movement, the Harlem Renaissance, and the Underground Railroad, just to name a few. One visit to the past led Dr. Coes to do a whole season of elf reports on the impacts and contributions of Black Wall Street. This daily act of play and learning continues to be a part of the Coe family holiday five years later, and it has had a ripple effect on Gabby as she, like her mother who modeled it for her, is creating *A Movement* of her own.

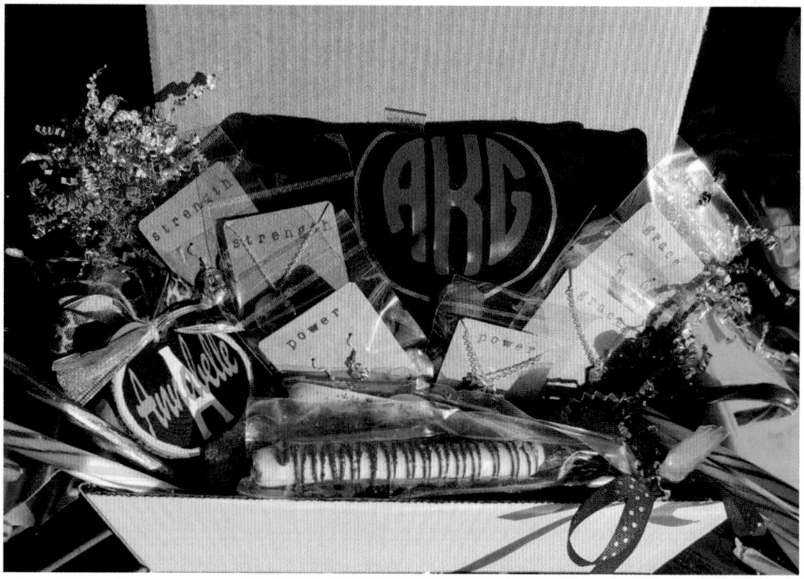

Black Girl Wall Street, a collective of intelligent, driven, and advocacy-minded Black female students (Gabby Coes being one of them), began its journey with a soft launch in late 2021. The goal of the group was to empower other girls of color to follow their dreams, become entrepreneurs, and impact change in their community. How are they doing it, you ask? It is all through the power of play! The girls joined together to create T-shirts, jewelry, scarves, keychains, baked goods, and more. They then marketed their wares on social media in a subscription box plan. Within hours, y'all, the boxes sold out! These young and gifted entrepreneurs, influenced by the teaching of their parents, along with Dr. Coes and Miss Georgia Roots, officially launched their small business in February, Black History Month, of 2022. If you would like to learn more about their work, search for the Facebook page Black Girl Wall Street.

Playfulness Leading to Advocacy Is Nothing New

When she was a student in the fifth grade, **Cassandra Lin** of Rhode Island learned that cooking oil could be used for biofuel to heat homes. We cheered as we read about her, because she likely learned this in some sort of education setting while participating in a STEAM (science, technology, engineering, arts, and math) experience, which is most definitely a moment of play. As of result of the new knowledge, Lin felt compelled to rally her classmates to action in hopes that they could create a plan to help their community and the environment with their newfound understanding about cooking oil. Eventually, after researching the needs in their community, the young people started their own movement, calling it Project TGIF (Turn Grease Into Fuel), which would help warm the homes of those who needed assistance with their heating bills. They students lobbied their Town Council to set up a grease receptacle at the transfer station where residents could recycle their oil. They asked local restaurants to donate their grease to the program, leading to over 120 businesses participating. They even drafted and helped introduce a bill in Rhode Island that mandates that all businesses must recycle their grease. If you are wondering how all of this was playful, and not work, check out our play personality chart to refresh your mind. These students were most definitely experiencing playfulness as they advocated for change in their community. We were unable to locate a social media page for their work, but an internet search of Project TGIF will connect you with their group if you'd like to learn more.

Ball4Good, founded by then 12-year-old **Adom Appiah**, (@weball4good) is a 501(c)(3) nonprofit supporting the community and other nonprofit organizations through sports. The organization began as a school project during the fall of 2016. Mrs. Kelsea Turner of Spartanburg Day School inspired her students to dedicate 20% of history period to a service project. Mrs. Turner called the project 20Time. Ball4Good is a result of Adom's seventh-grade 20Time project. Today, Adom is a high school senior, the author of three books motivating kids to change the world, and was a 2021 recipient of an ESPN Humanitarian Award. His mother, Marjorie Boafa, is featured in Section Six. Playful advocacy is a part of their DNA!

New York Times best-selling author **Peter H. Reynolds** (@peterhreynolds) uses his children's books, which are always playful, as a way to teach about acceptance, love, peace, diversity, and community. It is just one of the many reasons we were thrilled that he illustrated the cover of both this book and *The Playful Classroom*. He and his twin brother, **Paul Reynolds**, (@fablepaul) founded FableVision Studios, a creative company designed to produce media to enhance the world and move it to a better place. The sibling tag team has created *A Movement* of creativity and play around the world with their motto, "Create Bravely." Their work has had a ripple effect of advocacy-minded projects around the globe. Because of Peter's work *The Dot*, an educator from Iowa,

Terry Shay (@tjshay), started what is now known as International Dot Day. Students, teachers, and countless others celebrate the day by following in the footsteps of Vashti, the book's main character, and making a mark to see where it takes them. Sometimes the mark is an actual dot that leads to artwork. Others make a metaphorical mark and take the proverbial first step to make change in their corner of the globe. You can learn more about this world wide celebration of creativity at internationaldotday.com.

Our friend and fellow educator **Livingstone Kegode** (@lkegode) is changing the world for his students in Kenya and around the globe by creating playful moments via video conferencing with others while teaching them about the culture of his homeland. On almost any given day, you can find Kegode's students singing, dancing, laughing, and teaching their peers across the time zones about life in Kenya. In turn, the students who connect with Livingstone's classroom reciprocate the education about life in various parts of the world. These playful learning moments built a bond between the classes and their empathy was strengthened as a result. Their relationship led to a national project here in the United States to help raise awareness about clean water for all humans on Earth. After a call with American educator **Mike Soskil's** (@msoskil) class, his students in Pennsylvania raised money for water filters to send to their Kenya peers when they learned that 12 students in Kegode's school had passed away that week from Cholera. What began as a playful collaboration turned into a life-saving mission.

M. Judson Berry, actor, comedian, and internet personality, who's been acting since the age of 6 when he got his first laugh while playing a prince in *The King and I*, began making short videos on his social media accounts (@mjudsonberry) when the pandemic began in 2020. In full costume, and more often than not a glorious wig, he portrayed himself as the main characters of the popular sitcom *Schitt's Creek*, most notably, the show's matriarch, Moira Rose. As you can imagine, the people loved him. His already-thriving career and platform grew because of the playful videos and now he is using that notability to advocate for a variety of groups. Red Nose Day, a campaign with the mission to end child poverty by funding programs that keep children safe, healthy, educated, and empowered is one of the most recent endeavors that Michael has endorsed on his social platforms. He is also raising money and awareness for polycystic ovary syndrome, in support of his friend, by running the LA Marathon. As a member of the LGBTQ+ community, he also regularly advocates for the equality of ALL sexualities and genders.

Patty Rodriquez (@pattyrodriguez) and **Ariana Stein**, (@ariana_stein) lifelong friends and new mothers, found themselves disappointed at the lack of children's books representing their Latino community. When they began to research, questioning existing publishing companies about the lack of diverse books, they were told there wasn't a market for the books they were wanting. Thus began their mission to introduce bilingualism and Latin American culture through picture board books. Rather than let disappointment defeat them, they founded their own publishing company called Lil' Libros. Their books honor beautiful stories like the life of Mexican painter Frida Kahlo and Cuban music icon Celia Cruz in English and Spanish with rich and colorful illustrations while also introducing them to concepts like first words, numbers, colors, shapes, and biographies! We love how their story, which began as they read (played) with their own children, has led to over 1.5 million books being sold to children around the world! Follow them on social media and support their work: @lil_libros

Start with a Dot

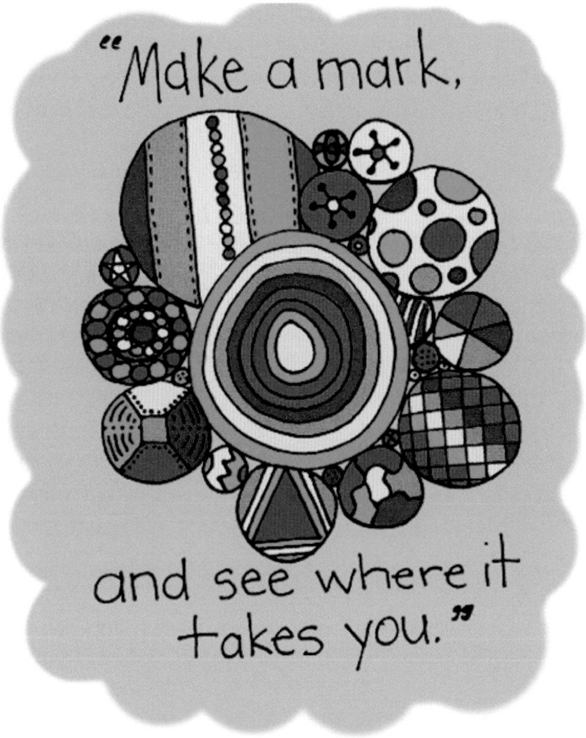

We mentioned Peter Reynolds's (2004) book *The Dot* just a few lines ago, but the story is too great not to mention again. As we shared, the main character is a young art student named Vashti. On the first page, she is in the worst of moods because she has been asked by her teacher to create. "I can't draw," she says. Her teacher, a master of educators, changes Vashti's mindset in a mere moment and the next thing you know, Vashti is the star of the school's art show and passes her gift on to others. We realize that some of you are likely reading these amazing stories of play and advocacy and all the while your brain is telling you, "You can't do that." We are here to counteract those curmudgeonly thoughts just like Vashti's teacher: "Make a mark, and see where it takes you." All of us have the ability to make that first little mark. When we reflect back on the stories of the humans we've shared, all of them had an idea, took one step that led to another step, and then another. Remember the process we shared with you in Section Four? Go back and read it again. Think of these people and think of the possibility that it could be you on the next list.

These are just a smidgen of our planet's playful citizens who are changing the world. We hope that their stories inspire you to take action in some way to bring about playfully inspired change for good. Remember, your playful impact doesn't have to be gi-normous—what makes a small impact can grow. Let it.

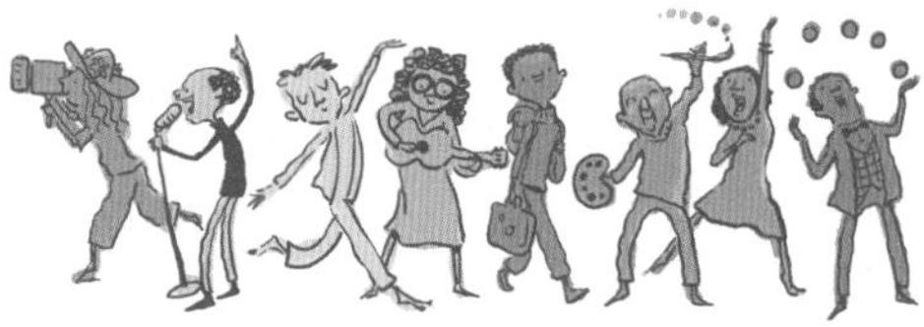

Play & Ponder

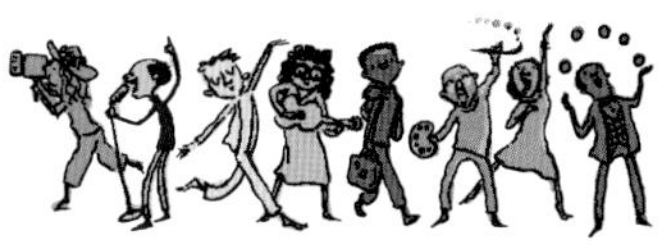

- Go outside. Move. That's it. Think about life while you are out there. Maybe skip a rock or climb a tree. Just be careful. We are not responsible if you fall.
- Take a good look at your social media feed. If you're a reader, take a look at your shelves as well. Do all the voices look like you? Do all the voices agree with you? Representation matters in all areas of our lives. We're not saying to start following folk who spit nonsense. No. What you read should fill you up, but it should also challenge you. In one of my scrolls recently, someone posted "Your Martin Luther King, Jr. quote for Black History Month is nice, but have you read the books these activists wrote?" That challenged me. Wow. I (Julie) am that person. I posted a quote. I believe in celebrating all voices; I seek the true stories. But have I (a reader!) read a book by Dr. Martin Luther King, Jr.? No. No, I haven't. Let your feed challenge you. Let it help you grow. In all ways.
- Find a copy of *The Dot* by Peter H. Reynolds. Online, your library, a bookstore. Read it. Enjoy it. Make your mark.

SECTION 6

Mojo

You've likely heard the word *mojo*, either from Austin Powers movies or if you're a 1970s era Doors fan.

JED: What are you talking about?

JULIE: Well, I looked it up . . . turns out, there's a Doors song where Jim Morrison wrote in an anagram of his name, "Mr. Mojo Risin'"—cool, huh?

JED: Your phone has Michael Bublé and Ella Fitzgerald on it. Never have I known you to listen to the Doors.

JULIE: Oh, I don't. But I'm sure someone does.

JED: (Sips beverage. Looks away.)

Anyway, do you know where the word comes from? You're gonna love this. The term as we know it today has Southern roots! Etymologists (those friends who study words) trace it to the 1920s Gullah word "moco," for magic. The term *Gullah* refers to a group of Black people who live on the coast and border islands of South Carolina; their language is also *Gullah*. According to the travel site for Beaufort, South Carolina, the Gullah are known for preserving more of their African linguistic and cultural heritage

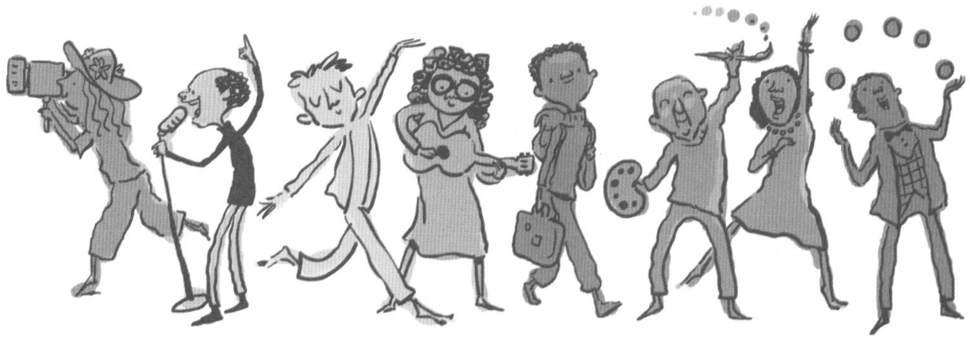

than any other African American community in the United States (Gullah Culture, n.d.). The original origins of the term *mojo*, which eventually shows up in jazz and blues music, originates from the continent of Africa—in Fulani, *moco'o* means shaman or medicine man. Full transparency, Jed and I both knew the term mojo from pop culture—not from its roots in the history of our home state nor from the continent of Africa. We challenge ourselves, and you, to dig deep into the history of our countries to fully recognize the contributions of all people.

We like to think of play and being playful as our own personal mojo—our magic juice that keeps us enjoying life. Julie's magic juice comes over ice in a to-go mug with fun stickers on the side. Jed's mojo is served in a Mason jar with a rainbow straw. The straw certainly lights up and shines bright like a diamond. (Julie (rolls eyes): I don't want to hear anything more about my literary puns.) Everyone serves mojo in a unique way. In this section, we'll explore mojo—the playfulness—of some of the most playful people in our circle. We sat down with them at our local coffee shop for a chat. Here is the result of our fun and deeply meaningful conversations about the power of play in their every day.

CHAPTER 27

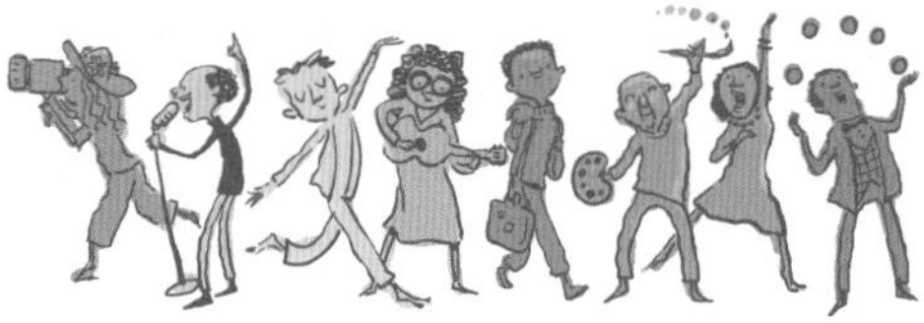

Ned Barrett

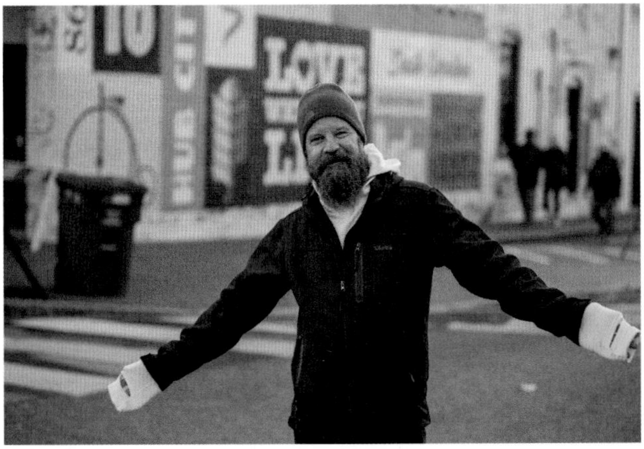

Social Media: @15minutesfromhome

The door chime is faint over the morning sounds of coffee brewing and local friends greeting each other, standing in pockets between our table and the front door. Ned is sporting worn jeans, a flannel shirt of blues and yellows, and his Covid mask cannot hold the facial beard energetically moving around as he greets everyone on his path to us.

"Ned!!"

"Hey y'all! How ya doin'?" *Hugs. Fist bumps.*

The conversation flows easily as we catch up. Ned is leaning back in his chair, one leg crossed over the other, ankle on knee, smiling with his eyes as we chat.

Jed: "Why do you think we reached out to you about being playful?"

Ned: "I employ mojo regularly. I have mojo all over the place."

Y'all. We had not even said the word mojo to Ned. He had no idea we were titling the section that way. Of course, we got all giddy as we explained that connection.

Ned: "No way!"

Julie: "Yep. How cool is that? We're in sync already."

Ned explains his play as a general approach—his intentional choices, but also his approach to life. A little background here—we both know Ned through the coffee shop, through his work with active events around town, through his biking photos, through documenting his runs on social media, through his volunteering at the bookshop.

"There are things I do for fun—running to me is play. It has never been exercise for me. It's always been my play."

Later, when questioned about his intentionality, Ned explains, "Like most athletes, I have habits—when I run in a race, I crumple my number. I keep crumpling it. Also, my socks (shows socks)." We both pause and lean over to inspect.

Jed asks (*perplexed*): "They don't match?"

Ned replies: "Yes, they do. They match by theme."

Today, Ned's socks display a duo of dancing skeletons on one and a sun on the other. He buys them in corresponding sets—another set he owns shows a shark and a peace sign. He likes to wear those in races: "I like to channel my inner peace-shark," he says.

Like us and likely many of you, Ned was known in his childhood as being the class clown. This label has changed as he's aged and progressed through various seasons of his life. Ned was a teacher at one point in his life—before his work as Trails Development Manager with PAL: Play, Advocate, Live Well (@palspartanburg). As a teacher, he was called immature by his professional peers. His colleagues were clearly the serious sort. Now, he's called childlike. We, however, see him as playful. Ned energizes us. He is the kind of soul who radiates happiness. One cannot remain stressed or sad if Ned is nearby.

Our conversation turns to parenting, and Ned reflects on the balance needed in his blended family. "Half of my job as a parent is to give my kids things to tease me about, and the other half is being able to take it."

A fun fact about our friend, Ned, is that he rides his bike to work. "I do it because it's super fun. Not because I'm on this climate-change mission. I'm not really saving much gas. I just do it because it's fun. Balancing on two wheels is magical. Getting into tight turns when you're going fast. . . ." He walks every morning, and runs often. When asked why he runs in the rain, he replies, "When's the last time you splashed in mud puddles?"

Ned recently took his fun to a whole new level, and decided to run every street in our city. This was a solitary mission, but he posted his runs on his social media, thus including us all in the playful experience. Ned explained:

> I borrowed this idea from another runner who ran every street in San Francisco. People have actually done this all over the world. So, I decided to do that here. It took me a full year. It was 385 miles. I used an app, G-map pedometer, that allowed me to plan the route and ensure I got to each street. One thing I really like about it is that every street gets attention—there's no priority of one over another. Never did I feel intimidated on those runs. People in the so-called "bad neighborhoods" tended to hang out on the street, and they cheered me on. It was incredible. I took pictures along my runs. I looked for the good stuff. When you look for the good stuff, you can find it.

Ned also hosts a podcast for PAL called *The Daily Required*. In each episode, rather than sitting down and interviewing guests, Ned takes them on a walk down one of our local trails. As we chatted together, Jed and I both agreed that Ned embodies the phrase *love where you live*. Toward the end of our conversation, Ned pauses and reflects, "I'm purposeful in each place I live to explore and find places to love. A quirky store, a museum. Every place can be playful."

Indeed, Ned. Indeed.

CHAPTER 28

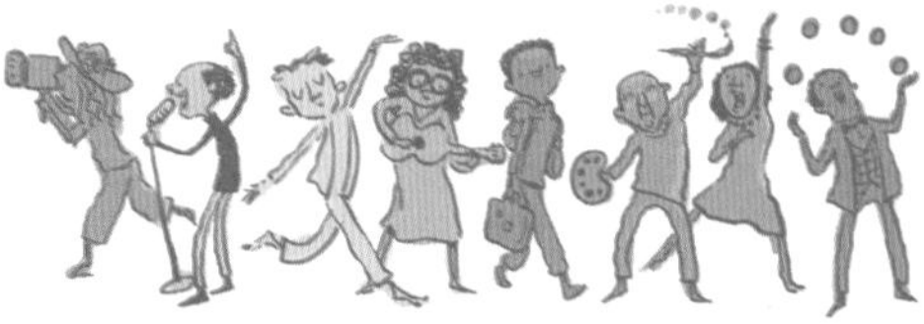

Tashma Glymph

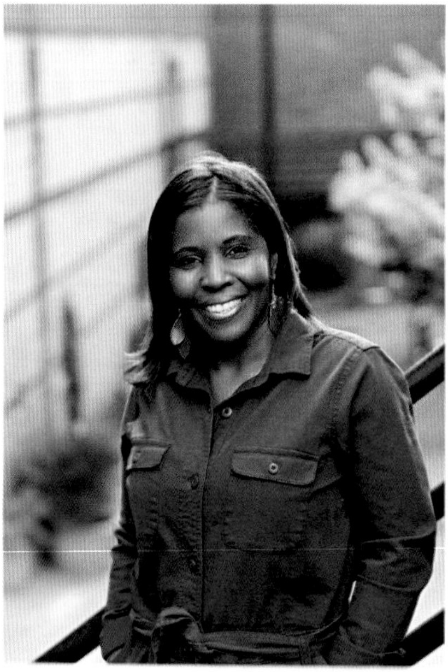

Social Media: @TashmaTalks

My cortado sits by my computer, and I'm laughing from something Jed has said. "Maybe the next book will be *Playful Livers* . . ." We are cackling. Chicken livers. Gizzards. Tears are in my eyes. That's when Tashma walks in. We tell her the story, and now she's bent over slapping her knee. Tashma has this way—everywhere she goes, she's a part of the group. If there's no group, she makes one. And everyone is included.

JULIE: Jed, I've known Tashma for a good long time. Our kids have swam, *have swum?*, together for years. But you know her from community work, right?
JED: Yes! In fact, this is the first time we've sat down for a real conversation. We follow each other online, so I feel like I know you, but I'm excited to really talk.
JED: (presses record)
JULIE: Okay, Tashma, why do you think we reached out to you about being playful?

Tashma explains that 98% of her work focuses on language development with infants and toddlers—she is a pediatric speech therapist, so it's natural for her to play all the time. She's also a mama. Her children, Karter (15) and Kirsten (11), are her joy. But as fun as we know her to be—the bringer of the party—Tashma describes herself as an introvert. "You know there's this new zip-up blanket—the swaddler? I want one. When I am not being *Tashma Talks, LLC,* therapist, community activist, board member . . . I'm on the couch with sweatpants and a blanket that my dad gave me." Like us, Tashma loves to read, and recharges with solo activities.

She interjects, "But y'all, I'm busy. I'm making moves whether as PTSO president or on a plane to Paris. I'm out there. I just came from a party at the middle school. It was so much fun." Tashma is telling us this story, but she's also spotting friends across the coffee shop and waving. "Hey y'all!" They wave. Everyone smiles. We're all a part of the fun.

JULIE: Tell us, Tashma. You do such great work in our community. What's a day in the life of someone as playful as you start like? When you wake up in the morning, are you playful then?
TASHMA: Oh, yes. I listen to the radio while getting ready. I love when the DJ tells jokes. Sometimes I need Anita Baker to feed my soul. Many mornings, I turn off the radio and listen to my son rapping. I tell my plants good morning. I talk to them.
JULIE: Wait. You talk to your plants every morning?
JED: I'm going to need to know more. Do they have names?
TASHMA: Oh yes. There's Vernon, that's my daddy—from his funeral. He's on the kitchen table.
Veronica is near the piano.
Otis is in the foyer.
Absalom is in my bedroom.
Uncle Leroy (from his funeral), Keitah, and Keitoh are in the family room.

Lee, our newest addition, is from Lidl. He's by the window in the family room also.
Uncle Zeb, he's not with us anymore . . . the plant nor the person.
We're giggling again.

Something I love, love, love about Tashma is her adventurous spirit. She travels. A lot more than other friends I know. Not just that, she will happily travel alone—to faraway places. Tashma models the kind of playful life I aspire to have. In January, she was in Charleston jumping high in front of the famed pineapple fountain and a couple months before that, she was in the tropics on a trip with her friends. Each month, Tashma intentionally plans trips with her children. Sometimes close, sometimes far. But the planning is intentional. She explains, "I plan for these experiences so we can have something to look forward to. Recently we participated in a progressive dinner in downtown Charleston, and now we're planning one here in town." As a partner with One Spartanburg, our local tourism group focusing on inclusivity in business, Tashma and her daughter are planning a progressive experience in town following the plot of a children's book. She says, "My daughter is a reader, and I wanted to provide experiences for her and others in our community that she would be interested in. I figured we could find a book she loves and connect that with local businesses and experiences."

JULIE: That takes so much planning, and that's one thing you're so good at! You always bring the party. Like, when we're at a swim meet, I bring bags of chips. But Tashma brings decorations and costumes and music. She takes an experience and makes it better for everyone.

TASHMA: Some of that is planned, but a lot is spontaneous. . . . Kindness is big for me. There are so many people out there who are sad. They don't know how to be included. Whether it's in the boardroom or classroom, they need moments that lift them up. I find joy by giving joy.

JED: But that can be draining, too. You do a lot of advocacy work with Tashma Talks, LLC, and that is heavy work. You clearly level up. But, as an introvert, how do you recharge?

TASHMA: Oh, I level down. On my couch. Sometimes I'm in bed at 7 p.m. I'm not sick. I just need that time, you know? My kids get it. When you give, give, give, you can give out—you need to refill.

Play is the fuel that allows Tashma to do the hard work required in social justice advocacy. Her company, Tashma Talks, LLC, is a communication business and so much more. It's social justice. It's advocacy for Black leaders. It's advocacy for female leaders. It's social justice tees and hoodies through her exclusive apparel line. In her most recent endeavor, she explains how the present available sign language videos for children don't showcase Black children signing. Some of her clients aren't able to see themselves in the instruction. Representation matters in all aspects of our life, and Tashma is making way for change through play and her playful spirit.

CHAPTER 29

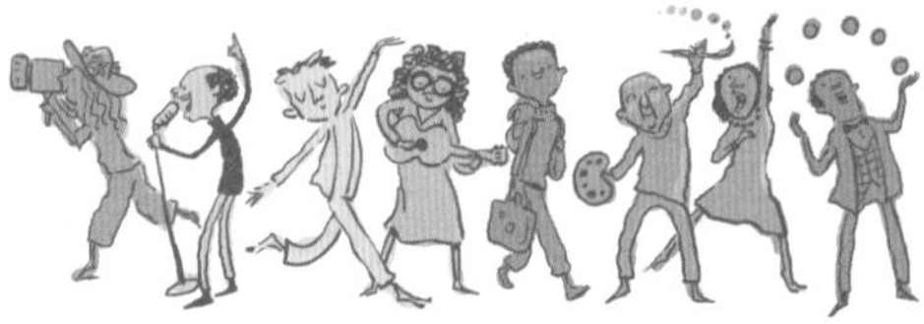

Sonia Aleman

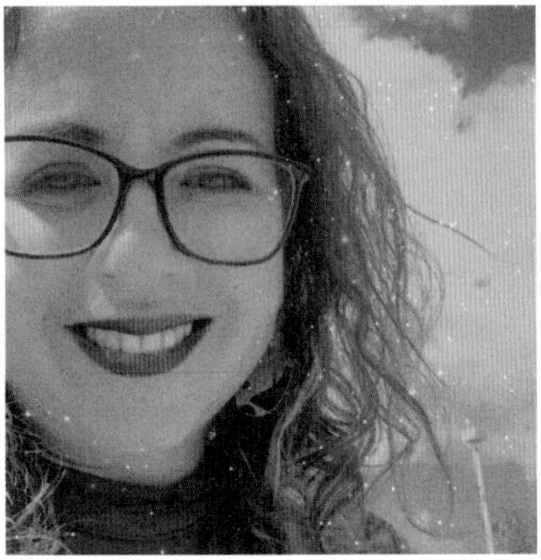

Social Media: @maestraalemanbilingue

It's Tuesday. Jed and I arrived to our writing space In. A. Mood. Both of us.

We stayed up late last night (me watching *Criminal Minds*, Jed at his niece's soccer game then later sucked into TikTok). We are tired. We're also having weird weather, and it's clearly having an impact on our moods. Rain last night. Oddly high temps today for February. The barometric pressure is off.

Suddenly, "Oh (bad word), (bad word). We're late to meet with Sonia!"

We scramble to get the Zoom call connected. Jed comes to my side of the table, and we put in the headphones. Sharing a pair of earbuds on a cord made us have to sit Waffle-House-sittin' kind of close. We hated it. Sonia is in Texas—she's a wonderful teacher, and she's taking time during her planning period to talk with us. We're apologizing profusely. She's smiling and waving us off. So kind. She's sitting in her school's collaboration space. Side note—the school is led by the playful administrators, Sheila, Courtney, Meagan, and Amy, who have adopted our book *The Playful Classroom* to guide transformative professional development for their faculty and staff this entire school year. At Belton Early Childhood School (BECS), Sonia teaches in a dual-language classroom.

She's wearing dangly blue earrings, and her eyes light up as we all easily hop into the conversation.

Jed: When I say, "Living a playful life . . . what does that mean to you?"

Sonia (smiling): Well, you know, in the summer, I can live a little bit.

We all laugh because we know how consuming the life of an educator can be. We are always planning, dreaming, creating experiences for our students. Then, later, reflecting and tweaking these creations.

Sonia explains how she is living a positive life. "You know how when there is a lot of bad around you, but you are positive—I feel safe when I'm playing. When I'm around people who don't like me, I don't allow them to impact me. I play. I escape."

Juile: What do you do to recharge?

Sonia: Well, I'm grateful. But, let me tell you—I don't feel very grateful today. I just want to cry. When I talked to my friend, she told me, "Begin the day with happy thoughts. Don't be a whiner. So (laughs to herself), you know, I interpreted that as happy thoughts and wine—at the end of my day.

Sonia also surrounds herself with people who help her recharge—people she cares about. "My family. We all have stressors, you know, but tonight, during dinner, we're going to pretend we're at a French restaurant.

Jed: Role play for dinner!

Sonia: Yes! (in her best Spanish-French accent) Today's menu is—they only have one choice—lol). In Spanish, we make up names all the time. In Puerto Rico, if Maria is Mommy, and Pedro is Daddy, the baby would be Maria-Pedro. So tonight we're having *Pavochon*: turkey that has a taste of pork. (She says this with a wave of her hand.)

Sonia explains how being playful disrupts the routine of life. "Having a playful mindset helps me break negative patterns. I'm flatlined on Friday. (Laughs—aren't we all?) On Saturday, I start having a heartbeat again. We love—my family—to go RVing. We drive to the RV park—it's only 10 minutes away, but we feel like we're in a different world. Even if it's only one day. It's good for my soul. But you don't have to go places. We sit in the backyard and play. I have games from Walmart. Cornhole. Candy. The kids are running around. And there's music—oh! I sing. Did you know?"

At this point, Sonia is clearly pulling up a song on her side of the screen.

Julie: Oh, sing for us!
Jed (adjusts to sitting up straight): It's about to get real.
Sonia: My go-to song is Gloria Trevi. Do you know her?

The music plays. Sonia is in character. Her head is moving to the beat. Her hands are taking control of the moment. "The lyrics are so good. So self-affirming. I am pretty. Everyone is looking at me, and I like it."

Later, Sonia is describing how being playful has given her the freedom to be herself. "Thinking in this way has made my play dangerous. I am a machine, I cannot stop."

Julie: Tell me about your earrings. (They are teardrop blue with a word written across them.)
Sonia: Oh, that's our resolution word. Resilient. I made these for my team to remind us of our goals.

The energy in this call is palpable. Both of us are keenly aware of the shift in our moods just from talking to Sonia. She explains, ". . . because I think in the world we're living in, we need more play in our teams. Depression is a growing condition, and having a playful mindset will heal us. We have to be multipliers. Just by looking at me—when I smile at you, the smile will spark something in you. Hey—this girl is wacky, but I want to be close to her."

Yes, we do.

CHAPTER 30

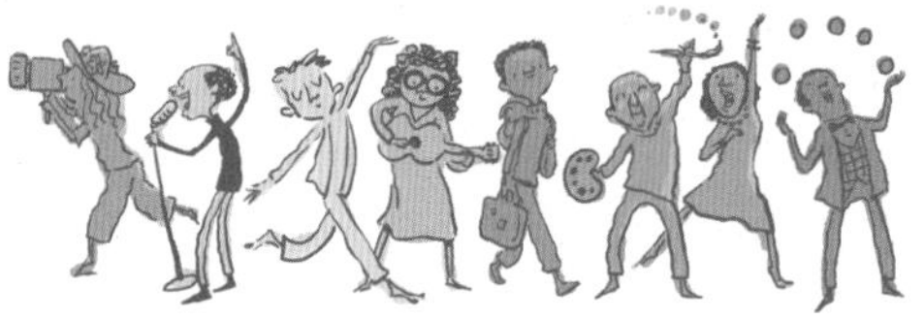

Joan Wheatley

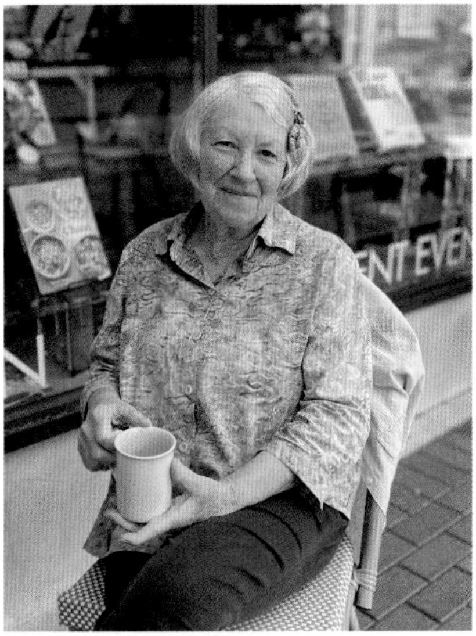

Social Media: @joanwheatlleyscreations

We've just hung up the Zoom call with Sonia, and we've not even had a full sip of our beverage when the doorbell jingles and Joan walks in. Her face lights up as she waves. Joan is wearing a tie-dyed T-shirt and black pants with her sneakers. Her wavy gray locks are pulled back to one side with a knitted barrette she made. (The exact one she is wearing in the picture above. They can be found worldwide in Art-o-Mat.) She claims a table by setting down her bag, her sweater, her wallet, two skeins of yarn, her iPad (complete in its new artsy skin and hand-sewn case), and her book of knitting ideas. After chatting with Tamara and Drew, our baristas for the day, she comes to stand by our table.

"I have to show you this," she says, as she opens her knitting book. "This damn dog. But, you know, I did the scarf. Let me show you his sweater." Joan pulls out a hand-knit creation, the perfect size for a real dog—maybe a toy poodle—and continues the story of her latest creation. Jed and I meet eyes across the table. He grabs his phone to record, and we say, "Joan, join us" (presses record).

When we think of playful people we know. . . (Joan nods as she sips the hot coffee Tamara has just brought her, raises a finger from the hand that's holding the handle of the mug.)

"Yes! You made the barrette you're wearing." Joan smiles.

"You have miniatures hanging from your jacket. What is this cute patch on your shirt? You did that too, didn't you?"

JULIE: Joan, where did we meet?

JOAN: Oh, at the coffee shop. We met at the coffee shop. (Sits back in the chair and sips again.)

JED: You are so playful, Joan. Every time we see you, you're creating or taking pictures. How old are you?

JOAN: Oh. Well. (Changes the subject.)

We're all giggling, knowing what just happened. Joan is taking control of this convo. She pulls out the new iPad, and scrolls—telling more stories.

Later, in the conversation, after at least two more failed attempts, Jed comes back to the topic of age.

JED: This is important. All the people we've talked with about play are of a certain age demographic, but that's not you. Joan, you are exceptional!

JULIE: Don't tell him, Joan. Keep it a mystery.

JED: Okay, let's do this: Would you consider yourself a senior citizen?

JOAN: Oh, yes. Most certainly.

Joan does not fit the stereotype of a senior citizen. She's adventurous. She travels. She creates. She never meets a stranger. She attends every function our town hosts and is named by us as the unofficial mayor of Spartanburg. She has met most of her playful circle of friends while she's been out and about—doing her thing.

JULIE: How did you find your playful people, Joan?

Joan begins with her story of living in the Netherlands. "In Holland, nobody does miniatures. When I lived there, I was the only one, but I didn't care. Here, well, there aren't a lot of people who create them either. You know, I joined the collective. And at the coffee shop, you know."

Joan talks to people. She finds connections. When you put yourself out there, you meet people.

One rabbit trail we follow in our fun ping-pong conversation begins: "My friend, Charlotte . . . we met at the Barnes & Noble. I told Charlotte about Art-O-Mat."

Another begins, "You know Ninfah—we cook, we knit . . ."

Later, Joan scrolls through photos: "Take a look at this card I made for Wendy."

Joan is having difficulty answering our questions. She shrugs off our comments on how wonderful she is. We know it's because Joan is *play*. Play is innate to her soul. Joan is EVERY play personality. She tells us, "You know, you can't say, *I have to wait*. You can always try. You can't wait until you're ready. You just do it."

Joan is also a poll worker on election days. "I do it because they need people, ya know. I want to be the person who hands out the stickers." In reality, there aren't that many people—you have to do all the jobs. And Joan does—all the jobs. While knitting. While connecting. While documenting the fun and sharing it with everyone on the socials.

Joan, for us, is the epitome of what Maya Angelo meant when she said of creativity, "The more you use, the more you have." And Joan has it flowing in her veins.

CHAPTER 31

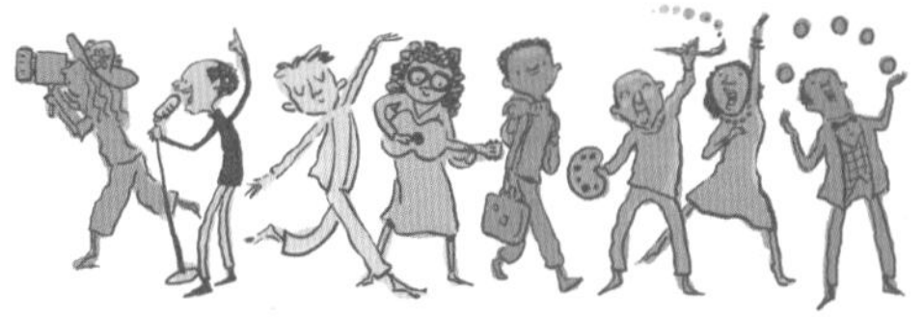

Marjorie Boafo Appiah

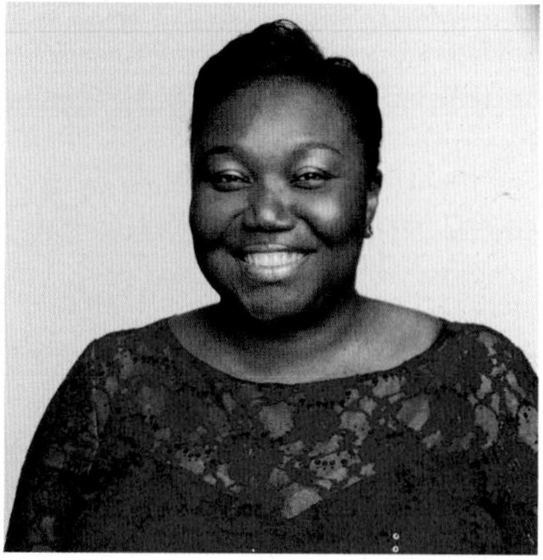

Social Media: @thismarjymarj

It's late afternoon on a weekday, and Jed and I have just claimed a table downtown. It was warmish earlier, but this breeze has a bite to it. I like a cortado after lunch hours—it's small enough to be cute, but has the pep I like to get me over the three o'clock hump. Except it's now 4 p.m. Marjy isn't here yet, but we're not worried. She'll be along soon—her schedule is always packed. I pull my puffer vest tighter around me, considering zipping it up, when a small black SUV drives by, slowing to inspect for parking. "There she is," I say. "Look at her jamming." Marjy whips into an angled spot across the street and pops out, head still bopping to the music. She is sporting a bright pink jacket and designer shades. There is no purse—instead, a backpack is slung across her shoulder. This is a woman on the move.

We hug hellos, and Marjy sits down, still dancing, now throwing up deuces. "Hey, hey, hey, my friends. How are you?" The mix of a West African and Deep Southern accent rolls off her tongue and makes us both smile. The initial conversation is serious and heavy. The school community where Marjy's son, Adom, is a student has just experienced a tragedy. As we discuss how children and adults cope with loss, we can see that the music still plays in Marjy's head. Her words are heavy, but still she sways.

Eventually, Jed pushes record and the conversation shifts. "Marjy," he says, "you know we're working on another book—this one for all people, not just educators. Why do you believe we called you?"

"Because I like to play." There is joy in each word, and a pause in between them. Her body is still as she speaks them, but then the snapping and swaying return. We all laugh. "Yessss," in unison.

Jed: Marjy, You are infectious. Your TikToks with Adom . . .

Marjy: There is always a song in my head. Sometimes happy. Sometimes it's a serious song. The happy songs are important because it gives me a sense of relief. You know, in the church offering line. You don't want to be behind me in the church line—you never know if I'm going forward or backing up. I'm dancing.

Jed: Well, the Lord does love a cheerful giver.

Julie: But you do a lot of heavy work, too. Your *Humanity Chats* show tackles difficult topics, but still is so playful. So energizing.

Marjy: Thank you. Yes. On MarjyTV, our goal is to talk about everyday issues that impact humans. So many people out there feel like they're alone. I want them to know there's someone going through the same thing. It's connection. I always ask my guests to share three fun things about themselves. It lightens the mood and brings that connection.

Jed and I jump in at the same time, having had the same question: "What are your three fun things?"

Jed: Wait, let us guess. You love to laugh.

Marjy: Yess (chuckling).

Julie: You love to dance.

Marjy: (Nods and begins swaying to her own music.)

Jed: And you love your son.

Marjy: Oh, yes. I am Marjy 1.0 and he is Marjy 7.0. He's so much better than me. I say God took the bad out of this one (points) and put the good in that one (points). You know, sometimes I cuss, sometimes I'm mad. But I look at Adom and I say, *God made this*.

JULIE: How did the TikTok dancing videos start?

MARJY: Oh, we did that first one for fun. You know, just for him. But every time I watched it, it made me smile. And I shared it. He was like, *Oh, Mom. I can't believe you did that.* But he likes it, you know. He keeps making them.

The conversation shifts to Adom, and his nonprofit Ball4Good. You read about his foundation in Section Five.

MARJY: You know, I got upset with him. He had decided to do his project on coding for the older generation. He turned in his proposal, and one day he calls me and has changed his project. We're going to play basketball. Oh, I was upset. He had done all this work, and now he's changing things. He was afraid of losing his points because he changed, and I said yes—because you wanted to play ball. But you know, you have to let them do. So I did. His teacher was giving the guidelines. He found his mentor. He arranged the meeting—forgetting he couldn't drive. So, I took him. The first event . . . he had reached out to people in his network (teachers, students, kids . . . community leaders) to build partnerships. His mentor encouraged him to reach out to all of these people—all while being in the seventh grade.

JUILE: Who says no to a seventh-grader?

MARJY: Well, some did, but they had good reasons.

JULIE: He has written books, too. All of this was while doing school, competing in the National Spelling Bee Championship, and playing ball. But you've modeled that for him.

JED: Let's talk about your books, Marjy. Which is your favorite?

MARJY: Well, *Shimmigrant* is about a young girl in Ghana. The story tells of her strong will—she survives against all odds. So many readers assume it's about my life, but none of these stories is my life.

JULIE: Oh, I thought your second book, *Same Elephants,* was you and your friends!

MARJY: Oh, no. But I know people, and I have had experiences that find their way into these stories. For example, my mother is from a polygamous family. So, I had seen this before—communal living, you know. And my books have had such a surprising impact. An immigration lawyer who works with the University of Maryland—she uses my book for advocacy in her classes.

Jed: That's it. Play leading to advocacy.

Marjy: We are humans from all around the world—one kind only. Human kind.

Those words hang in the air for a moment. We give them space.

Later, when we discuss the different roles play has in our lives, we turn to play that recharges us. To fuel herself, Marjy goes to the beach. "I might lay there and fall asleep for hours. I'll get up, and go in the water and jump around. I find the kid in me. If there is a show, I'll just go. I do the stuff that makes me feel better. If I see a guy dancing on the street, I'm like *Hey. Hold my bag*. Suddenly, my husband and son are dancing with us, and nobody's holding my bag" (laughs). We reflect. Why is this quality seemingly unique to a select few? Why aren't we all up jumping and dancing? Marjy says some people are more reserved. Some people are afraid of others' judgment. They feel like they have to behave a certain way.

Every day, Marjy wakes up and prays first thing. "If I don't, I've missed a step. Oh, and then I drink water. My mom told me if I drink water first thing, it makes me go . . . oh, we're recording!" After that, Marjy turns on the music. *Take the shackles off my feet so I can dance*. Mary, Mary. Oh, and Kirk Franklin—*Today's a new day, where are my blue skies. . .* Life is not perfect—there are times that aren't going well. You just smile through it—praising in spite of the sadness. Smiling through it.

Marjy ends her day with Afro beats. Right after *Jeopardy*.

Not five minutes later, Marjy's phone rings. "I have to take this. It was so good to see you both."

We hug our goodbyes, and Marjy dances to her car.

CHAPTER 32

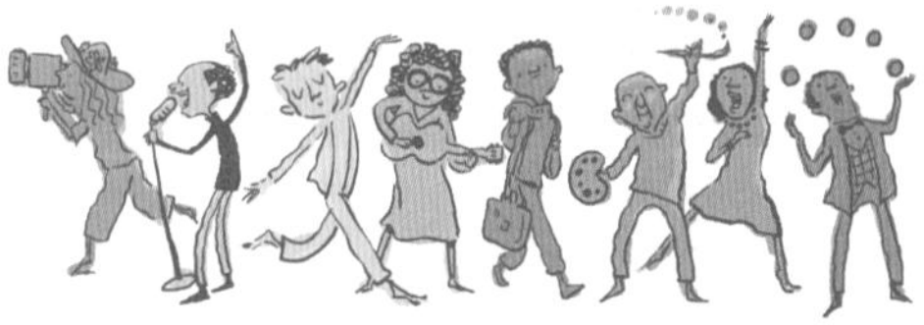

Tina Arenas

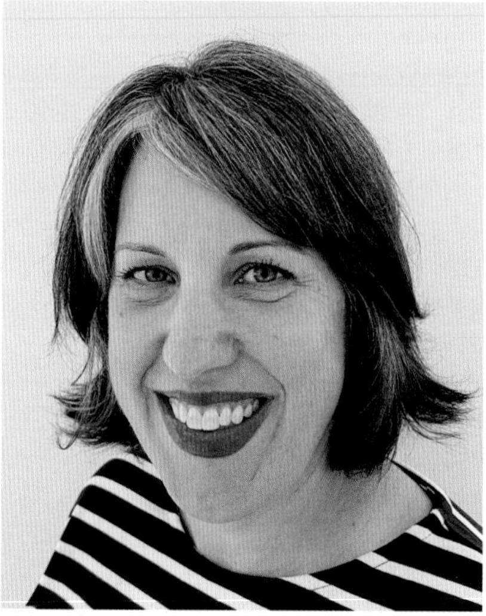

Social Media: @popupforplay

It's 10 a.m. on a Sunday morning in South Carolina, and Jed and I are at a chain-store coffee shop with our coats still on. It's freezing outside! Nine hours ahead of us on the other side of Earth is our new friend, Tina Arenas. When the Zoom screen connects, Tina bends under the table and "pops up" for our play conversation. We're all giggling.

JED: Tina, you know we're working on another book. So, we know you know why we wanted to chat.

TINA: I mean, I'm a little bit in shock . . . I'm like *why me?* If I had to guess, I think you see what is important to me and my community by what I share on social media.

Tina has just returned from her afternoon workout at her home in Dubai, UAE. But she could be Zooming us from across town. She's sporting a red sleeveless shirt, her hair pulled back, and a teal headband accessorizes her look. Originally from Oklahoma, Tina now teaches abroad, coming home to the United States only in the summer. Although her roots are international (her mom emigrated to the United States from Italy), she lived in the United States a long while before heading abroad—she didn't discover her love of travel until studying in Europe during college. She says, "I was obsessed with the music of other cultures, and the world was suddenly so big."

This love of exploration and music helped connect Tina and her husband. "You know, play brought us together. We met in a West African drum and dance class. I didn't need the class—I had already earned my degree—so I was just taking it for fun. We would go on these nerdy coffee dates, talking about education and music. I guess you could say *one beat led to another . . .*"

The conversation turns to how they got from Texas to Dubai. "My husband is Colombian American, so he experienced many cultures growing up. We had both been wanting to teach in another country for a long time. Eventually a friend of mine let me know of two positions opening in their school (Dubai). Our goal was only to do it for about three years, but we've been here for 10 years now. Speaking of playful, you know we moved here when I was 7½ months pregnant."

Jed and I both react with mouths open.

JULIE: Holy wow. You had to find new doctors and everything—so close to your due date!

JED: Talk about a playful mindset. But I can tell just from our conversations how your play history prepared you to handle new experiences that seemed to offer lots of curveballs.

TINA: Yeah, now my husband and I both teach music, and he often performs around the city.

JED: A playful musical family living in Dubai!

Tina continues, "My son is nine now. His playfulness is different from mine. He wants to play-fight. He's adventurous—you know, he does things to get a rise out of you. I'm an artist/creator, explorer, and kinesthete. I need to move around, and I like to discover new things. But sometimes, I need a push to take a risk. When we went to Georgia (the country), my son's play personality helped me to get out of my comfort zone and go zip-lining. He was four, and he remembers this vividly."

Reflecting on our play histories, Tina shares, "I think growing up, I didn't realize until now that this is a part of who I am. My parents weren't building castles with me or any of those stereotypical things we see. I was allowed time and space . . . and breadth. When I think back, play was expansive for me. It was and still is a way I recharge. Play wasn't an escape, really . . . no, it brought me into myself. It gave me a sense of belonging."

Jed: To someone who is needing time and space—what would you tell them?

Tina: I think we gravitate to what we need. Going to the gym on a Sunday afternoon is what I need. Those hard treadmill intervals? I call them my "Top 10" or the "Fab 15"—I make a game of it. You know, maybe the answer isn't carving out time, it's realizing what is integral to your life and making that your play.

Julie: What's it like, living in Dubai? I imagine life on the other side of the planet to be like some magical storybook.

Tina (laughs and adjusts her headband): Dubai has become just like anywhere else. When you first go somewhere new, you notice all the things that are different. But once you've seen all the differences, you're more attuned to all the similarities. Something I really love to do here is go to Expo every weekend.

Jed: You mentioned that before, what is that? Is it like a market?

Tina: No, it's kind of like the World's Fair, but it lasts for about six months. We have a season pass, and the kids get in free. They give you this cool passport (reaches across the table on screen and shows us her son's passport full of stamps), and you get a stamp each time you visit a new place.

Julie: Oh, it's like a game for explorers—you're collecting the stamps!

Tina: Yeah. It's like being in a big city. The people around you are representative of the world. When we go, we are immersed in so many cultures. Every four years there is a theme—this year it's all about sustainability, mobility, and opportunity. You visit these pavilions—these countries—and they showcase how the theme relates to their country. There are workshops on a

> variety of topics. I learned so much about Slovenia—co-creation and environmental issues. How the bees are so important. The connection—the relationship—it brought me to tears the other day. It was so beautiful. The cycle is essential to humanity.

As Tina tells the story of Expo, her music, her family, and their travels, you can see the compassion. Her words are full of reverence for all her experiences. She's weaving them like a symphony into her story of play. We're subscribing.

CHAPTER 33

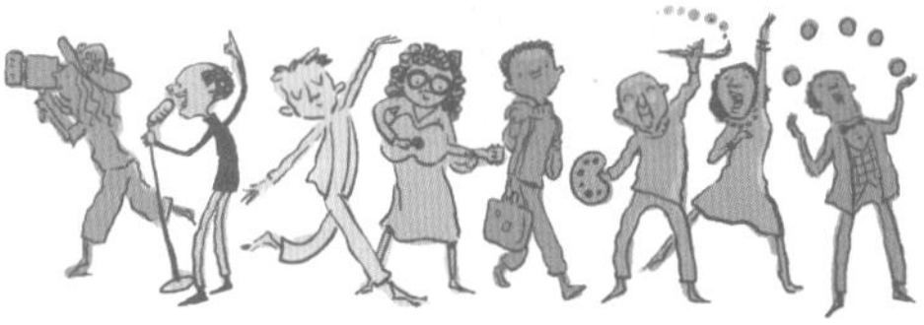

Matt Leung

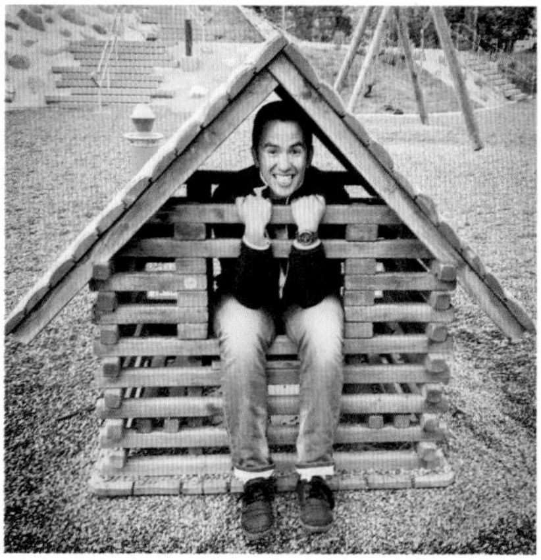

Social Media: @mattrleung

The last time we saw Matt was pre-pandemic at the 2019 Play Conference hosted by the US Play Coalition on the campus of Clemson University. He was on stage in neon attire, leading the entire room through a Jazzercise-like dance experience. Imagine a conference ballroom full of professionals, some in carefully pressed britches—hair just so—who are now *expected* to get all crazy. Matt was making us practice what we preach. Within the space of one minute, Matt had us role-playing superheroes and making connections all across the room. It's because of Matt that Jed and I have both literally danced with *THE Stuart Brown*, while pretending to shoot spider webs from our wrists like Spidey himself.

Matt laughs at our memories of neon and Spider-Man. It's been three years, but it was such a moment.

The conversation continues . . .

Matt: Play is a combination of movement—it's exciting. It's fun! And it connects people in a unique way. I am not the archetype for what a dance instructor is. It allows people to step outside their comfort zone and make connections and memories.

Julie: I will never forget that experience, Matt. Truly.

Jed: (Starts dancing in his Zoom square.)

Matt: I think the presence I'm able to bring catches people off guard just enough that it gets them involved.

Jed: It's almost as if dance is a form of storytelling.

Julie: Matt, what do you think it is that makes this happen?

Matt: Communication happens in so many ways. I think we overindex verbal and written communication. Movement is less formal . . . people don't often think of dance as a way to communicate.

Julie: Oh, dance as a form of nonlinguistic representation. . . . We write about that with sketchnoting and the power of images for learning, but we need to incorporate more dance in our lives.

Since we all were able to dance together, Matt has transitioned away from teaching dance full-time to managing a provincial health and prevention program. Now, he gets to integrate healthy living in his community. He shares, "When I took over, the work culture had room for growth, as do most organizations. I began to think—*how do I use play intentionally while also creating a positive workplace culture?* I was specifically focusing on the importance of positivity. I'm combating burnout through positivity. We're developing empathy through play.

One of Matt's favorite workshops helps participants think imaginatively and build empathy through their experiences. Our ability to understand behavior is our interpretation of what others believe combined with the level of safety we feel when we're with them. Matt explains that this is known as our unconscious bias. He uses optical illusions to help those in his workshops look from various perspectives. If you've not seen the illusion before (for example, the young or the older woman image), are you anchoring with what you see? If you have seen it before, does that experience help you see both sides? We use these experiences to help us consider what we can do with colleagues/kids to help them understand each other. It's all about feeling safe in the vulnerability. And the more we play, the more vulnerable we are willing to become.

What is the biggest aha for Matt's new coworkers? How play is both a behavior and a mindset. We adults are always the most difficult to convince about the benefits of play. Sadly, we still consider play to be the opposite of work. At this moment, all three of us on the call shake our heads. Jed and I do so in a *bless their hearts* kind of way. Not sure what the Canadian equivalent to this connotation is, but it wasn't lost in the non-verbal translation.

Matt continues, "When I started looking at play, it was through the lens of rec programming—you know, after-school programs—I just hate that the conversation of play stops with children. There are worldwide organizations that do incredible work in this area, but we all stop with youth. So, this area has become my niche."

Later, we reflect on the power of face-to-face meaningful conversations. How often do we have meaningful conversations with the people in our lives? Matt says, "Too often, I've found people rarely take the time to have these conversations with those who are close to us. If we're not practicing this with the people who are in our inner circle, it becomes really difficult to have conversations—meaningful ones—with people in other areas of our lives."

JULIE: Matt, how do you like to play? What do you do to recharge?

MATT: I love being outdoors. And, I watch far too much NBA basketball.

JED: Oooh—what team?

MATT: The Raptors. I also really love exploring. One of the classic tenets of play for kids is taking risks. Kids aren't afraid of getting lost—if they want to explore, they just do it. I live just outside downtown Calgary, and I love to put my headphones in, crank up the tunes, and get lost.

JED: Any favorite place you've gotten lost?

MATT: The one place coming to mind right now is St. Patrick's Island. It's a natural place—close to the river, and it has a great playground—developed by Richter Spielgeräte. There's a place where the walkway joins the river . . . it's the perfect place to take a book and sit and read. I'm still able to look at the city skyline, but I'm in the middle of nature.

It's like a secret place. I'm writing this section over a week after we hung up with Matt, and I'm still stuck on his secret reading spot. I need one of these in my life.

CHAPTER 34

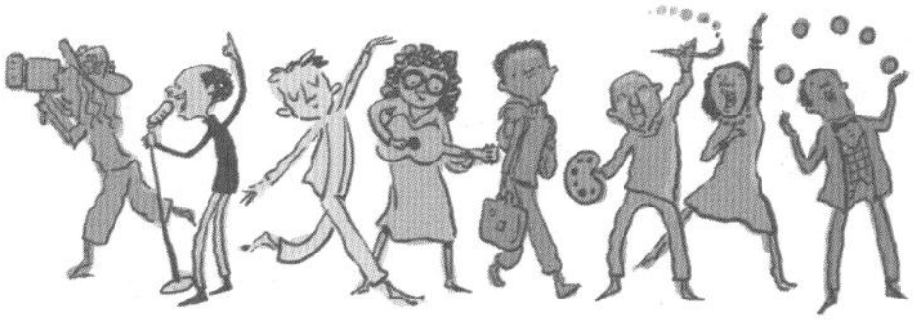

Balance

Something we hope you notice from these conversation stories is that these friends are not ON all the time. They have moments of up and moments of down. They sing in the shower. They talk to their plants. They dance across the street headed to meetings. Yet, these people are all making a difference in their circles. They are ordinary and extraordinary. They are serious and playful. They are balanced. In all aspects, their energy is contagious. Their playful actions mixed with their playful mindset helps them to tackle life—all of life—intentionally. In today's world, cultivating a balanced life like these friends is a skill that takes lots of intentionality and self-awareness.

Balance is evident all around us in nature.

The tides have a high and low.

The moon goes through its phases. Over and over.

Flow. DMN.

Inhale. Exhale.

Day. Night.

Bears eat. Bears sleep.

This balance spills into our daily routines.

Type. Type. Backspace. Backspace.

Make money. Spend money.

Dress up. Undress.

Coffee is hot. Coffee is cold.

Tea is sweet. Tea is . . . (we cannot even fathom the opposite).

A playful life is one that is seeking balance. There is a time for rest. There is a time for play. Sometimes rest is play as it meets both a physical need and an emotional one. Reading a book on the couch in the middle of the day brings rest, and it can also bring us joy. When life is out of balance, it is likely that our playfulness is the area that takes the biggest hit. Ironically, the neurotransmitters that are released from playing often act as personal assistants in helping us find needed balance. It is a vicious cycle, but one we must take notice of in order to level the scales. This is specifically true in American culture. Watching *Emily in Paris* recently, one character describes this mentality by saying, "Americans live to work, in Paris we work to live." No matter where you call home, we challenge you to examine the expectations of the status quo, and ask yourself: Are you living to work, or working to live?

Signs Life Might Be Out of Balance

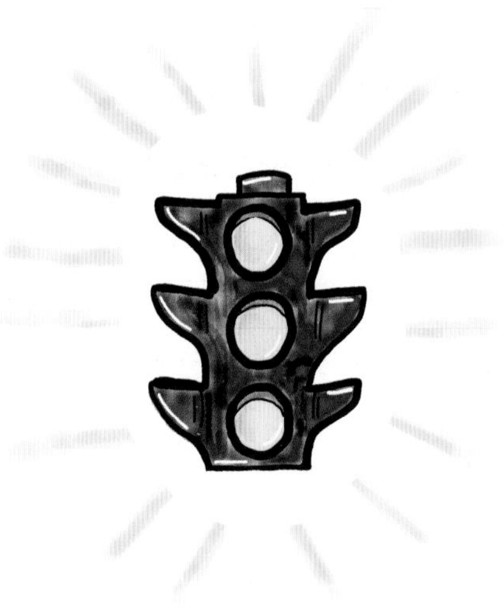

How do we know when our lives are teetering on the edge? Imagine the following as yellow flashing warning lights trying to tell us that change is needed. When I had a wreck once, the officer told me that yellow lights didn't mean slow down like I had always heard. He said they meant to proceed with caution. If the following is true of your life, we urge you to take a moment and examine how the following list resonates with you.

1. You're all kinds of busy, but you're not accomplishing much.
2. Your list of things to do is longer than the preacher's homecoming sermon.

3. You sigh a lot. You might be tired, overwhelmed, or just beat. That's stress, y'all.
4. The milk is clabbered. You don't feel like you're moving forward.

Y'all, full transparency. We've basically described ourselves here. And likely every other person who's not in a monastery on top of a mountain. Not that we aren't practicing what we preach in the book here, but gosh, life is so hard sometimes. Our to-do lists are certainly long, we often feel tired and overwhelmed, and sometimes we move in circles rather than forward. We're not seeking to eliminate these feelings entirely, but we do hope to lessen them. We want to create balance by recognizing our current state and move forward with caution, with intentionality.

Bringing More Balance in Your Playful Life

Daniel Pink tells us in *Drive*, both the title of his book and a synonym for motivation, that forward movement in life comes from autonomy, mastery, and purpose (Pink, 2009). **Autonomy** in feeling in control of our decisions, **mastery** in accomplishing our own goals, and **purpose** as a greater good. These three impact how we move forward. Guess what? All of this is talking about our mojo. This entire section has been dedicated to people who have their mojo, and it spills over onto others around them. We want you to have mojo just like that. As we consider the words of Dan Pink, we'd like to remind ourselves of a few tidbits that have helped us find and sustain our own mojo along the way.

1. **You cannot do it all.**

   This is number 1 on the list for a reason. While this isn't a hierarchical list, this one is indeed most important. Every single one of us has limits. We cannot do all the things all the time. You will hurt yourself physically, emotionally, and spiritually if you try. It is the reason you hear us say, start small, begin with a dot. The work of Peter Reynolds is a great reminder of this. Because he is our friend, we also know a little of his process and how he is able to continue as a creative person (doing the work) while also making a mark on the world. A playful life should be one filled with nooks and crannies of joy, not one that exhausts us.

2. **Trim. Trim. Trim.**

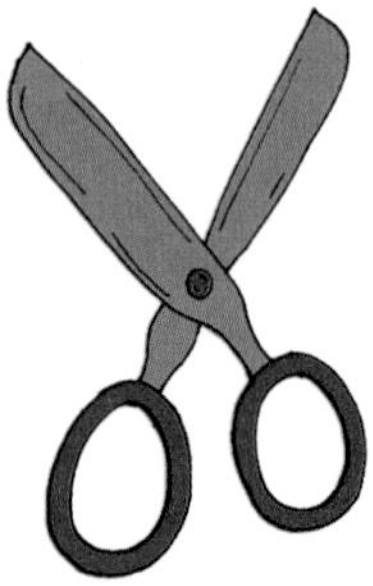

Some of us do too much. And we know it. There are aspects of our lives that need to go. Cut out what isn't helpful as soon as it's possible. Why do we try to do it all? Who are we trying to please? Channel your inner Elsa, and "Let It Go." With grace. With humility. With kindness. But know that choosing your playful path might involve trimming some of the fat. Our friend Jemelleh is great at this. Her story reminds us that we must rid ourselves of what society expects from us and seek out our own personal path to peace.

3. **Boundaries are good for people on both sides of the fence.**

   Dr. Henry Cloud and Dr. John Townsend explain boundaries as our personal property lines—marking those things for which we are responsible (Cloud & Townsend, 1992). These lines help define who we are and who we aren't. We have physical boundaries (who can touch us and how), mental boundaries (for our thoughts and opinions), emotional boundaries (helping us disengage with manipulative people), and spiritual boundaries (giving us awe for the higher power in our life). Tashma Glymph, and our mutual friend Stacy Brown, are both excellent at setting boundaries. Both women have modeled this for me, and I'm so much better because of their role in my inner circle.

4. **Schedule time for yourself.**

   Speaking of boundaries, how much of what we choose to do honors the need for independent, quiet, alone time? If you look at your calendar, at your to-do tasks, each block of the day should not be full. If it is, we risk limiting the opportunity for flow to occur, especially if we are of the creative play personality. I read somewhere that at least 20% of our day should remain unscheduled, and that rule has helped me so much with balance.

5. **Prioritize.**

   If you are a list-maker like we are, we highly recommend putting the most important task of each day at the top of the list. We have found that we are most productive in the morning. Thus, our writing times are always early and involve caffeine. We've learned this over years of collaborative work. Whatever you are working to accomplish, whatever play you are involved in, consider your optimal time for engaging in play. Making it a priority in your life will ensure that you include it.

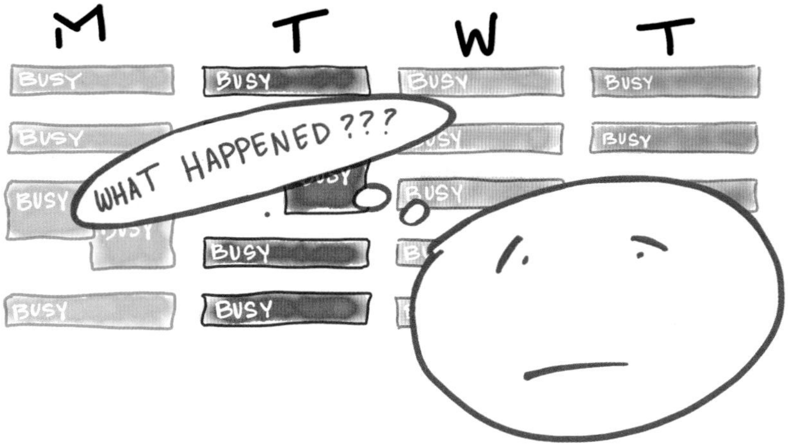

6. **Have reasonable expectations.**
   If your play personality is a competitor, you may want to start with winning *Monopoly* at the next family game night rather than setting the goal of being the quarterback for the next Super Bowl team. If you are a phenomenal football player for a university, then maybe that's a reasonable expectation, but for the vast majority of us, that ship has sailed. Making unattainable goals often leads to overworked bodies and defeated minds. Like Mama says, "Don't write a check you can't cash!"
7. **Relationships matter.**
   Don't ever let this become cliché, even when you have likely heard it numerous times. You hear it a lot because it is true. Developing and strengthening family bonds and friendships is a crucial part of nurturing the playful life. Think back to our friend Ned. With every walk he takes for his podcast, he is cultivating a relationship. Yes, he's making a podcast for his nonprofit employer, but he is also investing his time, resources, and energy in people who matter to him because the relationship matters.

8. **Pay attention to your health.**
   In Section Four, Jed shared how fear had a negative impact on his health. Often, an imbalanced life can lead to the same struggles he faced. If you notice a rapid change in your weight, abnormal mood swings, insomnia, and other signs of stress attacking the body, make adjustments and seek a doctor's guidance.
9. **Turn it off.**
   Work must have an ending time. The phone must rest too. That's so hard. How many times have you found yourself scrolling mindlessly without realizing how many minutes have elapsed? In the settings app of your device, there is likely a screen time monitor. I personally set 45 minutes a day for social media—Facebook, Instagram, Twitter, Snapchat—all of them. While that seemed like a lot of time to give myself (that's over five hours each week!), I find myself getting the alert daily. The reminder to close the apps is self-imposed and so helpful for me to keep my priorities in check. Instead of scrolling, I try to fill that time with what matters to me. Conversations, reading, painting, writing—none of which would have existed without putting the device down.

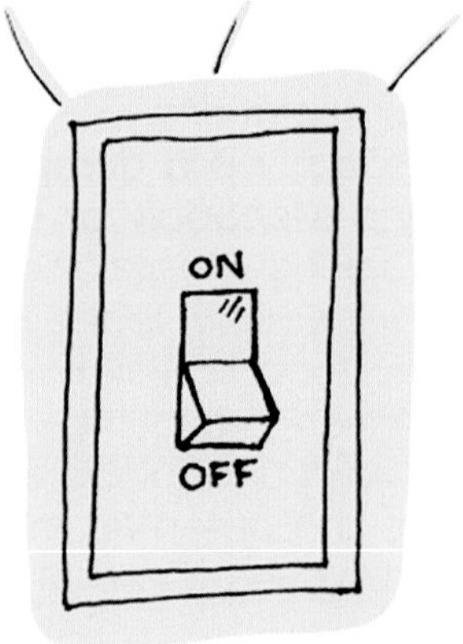

10. **Treat yourself.**
   Take the nap. Eat an extra helping. Get that ice cream cone from McDonald's (if you can find one with a working machine). Life is too short, y'all. We blink and it is over. Treating ourselves is okay. You hear us? It. is. *Okay*! You are the only one who can do the work you do, and you cannot take care of anything else without first taking care of you. There is a reason the flight attendant tells you to put on your oxygen

mask before helping the person beside you. You need air to do that. Without your air, you will die. We recently read the autobiography of superstar Will Smith. He made it very clear that in order to care for his family and to prioritize the well-being of his wife and children, he took care of himself first. Treating yourself is a must to caring for others.

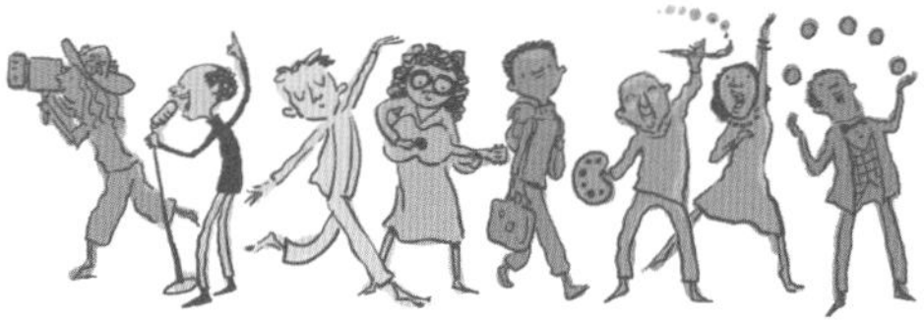

Play & Ponder

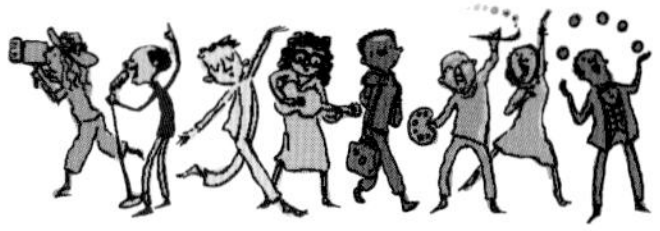

- We provided you with the social media accounts of lots of amazing people in this section. Why not send one, or all of them, a message to thank them for sharing their stories with us? Maybe something they said resonated with you. Playful living thrives through connections. All of these humans are ones you want to connect with. Don't be shy. They will love hearing from you.
- Every time we typed the word balance we immediately envisioned a seesaw. Is there one in a park nearby? If not, you could make one with a sturdy 2×6 and a concrete cinder block. Ask a friend to join you on the teeter-totter, whether at the playground or on the homemade one in your backyard. Talk about things that are causing imbalance in your lives as you seek to physically balance on the childhood favorite. We shall not be responsible if your board breaks. That's on you.
- Sing in the shower. Talk to your plants. Ride your bike to work. Take a walk with a friend. Dance across the street. Visit a new place. Create something new.

SECTION 7

Map

Hopefully, by now your tractor is cranked, and you are as excited as a fly in a cow pasture about inviting more play into your life. We have done our best to show its power, its benefits, the need for it in your life. Like any good journey, you need a map—or, in present-day terms, a GPS—to help you arrive at your destination. Think of this final section as your step-by-step guide to the playful life you desire. As you read, don't feel pressured to make changes too much too fast. As we mentioned earlier, mistakes will be made, but there's no sense in driving like Richard, and going too fast. Pace yourself. Enjoy the ride and see where it takes you. Let's get your popcorn a-poppin'.

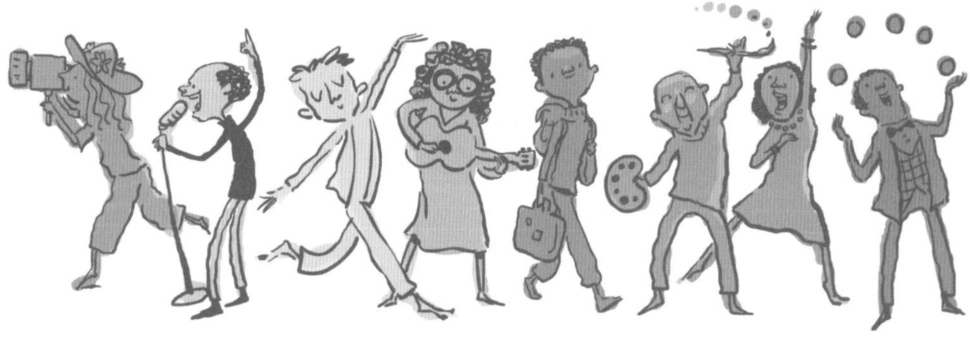

CHAPTER 35

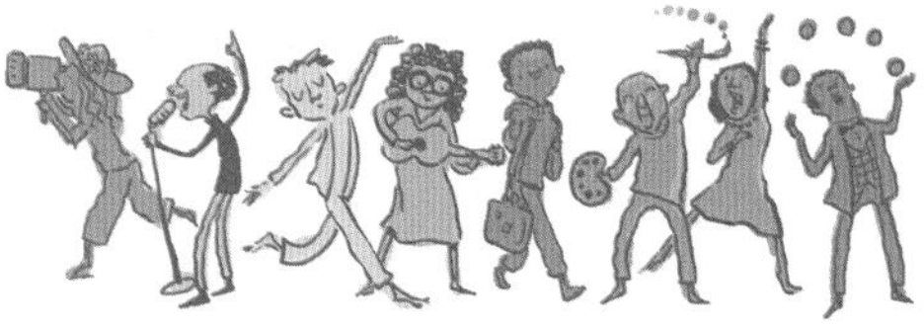

Play Alone

1. Map-a-Doodle Your Schedule or To-Do List

"Map-a-doodle" is something I do as a teacher to keep me on task during class. Basically, I doodle little pictures that help me remember what topics I want to cover while I am presenting the lesson. As I mention them during class or a workshop, I color each one to signify that I have talked about it. I often do this when presenting at a conference, and encourage the participants of the presentation to join me because it makes a fun little piece of art for me and them at the end of our time together. Sometimes, I do this for my grocery list. If I need a gallon of milk, a loaf of bread, and some oranges, then I doodle pics of them on a piece of paper or in my journal. No, I don't stop to color them in the middle of the aisle as I place them in my buggy, but the visual of the items on the list helps me remember them all while I am at the store. You can also do this with your errand list, things to do, vacation prep, etc. Just a free nugget of information here. . . . This is called nonlinguistic representation, which is the use of pictures, charts, graphs, etc. to communicate information instead of words. Also, don't fret if you are not an artist; doodles don't have to be perfect. Grab your favorite writin' stick (pen) and get started with your first map-a-doodle.

2. Take a Walk "Art"side

Years ago as I took a walk down a greenway trail, I took special notice of the cracks in the asphalt, the pattern of leaves along the edges of the path, the movement of the squirrels, and the rhythms of the birds. It hit me as I moseyed along that I was literally taking in all of the art nature had to offer. I was taking a walk "art"side. Get it? I was outside, but experiencing art as I walked. It may sound a bit cheesy to you at first, but when you get outside and take these new artful lenses with you, it will be surprising what-all is out there to see. You don't have to be an art museum curator to do this. The place to start is by noticing the trees around you. Their bark has beautiful patterns that will make pictures seem to appear before your eyes. If you happen to see a face in the knots and bumps, this is called pareidolia. Pareidolia is a trippy little trick our mind plays on us as it convinces us that we see faces in places they shouldn't be. Taking a walk "art"side will reveal lots of these fun little friends. There is a scrunched-up little face that I discovered in my neighborhood during a walk that I have named Mr. Grumps. He looks a bit annoyed. I imagine he is tired of being run over every day. I bet he has some cousins in your neighborhood. Let us know if you find them!

3. Read a Book

This may seem like a no-brainer for a way to play alone, but since we both are avid readers we had to include this here. Nothing is more fun for us than curling up on the couch with three of our favorites: a cozy blanket, a warm beverage, and a great book. Even as the words were typed just now, we both wanted to flee the coffee shop and read. Julie is currently reading about music and how it affects memory. She is clearly the academic in our duo. I am reading *A Star Is Bored,* by Byron Lane. It is a fictitious novel about the life of a celebrity assistant and it is *fabulous*! Alas, writing was the priority for the moment. But, you know what makes us better at writing? Reading! It takes us places we have never been to meet people we've never met and to experience things we've yet to enjoy. We get it, though, not everyone is a reader. I (Jed) wasn't until I was well into adulthood, thanks to the expertise of a very skilled librarian who helped me to find the just right book. If you aren't so excited about this type of play, you could skip it. Or, you could make a list of the top five things you like in life other than family, then take it to your local library and ask for books on the topics. For me, it all started with running and zombies! Once I found the dystopian genre, I was hooked! Thanks, Elizabeth Graham.

4. Organize the Junk Drawer

We were a bit hesitant to add this to the list of playful experiences because we are certain some of you will see this as a chore instead of a moment of joy that feels like play, but as we considered all the different play types, we felt it belonged here. We are confident you have a junk drawer. Inside it, you have batteries, safety pins, paper clips, buttons, scissors, an old phone charger, super glue, and probably a s*** ton of pens. The drawer is likely a hot mess and nothing in there is really functional because the mess is so deep that you cannot find anything without digging around. Maybe the digging is fun for you, but the sorting, the purging, and the organizing can bring lots of joy. We are both just Type A enough that a purdy junk drawer gets us excited. To make this more fun, put a tad of planning into it. Make a run to your favorite store in search of some just-right organizational baskets or containers, and while you are there grab a six-pack of your favorite beverage. When you get home, open said beverage first thing, then dump the whole drawer out on your counter. Of course, that will be a bit stressful so take another sip of said beverage and dive into the mess. We have no doubt that you will discover treasure as you do. The little note that a loved one gave you, a sticker from your favorite restaurant, a receipt from that movie you loved. Within moments you will be smiling as you think about all the memories that the junk drawer really contains. Have fun!

5. Tell Your Plants a Story about Your Life

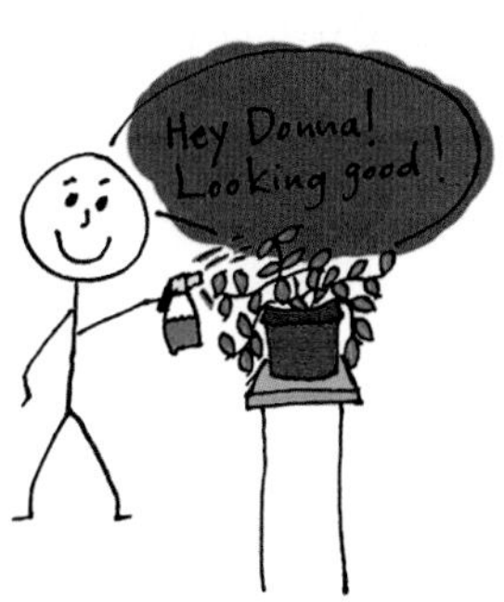

We assume since you are now reading this section that you read about our friend Tashma in the Mojo section. In case you don't remember, she loves to talk to her plants. She has many of them, and they are named for special people, places, and events in her life. Ironically, at the time we interviewed her, this list of playful experiences was already made. You can imagine our joy when she validated talking to plants as a way she was playful in her home. Talking to your plants, while not statistically proven in the scientific community as of yet, seems to have many benefits for our green children. The theory that talking to plants improves their well-being has been around since the 1840s, thanks to German professor Gustav Fechner, who believed plants might have the ability to feel human emotions (Fechner, n.d.). Regardless of the evidence to support either of these claims, many of us feel happy when we personify our African violet or fiddle-leaf fig. There's lots of science to support the power of having a pet; why couldn't that pet be a plant? If you haven't already, name that pothos plant (mine is named Donna, and she is fabulous). I named her Donna after Tabitha Brown's hair. You remember Tab, right? We mentioned her early on in the book. She too is fabulous as is her hair, thus the name for my pothos! After you name your plant baby, tell her/him/they all about your day. You may just find this moment of play is fun and a bit therapeutic.

6. Put Googly Eyes on Your Lampshade

Back in the initial phase of the Covid pandemic as the world began to shut down, many of us had lots of extra time at home and sometimes that led to a bit of boredom. Once our intrigue with the Tiger King subsided and we were left to figure out how to fill the down moments of our time, I turned to googly eyes for entertainment. Yes, the little plastic eyes that wiggle and shake when you move them. I am not sure why these little adhesive opticals excited me so; maybe it was my desire to see other people. Regardless of the reason, I began to stick the eyes on various objects around my house: pictures on the wall, the front part of the toilet tank, my laptop case, basically any surface that I felt needed to come to life. My favorite spot was a lampshade that sat just behind me when I was a participant in one of the gozillion Zoom calls that will forever be a part of the quarantine experience of the pandemic. I named him Mr. Tom—I have *no idea* why that name. Maybe because the lampshade reminded me of a top hat and the name Tom seemed like someone who would wear a top hat. Like I said, no idea. All I know is that once I named him he felt like comic relief in the madness that was the world. I would turn him on and off with a remote while on a video chat, and it was as if he came to life as he peered over my shoulder looking into the computer camera. More than once it brought a wave of laughter from those on the other end of the call. Tom is still with us to this day. I vowed to leave the eyes on the shade as long as the sticky held. If all goes well, he will be over two years old by the publishing of this book. Get some googly eyes, y'all. You won't regret it!

7. Paint a Rock

Humans have been creating artwork on rocks throughout our history on the planet. There is evidence of human cave drawings as far back as 36,000 years ago (Encyclopedia Britannica, n.d). Obviously this isn't a new idea, but the modern-day spin on it is quite fun and fairly inexpensive. You have likely seen painted rocks popping up in various places in your community for the past few years. This is largely due to a random happening that involved a sharpie, a kind heart, and a chance finding of an inspired rock created by Megan Murphy as she walked along the beach. Now known worldwide as the Kindness Rocks Project (2022), it all began when Murphy wrote encouraging messages on five rocks and left them along the way as she walked the beach reflecting on the passing of her parents. In a twist that only the universe could create, a personal friend of Murphy found the rock and felt inspired by the lovely message from a stranger. Ironically, it turned out to be her friend Megan who created the rock. The rest is now history and people around the world are painting kindness rocks and leaving them for others to find. You can order the nice smooth rocks online or you could just tinker around your yard and find some. The acrylic paint you need doesn't have to be the top quality. Most craft stores have a very affordable version. The best part of the whole experience is that playfulness and sharing kindness collide! You get the brain benefits that come from the playful painting and a stranger gets the kindness because of your work. It's a win-win!

8. Watch Videos Online That Make You Laugh

The options here are plentiful . . . YouTube, TikTok, Instagram, or any streaming service to which you subscribe. Our society has video content galore and some of it is super funny! There is nothing like a good belly laugh, and of course we always encourage you to do it with friends. But sometimes, the friends are busy and the schedules don't align. Online videos are a great way to get that deep guffaw out of your body and into the world. Seriously, sometimes at night I will be watching TikToks and laugh so hard I cry! I hate to admit it, but if there's a video of someone falling, as long as they don't get injured too badly, I go into hysterics as I watch gravity in action! One of my all-time favorites is watching people try a rope swing for the first time. I relate to these videos because it has happened to me multiple times. I imagine that I swing out over the pond, lake, or river and fall to the water as if an acrobat. The reality, however, is that I am much heavier than I realize and my strength fails me as I get dragged by the rope and tumble into the bank of said water. Watching others experience this gives me quite a chuckle. Whether it's a video of a failed baking experiment or a gender reveal gone wrong, the comic relief that these technological creations bring to us are incredibly beneficial. According to the Mayo Clinic (2022), the short-term benefits of laughter include enhanced oxygen intake, which helps your heart, lungs, and muscles, and, as we have already stated, the release of neurotransmitters from the brain increases, thus improving your overall mood!

9. Find a Class (So Many Are Free) and Join In!

Learning should always be an active part of our lives. It keeps us spry and increases the health of our brain. If teaching is done correctly, the learning should always be playful in some way. No, not every topic can be super fun, but if it is something you enjoy, then it most definitely is a form of play. Recently, I took a free class, titled *Metal Shaping 101*, from a local artisan co-op. I long to be some sort of visual artist beyond a writer, so I try to take advantage of free classes whenever I can. This particular one got my curiosity aroused because I had zero experience with metal. The class was a relatively small group of people, and not only did I learn a good bit about the metal-shaping process, but I also made a new friend named Robin. Who knows if I will ever see her again, but by participating in the class, she and I played together for a whole hour. We realize this is a section about playing alone, which I was fully prepared to do by taking the class. Meeting a friend was just a plus. If you are feeling a bit more introverted and want to learn alone, there are numerous online offerings, and many of those are free as well. If the idea of taking a class seems a bit more than you want, consider searching for a topic you'd like to learn about online. There are countless "how-to" videos that are waiting to be consumed.

10. Drive Down a Road You've Never Been

Remember back to our talk with Ned and he told us how he ran down every street within the city limits. That idea sounded so fun to us, but maybe running isn't your thing. Why not drive them all instead? Almost every single day I pass a road that I have never been down and I have lived in the same town my entire life. How is it possible that I would be so close to places, yet have never set foot or tire upon them? What surprises could you find if you just turned right instead of left one day? Could there be a restaurant you've never heard of? Is there a scrapyard full of metal that you could hammer into some artwork? There might even be a little house full of antiques for sale. You don't know what's down there if you never turn. Of course there could be a crazy dog that runs after your car, but chances are you will laugh and have a great story to tell your friends. I have found many times that taking the new road often leads to the discovery of something beautiful. Even if you pass a junkyard, there is beauty to be found. Those places are full of memories of times gone by if you open yourself up to the history that lies within. If you find yourself with just five minutes extra in the day and want to use it for something playful, take a detour and see what you find.

11. Beat Your High Score on Your Favorite Video Game

You read about our love for *Super Mario Brothers* earlier as we talked about leveling up, but that's not the only video game that has hooked us before. *Words with Friends* was quite an addiction for us a few years ago, and while we have somehow managed to stay clear of the *Wordle* craze, at least one of us (me, Jed) has recently become obsessed with *Fishdom*. Have you ever heard of it? It is a classic jewel-connecting game that when you link three of a kind they explode and more jewels fall down until the board is cleared of obstacles. It is similar to *Candy Crush*, but in this particular game each level you pass rewards you with coins to create your fish kingdom, *Fishdom!* Currently I have four aquariums full of fish. Maria, Don, Juanito, and Maggie are some of my favorites. Yes, they are named, just like my plants, but in this instance the computer coding of the game names them for me. I don't have the heart to change them because once I see their generated name, it sticks. You can also earn different decorations for your aquariums and the app allows you to connect with others to form a team. This is beneficial for many reasons, one being that they can share extra lives with you so you can conquer the super-hard level. There is a total rush of adrenaline when all the jewels finally align, the board is cleared of hurdles, virtual rewards are given, and a new level appears on the screen. I am certain that many of you will frown upon the use of screens for playtime, but there is joy to be found there, and I love my fish!

12. Complete a Whole Crossword Puzzle

There was a time in my life where I was more involved with crossword puzzles than with people. I had those little books everywhere. In the car, by the bed, on the coffee table, and of course on the toilet. This was clearly before the evolution of what is now the smartphone that keeps many of us occupied in all of the aforementioned locales. Anytime I sat still for very long, I wanted to be solving the next clue. This love affair started because of my grandma and her subscription to *TV Guide*. I spent many a weekend night watching her do them. I was probably the youngest person ever to know about jai alai, a sport involving bouncing a ball off a walled space using a wicker cesta (for whatever reason, that was a common answer in her puzzles). Seeing her complete the crosswords was so amazing to me. Her brain seemed so full of knowledge, and I wanted that for myself. Admittedly, I sometimes didn't know the correct response and would cheat by looking at the answers in the back of the magazine. But once I learned the answer I would always remember it for the next time it showed up. Still to this day I know a six-letter word that means withdraw is "secede," thanks to my days of self-competition with a devil of a crossword in the *New York Times*. I don't think of myself as a competitor when it comes to my play personality, but there was something mighty victorious about filling in those tiny squares. Dorothy in *The Golden Girls* once bragged that she was so smart she did her crosswords in ink. Far too often I used a pencil so I could erase my wrong answers, but one day, I aspire to be like Dorothy.

13. List All the Rhyming Words That Make You Giggle

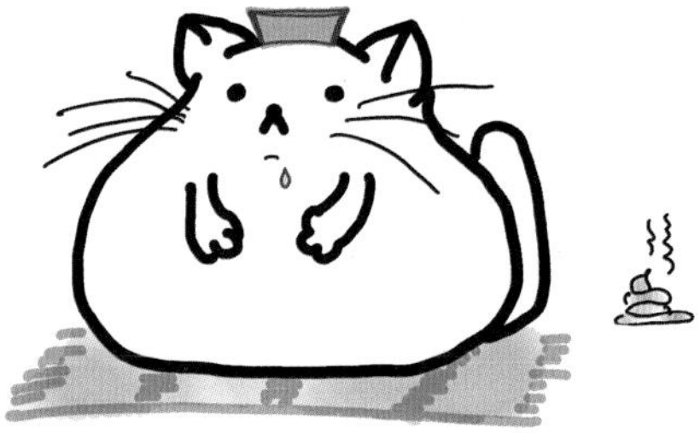

A fat cat was wearing a hat while he shat and spat, can you imagine that? We sure hope you laughed as you read about our feline friend. Lord knows we did. What about that doodle? It's quite the image, huh? The humor found in the sentence is definitely connected to the imagery we created in your brain, but the rhyming words aided in the comedy. The singsong pattern that rhyming words provide to our ears makes us happy. It's the reason so many songs are filled with rhymes. Read a children's picture book lately? A large number of them utilize rhyming words because it helps develop reading skills for beginning readers. If you are ever trapped in a meeting that could have been an email, take a moment to just jot down a list of rhyming words while the meeting leader who should've emailed drones on about whatever topic. Shoe, flew, through, moo, Whew! Try your best not to laugh out loud as you create the list; that might end poorly. We can almost certainly guarantee that your list of words will make you giggle and will likely release just enough good mood neurotransmitters to get you through the meeting. Remember, playful moments do not have to always be these grandiose experiences involving art, sports, board games, etc. They can be found in the nooks and crannies of life's most boring of experiences. If you do happen to make a list, please share it with us so that we can laugh with you. Bonus points if the words are actual words spoken in the meeting!

14. Make a List of All of Your Favorite Things

1. Crayons
2. Colored paper
3. Books and more books
4. Coffee shops
5. Fires in fireplaces
6. Paint
7. Play-Doh
8. Time with friends
9. Holidays
10. Snow days in the South

It is amazing how much fun it was to make a list of 10 things that bring joy into my life. Honestly, I could've kept adding more and more. Cracks in sidewalks, running, the beach, traveling to new places. All of the things on my list are connected to playful experiences, read memories. Think back to the first sections of this book. We wrote a lot about reflecting on your play history and your play personality. Creating this list can help you do that and double as a playful moment as you recollect why you enjoy all of the fun things you wrote. If you are up for it, mix this list making with the map-a-doodle at the beginning of the chapter. While you are doodling and writing, add the names of people who you've played with beside each item. I always think of my great grandma Maudie when I write the word Play-Doh. She introduced me to the modeling wonder many years ago as I sat in the floor on a plastic tablecloth creating masterpieces. The cloth was a must so the Play-Doh didn't get in her multicolored shag carpet. I must have had over 50 cans of it at her house. Every time we walked to the drugstore she bought me a new pack. This was before they had so many colors, so I had lots of the basics: white, red, yellow, blue. Gosh, I miss her. I am so glad I had all those years of playing and making memories. Thanks to this book and creating the list, I am smiling big right now. I hope your list will lead you to big smiles, too.

15. Turn Up the Tunes While You Wash Your Car, Your Dog, or the Front Stoop

Picture it: Your hometown, present day; winter has recently ended. The temperature is about 80 degrees, spring has sprung, and you are itching to get outside and soak up some of the warmth. You know there are chores out there that need to be done, but the beauty of the day is calling you just to lay out and drink in the sun. Then you have an idea: "Cutting grass is so fun, let's get out there and do it and get a tan at the same time!" Okay, okay, maybe it doesn't happen just like that. Lord knows I hate to cut grass. But any time I have to get outside tasks completed, I do my best to make them as playful as possible. Music is the way for me. Whatever the chore, I turn it up loud and sing and dance my way through the work. I have a playlist on my phone simply titled, "Fun." Any time I hear a song that makes me dance and smile, I add it to the list. Some recent additions are *Dance With Me Tonight* by Olly Murs and *Classic* by MKTO. I confess that both of these found their way into my music library thanks to lots of people dancing to them on the apps. Sometimes when these songs come on while I am cutting the grass, washing the dog, or cleaning the car, I try to remember all the steps. I am a better writer than a dancer, though. Maybe one day!

CHAPTER 36

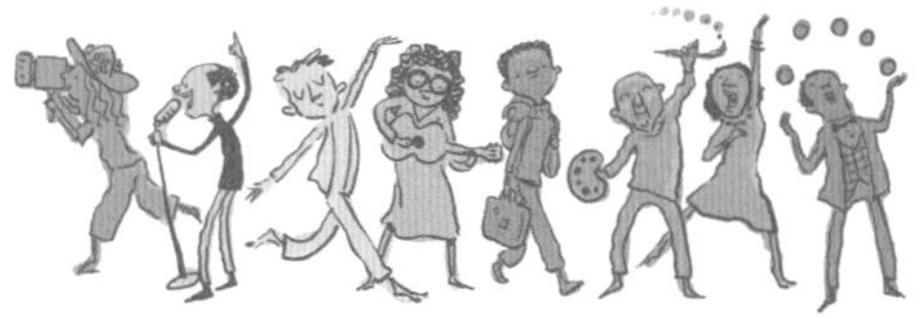

Play with Friends or Family

1. *Cow Poker* or *My Next House*

Y'all ready to learn a bit of Southern culture with these games? Okay, maybe they're not all Southern games, but we've not heard of them anywhere else. All three involve a road trip, short or long, and paying attention to what is around you as you move. Here's the skinny!

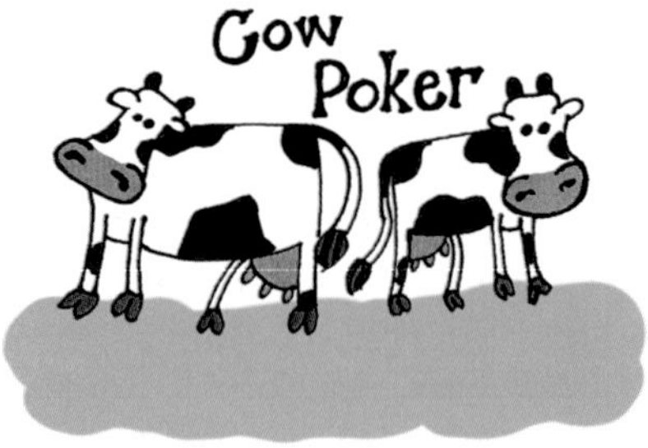

Cow Poker is played like this. First, divide the car into teams, passenger side versus driver side. Next, keep your eyes peeled for cows as you ride. See one on your side of the car? It's a point! See 20 on your side? It's 20 points! One point for every cow. But be careful as you make your way to your destination. If you pass a cemetery on your side of the car, you lose all your points. If you want to, you can add other animals and assign varying point values. Because we live in an area where livestock is common, we often count goats as five points, horses as 20, and if you see a deer, it's worth 50! None of them are immune to loss, though.

My Next House is a game Julie introduced me to on a trip we took to New England doing some research for this book. It's simple to play. See a house that you love while you're riding about? Claim it as your next house! Tell the car full of folks why you love it and who could live with you there. Be sure to note what time it is because you can't choose your next house for three minutes. This game works best if you are not in a "traffic-y" place. You might not move enough to pick every three minutes. Be wise with your choosing. You never know when the next fun place to live is right around the corner. What's fun about this game is that you can totally play it by yourself too. It's always fun to dream.

2. Game Night

This is certainly not a new idea, but one that has to be mentioned at the top of our lists guiding you to a more playful life. Game night is one of our absolute favorite ways to play. You and one friend can have a standing appointment to play *Rummy* and debrief about the week you've had while sipping your favorite beverage. My bestie and I once played all the way to 10,000 points thanks to a weekly appointment to play! Maybe that's not your type of game. Then, get your family or friends together for a rousing game of *Taco, Cat, Goat, Cheese, Pizza*! Don't know that game? Look it up right now. Trust us, it will invite so much laughter into your space, leaving your abs well worked out from all of the giggles and guffaws. Be careful not to flinch, though. You will lose miserably if you do. Besides just being a fun way to spend the evening, all that laughter is releasing the feel-good juice inside your brain and filling your body with a boost that you need to press through the next days and weeks ahead. Recently, a group of my friends has started gathering mid-week for a few hours of game time and it has done wonders for us all. We start around 6 p.m. and usually wrap it up by 8 since we all have to be up the next day for work. We usually choose games that are quick so we can play multiple times. We love *Telestrations* and *Codenames*. This isn't the night for *Monopoly*, but we do occasionally splurge on a round of *Settlers of Catan*. Got any wood? This weekly night of fun is such a valuable meetup that literally carries us through the rest of the week 'til the weekend arrives. While a Wednesday evening game night might not work for everyone, gather your friends/family together when you can and dig into your favorite game. Memories will certainly be made as you play together.

3. Progressive Dinner

When I was little, I read books in which the characters had elaborate dinner parties. They dressed up, they enjoyed each other. They enjoyed the cuisine. I still love to read food memoirs—Ruth Reichl writes the best ones. But you don't have to own a fancy dress or have fancy friends to enjoy an experience with food. Progressive dinners connect eating and experiences that move. Show up at location one for appetizers; location two for another small treat or meal; location three for dessert; location four for after-dinner drinks, leaded or unleaded. The locations can be restaurants or homes of those participating. A progressive dinner can also be a traveling picnic where each person is responsible for a portion of the experience in different parks or nature sites. The fun is in the planning and the connection that transpires.

4. Art Challenges

If you can't tell by now, Julie and I are big fans of the arts. Visual art, music, drama . . . all of it! At our hearts, creating and making is one of our favorite ways to play. Julie loves to paint, and I love to make stuff out of recycled materials. This is made even more fun for us when we create and make with others in a collaborative space. Those wine-and-paint classes were made for us. Sometimes when we are working together, Julie will scribble something in my journal and say "art challenge" as she asks me to add to the newly drawn image. I will usually give it some really cool eyes then pass it back to her to add the next doodle. Within a few minutes of passing back and forth we have created a new piece of art that has never before existed in all of humanity. Art challenges aren't always done with pen and paper, though. Sometimes we use Play-Doh, tinfoil, or colored masking tape. All of these are fun ways to create, and they challenge our minds at the same time. Another benefit of using unique tools like foil and tape is that we don't feel the need to be perfect when creating with those. Neither of us is the Picasso of those art media, and we can just relax and have fun. Don't believe us? Next time your friends and family are together, give everyone a foot-long piece of foil and ask them to sculpt a tree. You will all love it!

5. Play Calendar

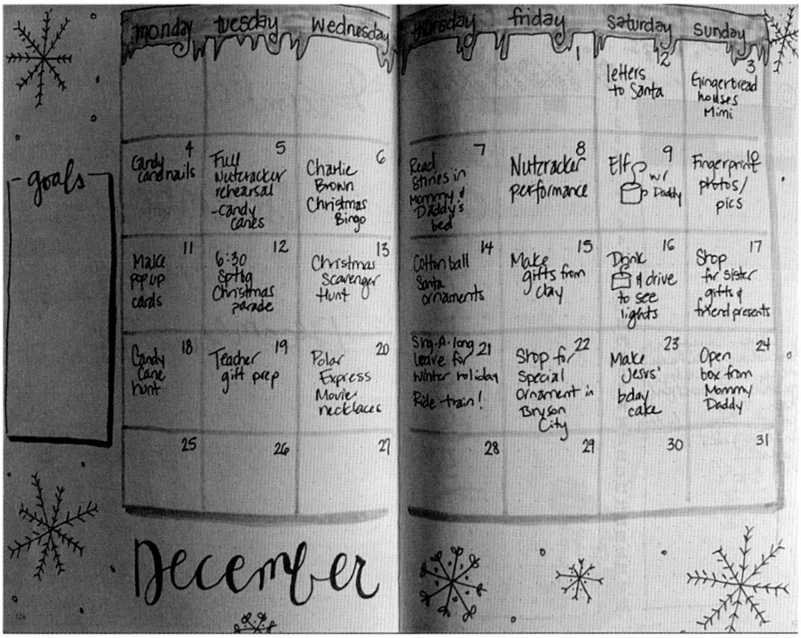

Every summer and on December 1, I (Julie) create a calendar of playful experiences for my family. In December, these events are totally a surprise; however, having done this for over a decade, there are many events that repeat, and we so look forward to them. Because these are a surprise, I write events on slips of paper and put them in our wooden advent tree. It has doors, so opening the door each morning to find out what we're doing that day is always a treat! Some days we make paper snowflakes, and other days we visit local businesses. I vary the days intentionally around our schedules and what's happening in the community. Our repeat events include: make snowflakes, read stories in bed, build gingerbread houses with Mimi, go ice skating, watch *Elf* wearing elf hats we made, and leave for our winter holiday. In summer, we have a less structured calendar—it's more of a list of all the events we collectively want to do. We grab a big piece of paper and make a checklist. That list goes on the fridge, and we check them off as we experience them. Some that always make it on our page include: catch fireflies, eat ice cream with friends, watch a movie in the park (our town hosts these), build sandcastles, tube on the river, lay outside and count the stars, paint rocks, and take a girls trip.

6. Butcher Paper Dinner Chat

Have you ever been to one of those restaurants that rolls out paper on the table and invites everyone to use crayons to create a unique tablecloth for the duration of the meal? We love those places, but we are sad that there are so few of them in our weekly/monthly schedule. So why not do this at home for your family meals? It's quick and easy to set up, and it would invite the dinner guests, kids, visitors, or otherwise to gather around the table rather than be in the adjacent room on their phones. It happens. We know because it happens in our houses too. To make the experience even more fun, you could have drawing prompt cards at everyone's seat like a place card. If that's a bit too structured for you, ask your meal companions to doodle things about their day and then share with the table what they drew. We can hear you now: "I don't have any of that paper they use at restaurants." No worries, we bet you have an old roll of wrapping paper nearby. The backside of it makes a great drawing surface. No wrapping paper? Give everyone a piece of a cardboard box. It could be a cereal box kind of cardboard or a piece of the box your recent online purchase arrived in. Regardless of the materials, gathering at the table to doodle and chat is a great way to spend an evening with family and friends.

7. Make Up Adventurous Stories about Everyday Events

Last night, after a school event, my youngest asked to go to Salsarita's. This Tex-Mex restaurant is her favorite. While in line, picking out what would go in our bowls, one of the workers brought over the cast iron pan and filled the serving bowl with shrimp. One of the shrimp got loose and fell into the bowl of ground beef. I started giggling, and my girls (who are used to my ridiculousness) gave me the side eye. This is the middle school version of *please-Mommy-don't-make-a-scene*. It didn't work. I said, "Did you see that? He escaped. 'I'm free, I'm free!'" When we sat down with our trays, we kept it going. Why did the shrimp jump out? What happened? Elaborate stories followed. Silliness. All-the-fun.

Yesterday, I was teaching my math teacher education course about how our number system is based on powers of 10. Thus, place value . . . base 10 blocks . . . 10 frames (you kindergarten teachers out there feel it, I know). At some point, I said the words "ten again." I stopped. Write that down. That's good. For the rest of the class, we kept a list of rhyming words. Silliness that is leading to a children's book creation. Just because we were paying attention.

8. Wish List/Challenge Board

Remember the calendar idea in number 5? Why constrain ourselves to a month? Why not make a list of all the things we want to accomplish or do in the coming season or year? This could be a personal list or a group list. Jed and I have such a list in our journals each year. This year we got a little playful with it and created a sketchnote vision board style entry. Some of the tasks on those pages have already been accomplished, and we know it's because in creating the list, we focused our vision. We knew in our hearts what we wanted. Writing it down, doodling it, helped us make it happen. On this, we also wrote the names of people we love and respect who might help us on this journey. They help via conversations and mentoring, but also with the content they put in the world. Tabitha Brown is on this list. I've never met her, but Jed has. She still fuels me with her positivity and authenticity.

9. Book Club and More

I (Julie) am in a book club. I didn't start it, but I look forward to our get-togethers each month. The person hosting picks the book, we all read it, and we bring book-themed food to the gathering. In our "meeting" we chat about the book, the characters, what we loved, and what we hated. I love that each month, my friend Kristina and I will disagree. We have opposite tastes in books. She loves true crime, and I love historical fiction. The fun surprise is when we agree. *How did that happen?!* For *Artemis* by Andy Weir, we brought food that could be eaten in space (lots of things on sticks), and for *The Haunting of Hill House* by Shirley Jackson, we brought spooky food—soup in a pumpkin shell, salad served with skeleton hands. Since the pandemic hit, we've continued to meet on Zoom. It's not the same, but we're powering through. Sometimes life gets to be too much, and we don't get around to a formal book club design. Enter literary circles. I heard about this on a podcast I love called *What Should I Read Next?* with Anne Bogel. Instead of everyone reading the same book, these informal gatherings ask friends to come and share what they've been reading or watching. From these conversations, attendees leave with a list of next-book or next-show ideas. There's no pressure to have done your homework, but all book lovers and/or binge-watchers get their fix.

10. Design a Scavenger Hunt

I (Julie) started these with my girls when they were small. We lived in a rural area with lots of yard space. The girls loved to run and play, were not afraid to pick up frogs, and had tea parties out of real dishes they purchased at the Goodwill specifically for that purpose. One day, I got a wild hair and made a list of things to gather in their plastic toy shopping carts. At the time, they pushed these kid-version buggies everywhere. The list read something like this:

Find:

- Something prickly
- Something soft
- Something blue
- Something that makes a noise
- Something that makes you smile

We had the best time—not only gathering the items, but also talking about our selections when we were done. Who says this is limited to kiddos? Why not design a scavenger hunt for your friends or community? We had a friend, Allison Ratteree (*God rest her soul*), who wanted to bring awareness to hula hooping. She put out a photo challenge with a prize drawing at the end. The challenge included photo opportunities like:

- Twin hula hooping
- Hula by the clock tower
- Hula while singing your favorite song
- Hula in front of your favorite local business
- Hula at the farmer's market

What's your passion? Can you make it into a scavenger hunt experience? Allison did. And we loved it.

11. Host an Art Party

Julie recently hosted a fantastic art party for some friends and it was so much fun. She invited a local artist, Joan Wheatley (who you met in Chapter 30), who makes the most adorable miniature ceramic mice, to join the group at her home and teach us all how to make *mice houses* out of recycled cardboard packaging material. As a bonus to the class, each of the participants got to have an original ceramic mouse for the house we created. None of the participants in the group had ever made such a dwelling, but thanks to Joan's patience and teaching, we all left with a quirky little piece of art for our homes and the memories and laughs that the party gifted to us. All of us walked away asking about the date for the next party. While this experience did cost us money as we wanted to compensate the artist for her time, these kinds of experiences don't have to be pricey. Art parties can literally be nothing but crayons, markers, and paper. Throw some scissors in for fun. The purpose of the party isn't necessarily the art that's made, but the conversations and giggles that are had while the art is being created. If you don't have any artsy supplies, revisit those cereal boxes and shipping cardboard we mentioned in number 6. Invite your guests to destroy the box and use the pieces to create some sort of structure. All you need for this is some tape and an open mind.

12. Connect with Nature

Nature and being outdoors has so many health benefits. We've given you some in this text, and a quick internet search will bring you more. Since the onset of the pandemic, connecting with the outdoors has grown in popularity—mostly because it's a safer way to play. The latest statistics of visitors to national parks in the United States were just released yesterday. Although they set visitation records in 2020, six parks broke that visitation record in 2021. The most popular national park? The Blue Ridge Parkway. In 2021, U.S. national parks saw a record 297,115,406 recreational visits, and 1,356,657,749 recreational visitor hours (National Park Service, 2022). Holy wow, right? Jed and I are blessed to live just an hour's drive from the Blue Ridge Parkway. There's a little company on my drive up the mountain that rents tubes for $10 each, and the price includes pickup from your ending spot back to your car. Don't want to get wet? Take a walk on a nearby trail and watch for movement in the trees. Birds, squirrels, and wildlife all come alive when you're patient enough.

13. Minute to Win It

Minute to Win It was a game show televised on NBC in 2010. The premise of the game was to complete a series of 10 challenges using household items. The host allowed 60 seconds per task.

Complete them all, and win a million dollars. Sounds fun, right? While the show is no longer in production, the lasting effects of its playfulness are still with us. The interwebs are filled with ideas for these games and the accessibility of them reaches far and wide because all of the challenges involve things most of us would find around our homes. They can be as basic as seeing which person can remove the full trash bag, tie it up, and get it outside the fastest. Want a bit harder of a challenge? Find an empty tissue box and fill it with tiny treasures. Then tie it to someone's waist. Ask them to shake the box until all of the treasure has been removed. It is hysterical to watch and makes for a great game night experience. If neither of these ideas suits you, there are seriously a ton of them out there. Use those, or create your own challenges as part of the play time.

14. Movie Night

Many of us have experienced movie nights with family or friends. While this idea is not new, we want to put a spin on it. Rather than pick a movie that no one has seen, which often leads to two hours of silence and someone likely snoring on the couch, pick a movie that everyone knows pretty well. Ask the viewers to come in costume, bring a prop, or make a poster of their favorite quote. If the movie has a common word that is said throughout, create an action that everyone must do when they hear the word. If you are feeling extra playful, make some snacks that are movie themed or plan a trivia game based around the feature of the evening. We have a great friend who hosted a night like this for his favorite, the 1975 classic *Monty Python and the Holy Grail*. The movie is filled with one-liners and actionable quotes that made it easy for viewers to act out. The night was so playful that the movie and the experience of playing with friends while watching it has been forever seared into my memory.

15. Role Play Dinner

Remember in Chapter 29 when we wrote about our friend Sonia? This idea is totally inspired by her. Prepare a meal for yourself, the family, and your friends, and ask all who will be joining you to dress as fancy as they can. Then pretend that the meal is being served in a faraway place. Use props if you have any. Pictures from the internet are absolutely suitable if you don't have real-life items. Name the food you are serving unique. You've heard of pigs in a blanket, right? Those are just weenies in a biscuit, but the latter sounds more fun. Get creative with what you call your spaghetti dish. This is like anything else in life. You will get out of it what you put into it. The more involved all participants are in making the event special, the more playful it will be.

CHAPTER 37

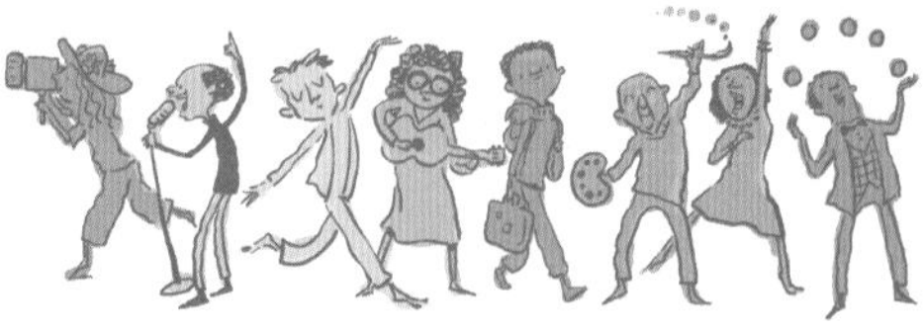

Play with Strangers

1. Join in on Neighborhood Events

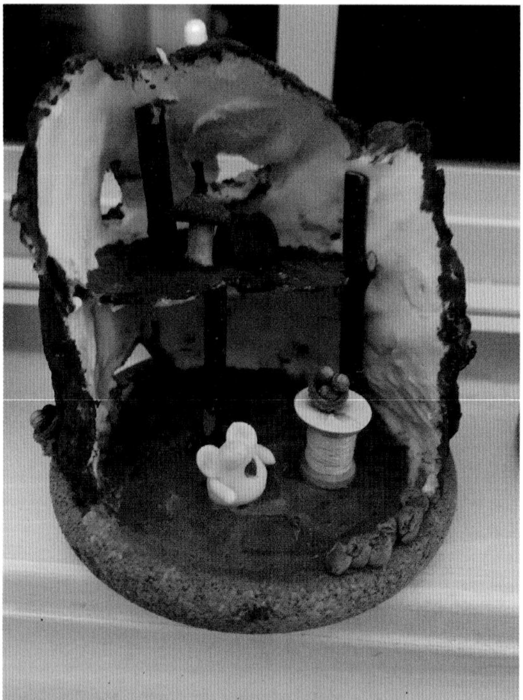

I (Julie) used to live out in the country. Lots of trees, wildlife—wild boar can be such a nuisance—and well water. There were no sidewalks, and the only paved road was the street. Mom fail: my kids don't know how to ride a bike because grass isn't as conducive to riding as the road, and I wouldn't let them do that. It took me 40 minutes to drive in to town. When the pandemic hit, and we had everyone on dial-up internet for school and work, change was essential. So we moved to town-ish. Our new neighborhood has matching mailboxes and an HOA. The board hosts events frequently—especially when it's warm. Since we've moved in, we've experienced ice cream socials, a food truck in someone's driveway, Halloween parties, and caroling. Each neighbor is free to host whatever they like and posts it to the social media group for the neighborhood. I've hosted an art party (remember those mouse houses you read about), and I'm planning more. I heard a bohemian-looking woman in flowy dress once stand at a microphone and say, "Life is a contact sport. You've gotta get out there and make it happen." I don't know her name, but in my brain it's something like Ismerelda. Why not start life in your cul-de-sac?

2. Visit Your Local Watering Hole, and Ask Strangers to Doodle in Your Journal

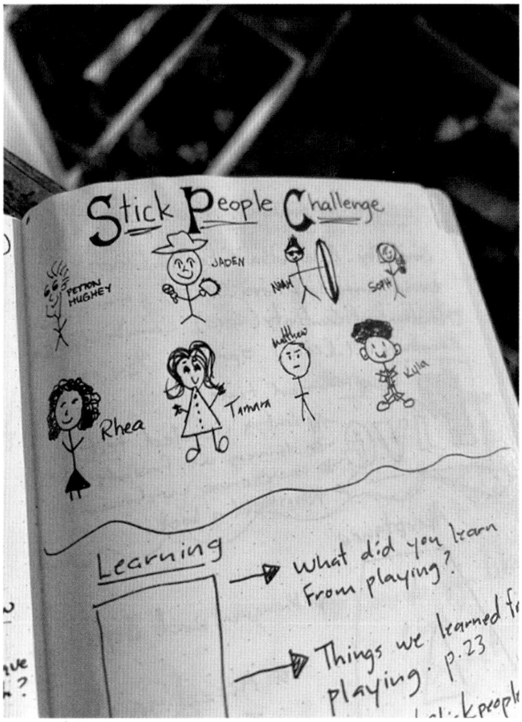

I (Jed) did this one day while getting work done at my home office, Little River Coffee Bar in Spartanburg, South Carolina. I was prepping for a class I was teaching at the university and needed a page of stick figures for part of the lesson I wanted to use. I didn't have access to a printer at the time, so I couldn't just print off a page of them I found online. So, I decided to just ask the folks around me to help out and doodle an image in my journal. Every single person I asked was so eager and excited to add their stick person to the page. It quickly became a communal event where everyone was talking and laughing. Just moments earlier we were all sitting in silence working on respective tasks via a laptop, phone, or notebook. It didn't last long because all of us were in the middle of our various projects and needed to finish, but for a brief moment, we all played together. I am confident that many of them told their friends about the guy at the coffee shop who asked them to doodle, and they most likely laughed, and maybe called me a weirdo, but what a great memory for us all. And, to make the whole experience better, I met a fantastic person who is now my chiropractor. She happened to be one of the people who drew for me that day, and she has been a part of my life ever since!

3. Pillow Fight

When I told Julie to add pillow fighting to our list of playful experiences we could have with strangers, she gave me one of the most puzzled looks I have ever seen from her throughout our entire friendship. But alas, this is a thing, and we think it is uniquely playful and wanted to share it with you. These are relatively new occurrences in the history of humanity, but on March 22, 2008, we were all gifted with the very first World Pillow Fight Day. On that day, people in more than 25 cities from all over the planet met in their public common areas, armed and ready to clunk each other with fluffy goodness. According to the *Wall Street Journal*, an estimated 5,000 New Yorkers participated in the city (Athavaley, 2008). Feathers and hypoallergenic stuffing galore were the centerpiece of the whole event! The day has since moved to the first Saturday in April, but a real day nonetheless. Our friends at National Day Calendar, a website that keeps track of the unique "holidays" around the country, share with us some important guidelines for such an event.

Essential rules are:

- Swing lightly
- Use only soft pillows

- Remove glasses before beginning
- Do not swing at people who don't have a pillow
- Do not swing at people with cameras
- Bring a bag to help clean up after

Does your town host a community pillow fight? Let us know if they do. Who knows? We may show up for the fun! Want more information about this? Search International Pillow Fight Day on Facebook.

4. Flash Mobs

Flash mobs, a sudden gathering of people in a public place for the purpose of singing or dancing in unison in what seems a spontaneous manner, have been around since 2003. According to the *Guinness Book of World Records* (2022), the first one was organized in New York City by a writer and cultural critic named Bill Wasik. Apparently authorities in the area thought it was a crime and thwarted the playful event. Mr. Wasik and his group of some 130 people tried again and were successful on June 3, 2003 at a Macy's in the city. Since that day, according to the National Communication Association, the use of this form of performance has multiplied exponentially. All sorts of public performances, dances, and even the pillow fights we mentioned previously, seem to fit this new category of performance art. Today, flash mobs are often seen as elaborate in-jokes, outright protests, and have made their way into pop culture via movies and television. We love that the National Communication Association (2013) says this about this creative way of playing: "The worldwide embrace of the flash mob points toward an interesting and ever-expanding fusion of performance, culture, and new technologies." While we have never been a part of one, we really hope that we are one day witnesses to this spontaneous moment of joy. If you have never heard of a flash mob, an internet search of the term will yield you hours of videos to enjoy until you can become a part of one. Happy viewing!

5. Curiosity Conversations

Brian Grazer, an Academy Award, Golden Globe, Emmy, and Grammy winning producer and *New York Times* best-selling author, wrote a book with his buddy, Charles Fishman, called *A Curious Mind* in 2016. We were both greatly impacted by the work, specifically due to Grazer's innate ability to connect with his fellow humans through conversation. Although we both crave alone time to recharge, we love talking to people. As you know, storytelling is one of the eight play personalities, and throughout the book, Grazer shares his own stories of conversations he had with people all around the world—most of them complete strangers. Julie and I apply many of Grazer's communication strategies with people we meet in our work, and almost always it leads to playful moments. Grazer calls these curiosity conversations. Often, when talking with folks, we learn about people's hobbies, the latest book they've read, or an upcoming special moment. Sometimes we learn about their Aunt Cheryl who lives on a farm and has a pet pig named Percy that likes to take walks on a leash and have warm baths in the tub. As you can imagine, these chats with strangers are often funny, but they consistently lead to moments where barriers are broken and differences put aside as we experience playfulness together.

6. Rock, Paper, Scissor Challenge

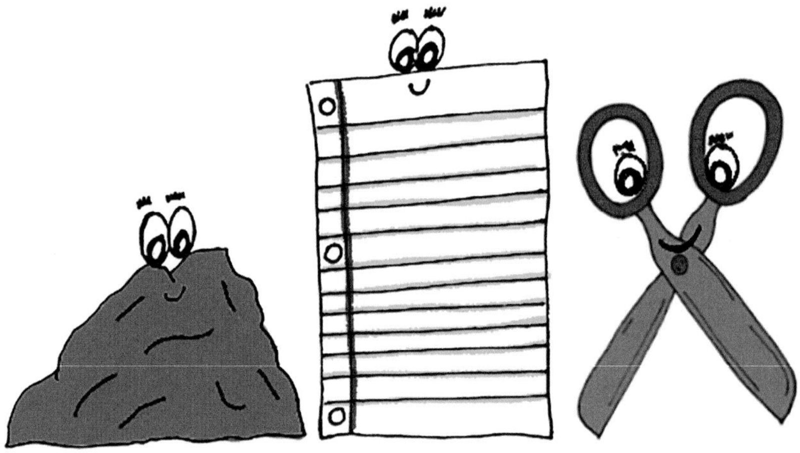

Okay, y'all. We admit it. This idea is not for the faint of heart. But, if you really want to invite more playful living into your life, we beg you to give this one a try. We first saw this idea on YouTube. Someone was stopped at a red light when a car pulled up beside them. Instinctively, the drivers of both cars turned to look at the other beside them. We've all been there, right? But one of the drivers was fully living their best playful life and he pounded his fist into the palm of his hand in the manner that signified he wanted to play a round of Rock, Paper, Scissors while waiting for the green light. It took the other driver a moment to figure out what was happening, but within seconds, both drivers were shooting their shot.

One rock, the other scissors.

Rock won.

Again. Shoot.

Paper. Rock.

Paper wins.

Again. Shoot.

Scissors. Scissors.

A tie.

The light changes and off they go, never to see each other again. But how amazing that the whole experience was captured and is now impacting us all here in this book. So much so that during the writing of this section, I turned to a complete stranger in the coffee bar and pounded my fist three times to signify the start of the game. Of course she looked at me funny the first time so I did it again. The next time she was aware of the happenings and jumped right in. She was rock. I was scissors. She beat me. Defeated, I went back to typing, and she returned to her studying; all the while Julie laughed hysterically.

7. Finish the Lyrics

There's this guy on TikTok, username @erichowl, who we love to watch. He ventures around the streets of his city singing popular songs that most people know at the top of his lungs, all while videoing himself, and then at just the right moment, he stops singing and gestures for random people around him to finish the lyrics of the song. Sometimes people look at him like he has lost his mind, but more often than not, the strangers he encounters jump in and finish the next line. As of now, he's got almost three million followers so it's becoming less and less weird for him to ask people on the street to sing with him, but through his work, he's inviting all of us to relax a bit and enjoy playful moments that come to us. If he came up to you, what would you do? Gosh, I hope I would sing. Instinct may keep me quiet as I could perceive it as a threatening moment, but I really wanna be the person who belts out right along with him. Ironically, *Sweet Caroline* by Neil Diamond is playing in my headphones as I type this. I almost bet most of you sang "Bump Bump Bum" just at the mention of the song didn't you? Maybe you aren't ready to try this with complete strangers on the street, but give it a go at the office, at your next class, or your next group social event. The worst thing that can happen is that they won't finish the lyrics.

8. The Conference on the Value of Play

The Play Conference, as it is commonly known, is an annual professional conference presented by the US Play Coalition. Since 2009, the latest research and practices in the field of play are presented at the conference, which brings together play researchers, educators, health scientists, architects, landscape architects, designers, planners, parks and rec professionals, business and community leaders, psychologists, physicians, and parents from across the US and beyond. The US Play Coalition is an international network of individuals and organizations that recognize play as a valuable and necessary part of a healthy and productive life. The coalitions hosts conferences and educational trainings, encourages and conducts research, and provides avenues of communication about the value of play worldwide. Membership is free, and simply requires a declaration of shared commitment to the value of play. While their annual conference does cost, the learning experience and connections made with others who are living a playful life are invaluable. Remember that class we took with *Animal Moves* author Darryl Edwards, we mentioned earlier? This is the conference where that happened. We would love for you to come play with us there. You will be a stranger when you get there, but will leave as a friend.

9. Community Classes

We mentioned this one earlier as an option in Chapter 35 because you may have to attend a class by yourself, but it must be repeated here because of the invaluable work of folks in our own community who provide free learning experiences for anyone who wants to learn. We are almost certain that there are numerous options like this somewhere in your town. If not, maybe you are the director play personality and you could organize one. Do you have a hobby or skill that you could teach someone about? Of course you do. You are nearing the end of a book all about the playful life. You are ready to help others learn all about the power of play. Why not organize a play club for adults, for families, for college students at a nearby campus where you teach them how to be more playful? After the years of pandemic stress and worry, people are longing for these kinds of moments. Maybe it's you who needs to start it? Mention it to those in your friend group and see if there is an interest. Ask them to bring others whom you may not know so that more can learn. Julie is currently planning to organize a monthly game night in partnership with a locally owned toy store. She is gonna teach participants how to play the games and at the same time she'll be educating them about the power of play in their lives. Using this book as a resource, we are confident you could do the same of those in your own community.

10. Reading Clubs at a Local Bookstore

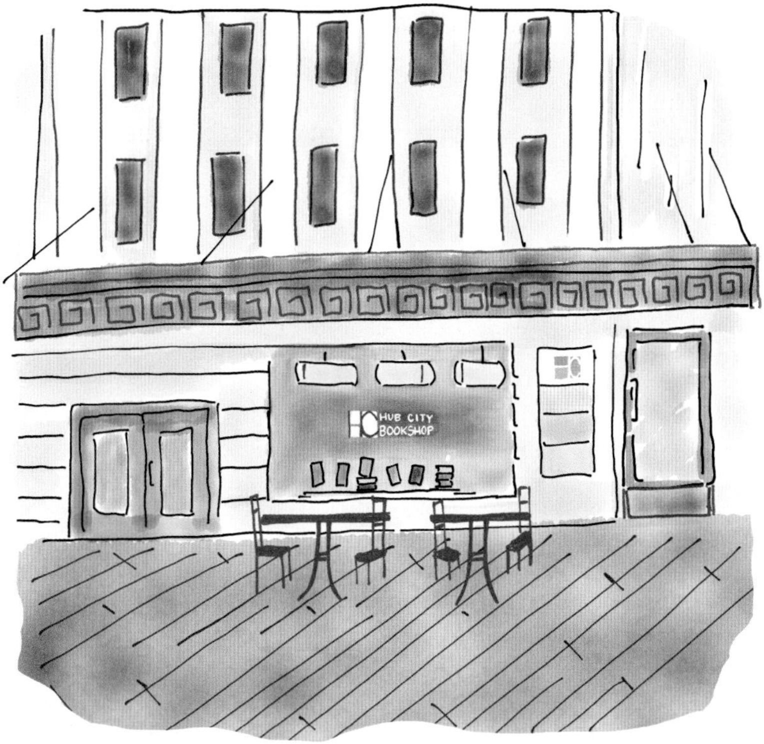

We have mentioned our local bookstore, Hub City Books, a few times throughout this book. Its impact on us cannot be measured. It is often a place we write and meet with others about our work, but it also serves as a place of learning and connection for us. Those who work there feel like family to us, and Anne Waters is a gem to all of Spartanburg. One of our favorite offerings they provide to our community is their reading clubs. There is always a shelf full of books displayed there at the store that various groups of people around town are meeting to discuss. To join in, you just simply read the book and show up to the meeting. Most of them are held right there in the store. Sometimes there's a snack or the author comes to participate. For those of us with social anxiety, that can sound intimidating, but the nature of these groups is very open, friendly, and accepting of all who come. Everyone there has the common thread of the book to bring them together. If your local bookstore doesn't have anything like this, mention it to the store owner/manager. They would probably be thrilled to host an event. Maybe even use this book as a launching pad. Create a night of playful experiences connected to talking all about the nuggets of playful wisdom you took away from the reading. Remember the play types and think of a variety of experiences for the group. If you choose this, send us a message on social media and we may join you via video chat.

11. League Sports for Adults

Back when we were in college, intramural sports were often the highlight of the week for so many on campus. Even if you didn't participate on a team, it was still a function that lots of students attended as spectators. It wasn't just a place for sports, but a social event. It was where you met new friends and cheered on old ones who were playing. For whatever reason, once we leave the confines of school, opportunities like these seem to diminish as the throes of adulthood take over. But, for those of us who enjoy this kind of play and long for it to be a part of our lives, there are possibilities. A few years ago we learned about a local kickball league for grown-ups that started in our area. The excitement I felt about learning this was not a normal feeling I experienced in relation to sports, especially kickball. I was always the last one picked for a team. I never really understood why because I was a great kicker, but alas, I was last. Regardless, I can smell the red rubber ball even as I type this and I would love to sign up for a team. The last time I looked into it, their practice schedule was a bit more than I could commit to at the time. Maybe kickball isn't your thing. My mama was in a bowling league for years and years. Take a trip to the local alley and sign up soon.

12. Organize a Rainbow Ball

A nonprofit organization in our community, the Uplift Outreach Center, is a safe and inclusive space for LGBTQ+ youth. For their yearly fundraiser, they host an event called the Rainbow Ball. It is an evening full of fun and frolic with acceptance as its theme. The goal of the event is to raise money for the organization while encouraging and empowering the queer community in our small Southern town. You don't have to be a member of the gay community to go. It is for everyone! You can certainly attend with your straight partner as a show of solidarity with those who must still continue to advocate for their equality. Parents can take their children for a parent–child event of advocacy. Many of us model advocacy and support in our homes—just think of what that can look like if we join forces with other families in support of love's many forms. The first time I (Julie) took my daughters to the Pride Festival in our town I wanted them to see the diversity of love, friendship, and community that is alive in our small town. We saw so many friends. We hugged, we sang, we marched. When our friends came on stage, we stood and yelled for them. We supported them—all of them. A rainbow ball isn't a festival with parades and floats, though. Instead, it's glamorous. It's elegant. It is a night of celebrating the beauty of *all* of our community.

13. Poetry Slam

I love rhyming words. I do. Every time I hear them, I stop and say, "Hey, that rhymed!" Sometimes I write bits of poetry on beverage napkins, and sometimes I get my car passenger (whoever is unlucky—lol—enough to be sitting there) to write the verses I come up with as we drive. I know, I know. Not all poetry rhymes. But, I happen to be in tune with the rhyming ones. I love a poetry slam. *Snap Snap Snap.* Our local Hub City Writer's Project used to host one in an old building above what used to be the city's founding shoe store. Now, the coffee shop we frequent hosts their own. People gather, people sip beverages, brave souls approach the mic and spill ideas in the air. It's wonderful. If this is not a thing in your town, why not make it one? Invite friends to have drinks. Get the microphone ready. Level up and use your event to bring advocacy and awareness to a group or a cause.

14. Karaoke

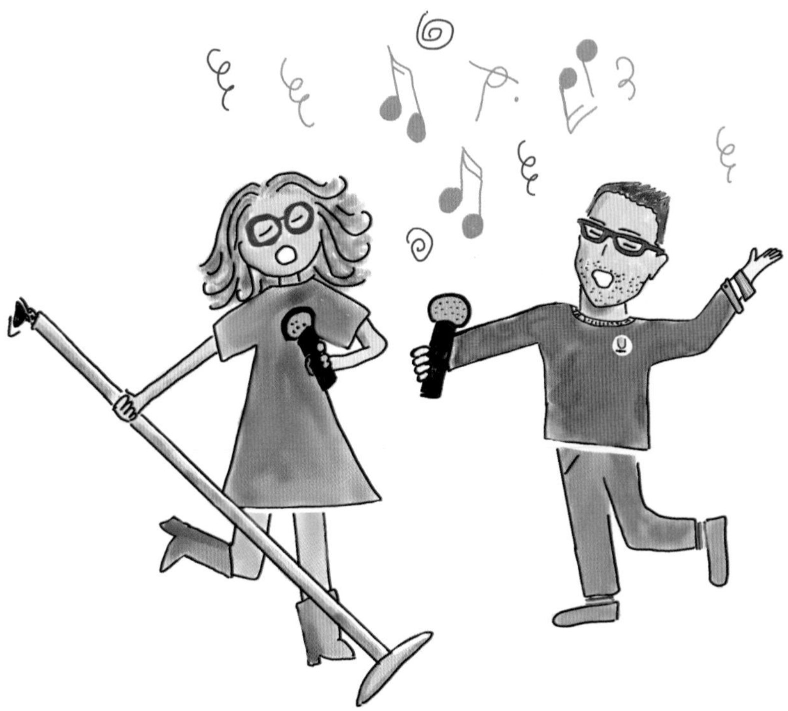

Let it go! Let it go! I can't hold it back anymore! Oh. My apologies. I saw the word *karaoke* in the list and lost all my control. My go-to song from a favorite movie about an icy princess—I just belted it right out. No, it wasn't in perfect pitch, and I didn't have the dance moves down just right, but man did I sing it with all of my heart right smack dab in the middle of this coffee shop. I am sure that you are not surprised to hear this isn't the first time I have sung these words loud and proud! My favorite time ever was when the dueling piano players invited me on stage at *Jelly Rolls*, located at Disney's Boardwalk Resort. A standing ovation was well received as I *threw down*, y'all. I fully realize that karaoke is not a playful experience for everyone. Singing in front of others can be terrifying. But watching others do it is a piece of cake and sometimes can be hysterical to see. Just ask those who have ever watched me sing. Whether you are singing or watching, at a karaoke bar or at home with lyrics on your TV, this musical form of play can provide hours of entertainment. When I once lived in Cebu, Philippines, karaoke was a daily form of play for almost everyone and it brought so many people together. It wasn't just the music that entertained us, but the joy of being together, the freedom to be silly, and the human connections made through song.

15. Barista Bop

Okay, we made this one up on the spot while sitting in a local Starbucks. This isn't our normal coffee shop but it is the only one open on Sundays and we had a writing deadline. It is about 7:30 a.m. and these incredible employees have been here since before 5:30. They have been caffeinated for hours and we are just now warming up. They are singing and dancing behind the counter. I want to be annoyed because they are so cheery, but I can't. They are the embodiment of the playful life we all should long for. I find myself being drawn to their energy. I literally stopped typing this so I could go to the counter and engage with their moving and grooving. They are definitely infectious with their playful spirit. While the place is known for its caffeine assistance, Taylor and her friends from the Pine Street location just boosted our entire morning with a playful interaction as I ordered my bacon, egg, and cheese sandwich with a venti vanilla latte. They could have just taken the order and handed it to me, but every interaction from the register to the pickup was playful. Visit your local coffee spot soon and engage with your baristas. They are a bop!

CHAPTER 38

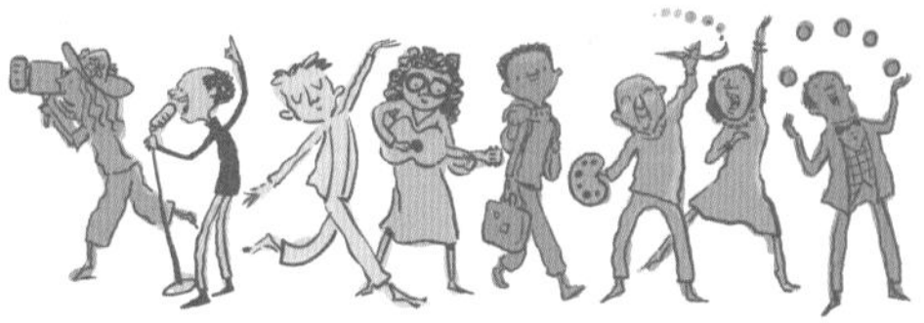

Play as a Community

1. World Play Day

Sponsored by the International Toy Library Association, World Play Day is an annual event occurring on May 28th, with a focus on celebrating the power of play throughout humanity. The day is meant to encourage an attitude of connecting with others through play rather than an official schedule of events. Started in 1987, this day serves as a reminder to us all that play is inherent to our existence as a people. It's part of our DNA. Regardless of where you exist on the planet, playfulness is beneficial to us all. We hope that on this date, you will find someone to connect with in a playful manner and celebrate the awesomeness of play in our lives. Find out more at https://www.pgpedia.com/w/world-play-day.

2. Music on Main/Jazz on the Square

Who doesn't love to unwind after a long day with a beverage and some jazzy tunes? Whether or not jazz is your thing, music is often integral to our mood. John Powell, a professor of physics with a master's degree in music composition, tells us, "Listening to calming music has been shown to diminish the adrenaline and cortisol levels in the bloodstream and therefore reduce stress" (2020). How can you bring the health benefits of music to your community? If you're an artist/creator of the music type, you likely have many like-minded musician friends. Why not get together and host a weekly event in your town's common area? Spartanburg, South Carolina, the place Jed and I both call home, hosts these such events. Coined Music on Main and Jazz on the Square, these gatherings do more than provide entertainment. They also serve as fundraising opportunities for our local civic organizations. Clubs who volunteer at the event can earn for their cause a portion of sales to support their charities. What is sold? Food, beverages, crafts, art—you name it. What are you waiting for? Call your buddies and make this happen in your community too.

3. Duck Derby

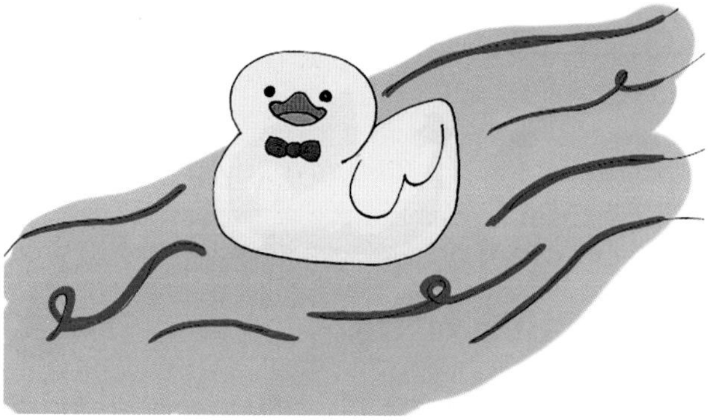

In Tempe, Arizona, in 1988, the first-ever Duck Derby occurred, ushering into being a fun, playful way to raise money for a worthy cause. Since that day, the founding organizer, GAME, has partnered with over 2,000 groups worldwide for fundraising collaboration by providing a unique, family-friendly event for the entire community. Participants in the event pay money to sponsor a rubber ducky that is then launched into a local river with thousands of other duckies. Each ducky then fights its way to the finish line to be crowned the winner of the Duck Derby. Along the banks, hundreds, sometimes thousands, of people line the race route to cheer for their duck. Of course they have no idea which one is theirs, but the cheering frenzy is often intense nonetheless. The ducks are numbered so the winning duck can be connected with its sponsor, but until the winner is announced, the suspense is electric. Who knew screaming and yelling for a little rubber duck could be so much fun? Have y'all ever been to one? Does your community host one of these events? We love them so much! It reminds us both of times when we would drop a leaf or a stick into a stream and watch it float down with the currents. Such a good time! If you wanna learn more about hosting a Duck Derby in your town, visit game-fundraising.com.

4. Yarn Bomb

No, not exploding sweaters. Yarn bombing is a street art movement. Have you ever passed a city bench wearing a crocheted accessory? The first time I saw this, I was confused. It was at the local library here, and all the handrails were wrapped in what must have taken someone a lot of time to create! Once I saw the one, I started seeing them everywhere—and what a happy surprise it was. When we say yarn bombing, we are referring to the "covering, wrapping, or decorating objects in pieces of knit or crochet" (Rosenburg, 2020). Instead of a permanent form of street art, this form of fabric art can be removed rather easily from its location—a fence, a tree, a light pole, a sign . . . the possibilities are endless. Are you a fan of fabric arts? Why not start yarn bombing in your village? Level up by using your art to advocate for a cause.

5. Collaborative Murals

In the summer of 2020, as the pandemic raged and the advocacy for equitable and fair treatment of Black people took center stage because of the unjust murder of George Floyd at the hands of law enforcement, many communities began to rally together to announce to the world that Black lives mattered in their town space. In Spartanburg, South Carolina, where we call home, on the day after the celebration of Juneteenth (June 19th), 16 artists collaborated to create our very own Black Lives Matter mural. It was a grassroots effort led by artists Frankie Zombie, Adrian Meadows, and Bleu Cooper. The only one of its kind in the Palmetto State, the painting of the mural was a community-wide event. Over a span of two days, volunteers worked alongside the artists to create a one-of-a-kind piece of artwork on our city street. The mural stretches 240 feet, facing Spartanburg City Hall and the Spartanburg Police Department headquarters. The mural was fully funded by private donations but had the support of city council and the city police. The beauty of the mural is only made more inspirational knowing that the artists who created it did so without compensation and in partnership with those in the community. Throughout our small town, murals have become a regular playful experience for the community to join in. Take a drive around your town to scope out where you could create your own neighborhood art collaboration. Of course, be sure to get permission before you start.

6. Mice Hunt

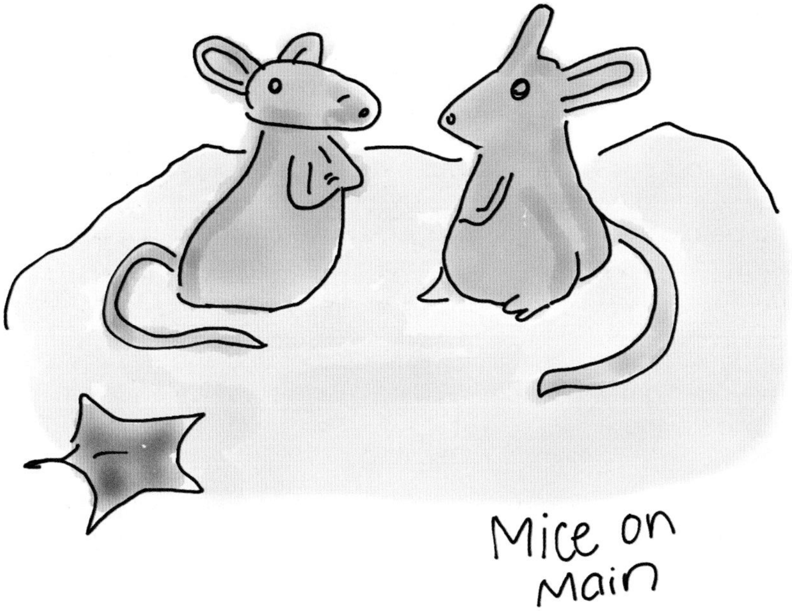

On the front porch of my home, there is a metal mouse. He's about four inches high, and just barely blends in to the brickwork. When visitors see him, they're always pleasantly surprised. He was a gift from my stepdad, who knows how much I love the mouse hunt in our neighboring city, Greenville, South Carolina. Inspired by the children's book *Goodnight Moon*, the mice were brought to life by local sculptor and illustrator Zan Wells as a service project by local high school student Jim Ryan. Visitors to the area travel Greenville's Main Street and check off their mouse-scavenger-hunt list as they visit the area. Some are hiding by the wall, and others are perched high on light poles. You can download a PDF of all the clues by searching Greenville Mice Hunt. Does your city have such a fun playful opportunity? If not, why not create one? It can be temporary with art displayed at various locations, or it could be more permanent like the one we've described here.

7. Online Games (*Wordle, Farmville, Candy Crush*)

We probably don't need to do a lot of splainin' with this one due to the fact that smartphones and their gaming ability is as common as breathing for many of us, but the connections that are made through these shared games is worth noting in a book about play. According to *PlayToday*, these are a few current stats about mobile gaming (2022):

There are more than 2.6 billion mobile gamers worldwide.
The average age of mobile gamers is 36.3 years old.
50% of mobile gamers play while using the bathroom.

That last one sure made us chuckle. We laugh because we know it's true. Whether you play on the couch, the toilet, or in bed before you sleep, online gaming communities are definitely a part of the playfulness of humans in the 21st century. While we certainly advocate for in-person experiences, playing online with friends became an integral part of our lives when the COVID-19 pandemic forced our social experiences into the virtual world. Many a night we spent playing games with friends via our mobile devices.

8. Community Chess

During the summer of 1994, I was very fortunate to travel to Europe with the Spirit of America National Honor Band. I was selected to play trumpet with the group as one of 105 students from across the country. We toured seven countries, performing in multiple cities as a goodwill gesture, for three weeks. In almost every city we visited, there was a giant community chessboard built into the city square. The board was roughly 20×20 feet and the pieces were about three feet tall. They weren't too heavy, but they were definitely sturdy enough to withstand any wind that might seek to carry them away. I remember how groups of people surrounded the board to watch the match of two complete strangers who volunteered to play. It was almost like being at a sporting event. When player one would make a move, the crowd would cheer. Player two would counter that move only to bring more applause. I admit it. I was only 16 at the time and had no inkling of an idea about the rules of chess. What I did know, even then, was that these people were playing—obviously the game players, but also the people watching intently, the walkers who casually sauntered by, the nearby shop owners standing on the curbs in front of their bodegas. All of those who got a peek of the game were joining in on this communal play experience. I wish our town had one of these. We have communal play spaces, of course, parks, trails, etc., but there was something about this oversized board game in the middle of town that just brought people together.

9. Connect the Dots

Not every idea here needs to be shiny and new. Your town might already have a few playful aspects. Have you considered how your current playful opportunities might be connected? Consider what has been done in Pittsburgh's Hazelwood neighborhood. Here, the Playful Pittsburgh Collaborative connected the dots in their community, leveraging the assets of play that already existed. They created the Hazelwood Play Trail, weaving together a chess club run by a police officer, a produce stand with a game on the outside wall of the store, and a mural capturing the history of the community. Cara Ciminillo, executive director of Trying Together, says, "I think what is important when it comes to community work is . . . elevating assets that exist in the community" (Hadani & Vey, 2021). PAL: Play, Advocate, Live Well, is a small nonprofit connecting the dots in Spartanburg, South Carolina. Their goal is to improve health and wellness throughout the area by creating an environment and culture that fosters physical activity and healthy eating through an equity lens. While this is an organization specific to our hometown, what could a similar group look like in your town? Are there running or hiking trails nearby that you could promote? Does anyone in your circle like to host 5K road races? Could there possibly be a yoga teacher on your friend list that could help get neighbors in your community stretching their mind, body, and spirits? How could you help connect those people with the community at large?

10. Playful Sidewalks

Concrete, meet chalk.

Chalk, meet concrete.

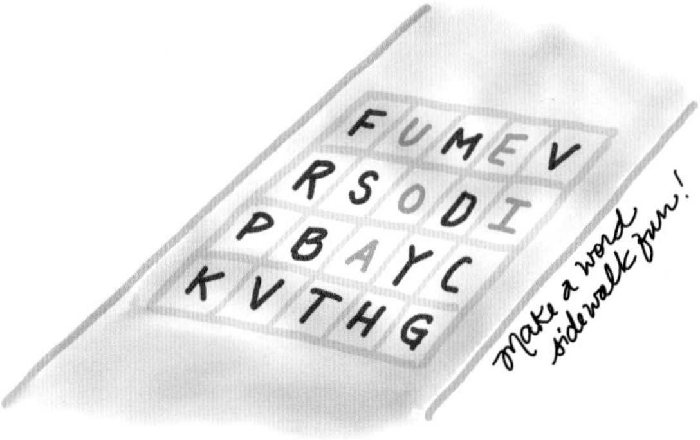

Imagine how we might be able to take sometimes as simple as a sidewalk and make it playful for pedestrians in our communities. Not only can imaginative art transform the walking experience, but it can also encourage people to get out and get moving, thus benefiting the local economy and public safety. Invite your friends to join in the creation of sidewalk games along a particular path. Want to level up? Incorporate art and history of the area into your creations. Chalk is a great medium for this kind of play because of its temporary state. When the rains come, the slate is clean for the next creation. If you find a particular design is popular, consider making it a permanent addition to the community space (with permissions, of course).

11. Photo Challenge

Have you ever played chicken in a swimming pool? Or had someone carry you on their shoulders while dry? In either situation, you've had an opportunity to see how super-tall humans view the world. I'm not very tall (five feet and half an inch, to be precise), so these differences in views are always so interesting to me. To see the world from someone else's height is such a new experience. Why not let this be a metaphor for perspective and diversity where you live? A few years ago, a local group passed out disposable cameras to people downtown and challenged them to take photos of Spartanburg throughout their week—the people, the places, the views. Once they were full of photos, the cameras were dropped off at a predetermined location and the film was printed on artist paper. Photos were displayed for public viewing, and they were later made into a book. What perspectives exist in your area? Are you seeing them all? Are you really?

12. Start a Community Garden

Do you have a green thumb, but no space to cultivate your talents? Consider partnering with your town to begin a community garden. Not only do these spaces provide space to grow fresh, healthy food or flowers, but they can also contribute to the accessibility of food. These garden spaces can also include shaded seating for gathering—imagine shared meals, meetings, classes, conversations, or even performances in this transformed space. Our town has several of these gardens—one is a partnership with the local farmer's market and fees are less than $100 per year. Another is an extension of the environmental studies program at a local college, housing a vineyard, a garden, classrooms, and walking trail. We highly recommend taking a good look at the spaces around you. How can you channel your skillset, putting your gardening talents to work for neighborhood-level social change?

13. Organize a Movie Night for Your Community

In the warmer months in South Carolina, when the sun stays up longer than the moon, we like to be out and about longer. Down here, these lazy days of summer usually involve ice cream, lightning bugs, and water—either a swimming pool, a lake, or a creek. But, we know that not everyone wants to be wet and messy. Some folks like to feel cute while eating boiled peanuts and a Coke Zero while sitting in a lawn chair with friends. In the past few years, various groups in our town have sponsored a movie night in the park. Sometimes there are drawings for gift cards to local businesses. The movies are family-friendly and fun; the past few years' showing list includes titles such as *Despicable Me 3*, *Peter Rabbit*, *Paddington 2*, and *Back to the Future*. If you want to get this going, you don't have to do it alone. Seek out sponsors to showcase movies that align with their mission. For example, *Back to the Future* was sponsored here by our Science Center. What a beautiful opportunity for play to lead to advocacy. If you build it, they will come.

14. Pop-Up Yoga

No, not exploding yoginis. Pop-up yoga refers to the practice of yoga in nontraditional spaces. Whether it's in a public park, a coffee shop, a cow pasture, or a beach, hosting a pop-up yoga session makes fitness accessible to the community. Sessions are often free, and always open to everyone—adults, kids, pets, you name it. Many times, pop-up yoga sessions are meant to entice people to try yoga for the first time. But they can also be themed sessions meant to bring people together for fun. Don't freak out here: you don't have to be the leader of this vinyasa, but one who is gifted with the idea is expected to take action—even if the action is spreading the idea to those with the skills. Namaste.

15. Cooter Fest!

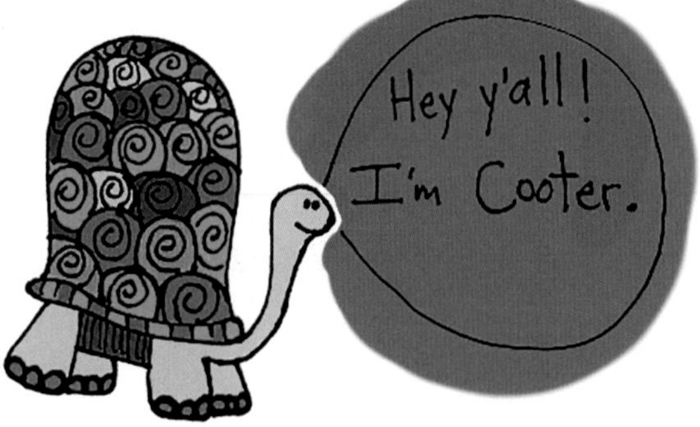

South Carolinians know how to have a good time. Sometimes, that involves cooters. I suppose it helps to know that a cooter is a class of freshwater turtles, with eight different species across the Southeastern United States. In our home state of South Carolina, cooters like to live in quiet ponds and ditches. These turtles aren't known for their speed, but that hasn't created a shortage of love from the good folk down in Allendale, South Carolina. Here, they hold cooter races each spring at the Cooter Bowl in front of the Allendale County Courthouse. Are you intrigued? Why not try to catch a winner, and enter the races? Are you anti-turtle-trapping? No worries—you can rent one at the "Rent a Cooter" booth, and then set that sucker free! If this ain't playful, we don't know what is, y'all. We have never been to the famous Cooter Fest, but after learning about it for this book, we *must* take a trip to experience this with our neighbors in the southern part of South Carolina. These fun, quirky celebrations and festivals aren't unique to our state. All 50 of the United States and numerous countries around the globe have events to honor their local history and traditions. On our must-participate bucket list is the Water Gun Festival in the Sinchon district of Seoul, South Korea, the Cheese Rolling Festival in the South West England Gloucester region, the Annual Avon Heritage Duck Tape Festival in Avon, Ohio, and the Hollerin' Heritage Festival in Clinton, North Carolina.

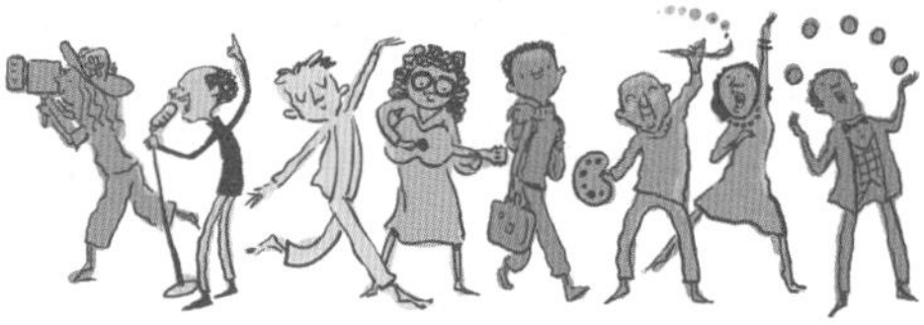

Play & Ponder

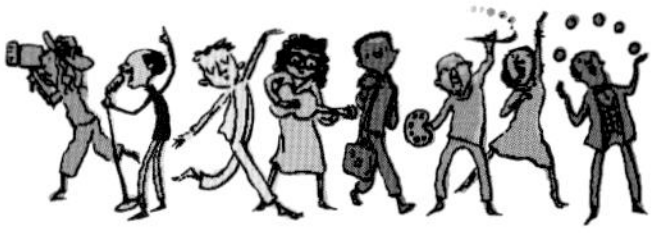

Well, y'all. Here we are. If you have made it this far with us, there is no doubt in our mind that you are hearing the words of grannies that we shared near the beginning. "Play purdy," they'd say. Their words will forever be etched into our hearts and minds and we hope that they are now part of yours. Just as it was their desire for us to get along, be nice, work together, treat others with respect, value others as ourselves, love one another, talk through our differences, and join together in play because it is good for our lives, it is our desire that somewhere within these pages you have found a new meaning to the word *play*. Maybe your memories led you to rekindle a love for a long-lost hobby that brings you joy. Hopefully you learned something new about how play impacts the mind. Surely you heard us all but yelling that mistakes would be made. Gosh, how we hope you start *A Movement* in your community. We tried to give you as much mojo as we knew how, and you have a map if you need it. You also have us. We don't have all the answers and we certainly aren't the only ones encouraging the world to play, but we are here to cheer you on as you journey deeper into a playful life.

Southernisms and Their Meanings

Section One

1. Mule wants a pickle patch: This isn't something we say regularly, but it is colorful and paints a purdy picture. Don't y'all think that a mule would want a pickle patch? Certainly he'd love it, right? Exaggerated speech is part of who we are. Roll with it. :)
2. In the floor: Some of y'all might say *on* the floor, but we say *in* the floor. We recognize that one is not really inside the floor, but "in" implies that you are not out. And in the floor means you are on it.
3. Lawsy: Good grief.
4. Bless his heart: This one deserves its own book, but the short and skinny of it means that we pity you, but with the utmost kindness.
5. So confused we don't know whether to scratch our watch or wind our butts: This quote was made famous by none other than Dolly Parton in the movie *Steel Magnolias*. Quite simply, it means you are very, very confused.
6. Whatever cranks your tractor: What gets you really excited.
7. We ain't perfect: This isn't a Southernism per se, but we do love the word *ain't* from time to time and just want you to know it wasn't a typo.
8. Didn't just fall off the turnip truck: We weren't born yesterday.
9. Since Moses was a baby: A long, long time ago.
10. To tide you over: Something to keep you occupied for a bit.

Section Two

1. Put your fur down: You know how when a dog or cat gets angry the fur on their back raises? This is a reference to that. Put your fur down means don't get mad.
2. Dollop of mayo: A spoonful of mayonnaise; Duke's is the ONLY kind.
3. Soft eyes: Look with grace and mercy upon someone's mistake.
4. Want to hear you crow: Don't brag too much.
5. "Y'all play purdy": Be nice, don't argue.
6. Coming up: Growing up, getting older.

Section Three

1. Working harder than a mule in May: Anytime between April and May, mules worked hard to get the crops planted.
2. What to and how for: If someone gives you the what to and how for, they are basically telling you how it is. Setting you straight, so to speak. Correcting your misunderstanding and putting you on the right path as forcefully, but as nicely, as possible.
3. Weedin' a pretty wide row: Being efficient at a task.
4. Hunky-dory: Everything is great . . . everything is fine.
5. Show you the weeds in your garden: Reveal the bad parts we would like to keep hidden.

Section Four

1. Get to gettin': Start moving, get to work.
2. Buggy: This is what we call a shopping cart and we shall not be convinced to change our minds.
3. Oh Law: Good grief.
4. Underpinning: The official name of the metal skirting that is often used to conceal the underpart of a mobile home. It is also used to refer to underpants.
5. Fuller than a tick on a dog's ear: After a long day of sucking blood from a dog via its ear, a tick is pretty full and about to explode. Nothing is fuller.
6. A-wondrin' what in tarnation: We really have no idea what tarnation is, but the expression is often used when something really confusing happens.

7. Grow faster than a milkweed in June: Nothing grows as fast as a milkweed in June.

Section Five

1. Struck my fancy: If something struck your fancy, it made you happy.
2. Peddlin': You may have seen lots of words in the book that are supposed to end with "-ing" but we Southern folk love to drop that "g" off the end.
3. Mind ya own beeswax: Mind your own business.

Section Six

1. Get a rise out of you: When someone says or does something simply to see if they can get a response from you.
2. Longer than the preacher's homecoming sermon: Trust us, this is a long, LONG time!
3. Milk is clabbered: This is a Southern way of referring to curdled milk.
4. Trimming some of the fat: Getting rid of things that aren't important.
5. That ship has sailed: The time, the opportunity, the idea has moved on.
6. Don't write a check you can't cash: Do not commit to doing something that you are not capable or willing to do.

Section Seven

1. Excited as a fly in a cow pasture: Flies like poop and cows poop a lot. Imagine how excited flies would be here!
2. Richard: A reference to Richard Petty, who is known as the king of NASCAR.

REFERENCES

About Jazzercise. (n.d.). Jazzercise. https://www.jazzercise.com/About-Us

Ackerman, D. (2000). *Deep play* (Illustrated ed.). Vintage.

Altschul, D. M., & Deary, I. J. (2019). Playing analog games is associated with reduced declines in cognitive function: A 68-year longitudinal cohort study. *The Journals of Gerontology: Series B*, *75*(3), 474–482. https://doi.org/10.1093/geronb/gbz149

Anyangwe, E. (2015, August 10). Sports for development: More than just fun and games? *The Guardian*. Available at https://www.theguardian.com/global-development-professionals-network/2015/aug/10/sport-for-development-charity-ngo-effective-change

Anyangwe, E. (2017, October 6). Sports for development: More than just fun and games? *The Guardian*. https://www.theguardian.com/global-development-professionals-network/2015/aug/10/sport-for-development-charity-ngo-effective-change

Athavaley, A. (2008, April 15). Students unleash a pillow fight on Manhattan. *Wall Street Journal*. Available at https://www.wsj.com/articles/SB120814163599712081

Badenoch, B., & Kestly, T. (2016). Exploring the neuroscience of healing play at every age. In D. A. Crenshaw & A. L. Stewart (Eds.), *Play therapy: A comprehensive guide to theory and practice*. Guilford Press.

Basso, J. C., & Suzuki, W. A. (2017). The effects of acute exercise on mood, cognition, neurophysiology, and neurochemical pathways: A review. *Brain Plasticity (Amsterdam, Netherlands)*, *2*(2), 127–152. https://doi.org/10.3233/BPL-160040

Bateson, P. (2015). Playfulness and creativity. *Current Biology*, *25*(1), R12–R16. https://doi.org/10.1016/j.cub.2014.09.009

Becker, I. (2008). Uses of yoga in psychiatry and medicine. *Complementary and Alternative Medicine and Psychiatry*, *19*.

Behncke, I. (2015). Play and the Peter Pan ape. *Current Biology*, *25*(1), R24–R27. https://doi.org/10.1016/j.cub.2014.11.020

Bjorklund, D. F., & Pellegrini, A. D. (2000). Child development and evolutionary psychology. *Child Development*, *71*(6), 1687–1708. https://doi.org/10.1111/1467-8624.00258

Brown, C. (2017). *The default mode network and executive function: Influence of age, white matter connectivity, and Alzheimer's pathology*. Doctoral dissertation, University of Kentucky. Available at https://uknowledge.uky.edu/neurobio_etds/18/

Brown, S. (2009). *Play: How it shapes the brain, opens the imagination, and invigorates the soul*. New York: Penguin Group.

Brown, T. (2008, November 6). *Tales of creativity and play*. TED Talks. https://www.ted.com/talks/tim_brown_tales_of_creativity_and_play

CBS. (2021, November 14). *Adele one night only*. https://www.cbs.com/shows/adele-one-night-only/video/BoW36T84IPNYyOfJv7a0UK-064wALi3Of/adele-one-night-only/

Chaouloff, F. (1989). Physical exercise and brain monoamines: A review. *Acta Physiologica Scandinavica*, *137*, 1–13.

Cloud, H., & Townsend, J. (1992). *Boundaries: When to say yes, and how to say no to take control of our life*. Zondervan.

Covey, S. (1990). *Seven habits of highly effective people*. Simon & Schuster.

Cuthbert, B., Kristeller, J., Simons, R., Hodes, R., & Lang, P. J. (1981). Strategies of arousal control: Biofeedback, mediation and motivation. *Journal of Experimental Psychology*, *110*(4), 518–546.

DeBenedet, A. (2018). *Playful intelligence: The power of living lightly in a serious world*. Santa Monica Press.

DeBenedet, A., & Cohen, L. (2011). *The art of roughhousing: Good old-fashioned horseplay and why every kid needs it*. Quirk Books. *Definition and etymology of play*. (n.d.). Etymonline. https://www.etymonline.com/word/play

Delagran, L. (n.d.). *Impact of fear and anxiety*. Earl E. Bakken Center for Spirituality & Healing, University of Minnesota. Available at https://www.takingcharge.csh.umn.edu/impact-fear-and-anxiety#:~:text=Fear%20weakens%20our%20immune%20system,ageing%20and%20even%20premature%20death

Dewar, G. (2014). The cognitive benefits of play: Effects on the learning brain. *Parenting Science*. Retrieved from https://www.parentingscience.com/benefits-of-play

Doyle, G. (2020). *Untamed*. Dial Press.

Dubuc, B. (n.d.). *The amygdala and its allies*. Available at https://thebrain.mcgill.ca/flash/d/d_04/d_04_cr/d_04_cr_peu/d_04_cr_peu.html

Duhigg, C. (2014). *The power of habit: Why we do what we do in life and business*. Random House Trade Paperbacks.

Eby, L. T., Cader, J., & Noble, C. L. (2003). Why do high self-monitors emerge as leaders in small groups? A comparative analysis of the behaviors of high versus low self-monitors. *Journal of Applied Social Psychology, 33*, 1457–1479. doi: 10.1111/j.1559-1816.2003.tb01958.x

Eckert, J. (2016). *The novice advantage*. Corwin.

Edwards, D. (2018). *Animal moves: How to move like an animal to get you leaner, fitter, stronger, and healthier for life*. Explorer Publishing.

Encyclopedia Britannica. (n.d.). *Rock art*. Available at https://www.britannica.com/art/rock-art

Engelen, E.-M. (2021). *Empathy and imagination*. Conference paper, American Philosophical Association, Pacific Division, San Diego. doi: 10.13140/2.1.1372.8808

Fechner, G. (n.d.). *Nanna oder über das Seelenleben der Pflanzen*, 1848. Referenced in https://plato.stanford.edu/entries/fechner/

France, V. A. (1991). *Window on Main Street: 35 years of creating happiness at Disneyland Park*. Stabur Press.

Frank, S. J. (1978). Just imagine how I feel: How to improve empathy through training in imagination. In J. Singer & K. Pope (Eds.), *The power of human imagination: New methods in psychotherapy* (pp. 309–346). New York: Springer.

Gardner, H. (1983). *Frames of mind: The theory of multiple intelligences* (1st ed.). Basic Books.

Gardner, H. (2020). *A synthesizing mind: A memoir from the creator of multiple intelligences theory*. MIT Press.

GI Society. (2022). *Irritable bowel syndrome (IBS) and serotonin*. Available at https://badgut.org/information-centre/a-z-digestive-topics/ibs-and-serotonin/

Gilbert, E. (2015). *Big magic: Creative living beyond fear*. Riverhead Books.

Gladwell, M. (2008). *Outliers: The story of success*. Little, Brown and Company.

Golde, C. M. (2019, February 4). Careers go in chapters. *Inside Higher Ed*. https://www.insidehighered.com/advice/2019/02/04/phd-students-and-postdocs-should-view-their-careers-chapters-book-opinion

Gordon, N., Burke, S., Akil, H., Watson, S., & Panskepp, J. (2003). Socially induced brain "fertilization": Play promotes brain derived neurotrophic factor transcription in the amygdala and dorsolateral frontal cortex in juvenile rats. *Neuroscience Letters, 341*(1), 17–20.

Gov.UK. (2016). *Using sport to tackle games*. Available at https://www.gov.uk/government/news/using-sport-to-tackle-gangs

Gray, P. (2013). *Free to learn*. New York: Basic Books.

Grazer, B., & Fishman, C. (2016). *A curious mind: The secret to a bigger life*. Simon & Schuster.

Greenough, W. T., & Black, J. E. (1992). Induction of brain structure by experience: Substrates for cognitive development. *Developmental Neuroscience, 24*.

Guadagni, V., Drogos, L. L., Tyndall, A. V., Davenport, M. H., Anderson, T. J., Eskes, G. A., Longman, R. S., Hill, M. D., Hogan, D. B., & Poulin, M. J. (2020).

Aerobic exercise improves cognition and cerebrovascular regulation in older adults. *Neurology, 94*(21), e2245–e2257. https://doi.org/10.1212/wnl.0000000000009478

Guinness Book of World Records. (2022). *First flash mob*. Available at https://www.guinnessworldrecords.com/world-records/first-flashmob

Gullah Culture. (n.d.). Visit Beaufort. https://www.beaufortsc.org/things-to-do/gullah-culture/

Gulzhaina, K., Aigerim, K., Ospan, S., Hans, S., & Cox, N. (2018). Stress management techniques for students. *Advances in Social Science, Education, and Humanities Research, 198*. 47–56.

Hadani, H. S., & Vey, J. S. (2021, April 1). *Infusing playful learning in cities: How to partner with communities for impact*. Brookings. Available at https://www.brookings.edu/blog/education-plus-development/2021/04/01/infusing-playful-learning-in-cities-how-to-partner-with-communities-for-impact/

Hao, H. (2022, April 13). *Michelle Obama: Daily routine*. Balance The Grind. https://balancethegrind.co/daily-routines/michelle-obama-daily-routine/

Harvard Medical School. (2020, July 7). *Exercising to relax*. Available at https://www.health.harvard.edu/staying-healthy/exercising-to-relax

Healthdirect (n.d.). *The role of cortisol in the body*. Available at https://www.healthdirect.gov.au/the-role-of-cortisol-in-the-body

Hui, B., Ng, J., Berzaghi, E., Cunningham-Amos, L., & Kogan, A. (2020). Rewards of kindness? A meta-analysis of the link between prosociality and well-being. *Psychological Bulletin, 146*(12), 1084–1116. doi: 10.1037/bul0000298. Available at https://www.apa.org/pubs/journals/releases/bul-bul0000298.pdf

Jensen, E. (2005). *Teaching with the brain in mind*. Alexandria, VA: ASCD.

Johnson, S. B., Blum, R. W., & Giedd, J. N. (2009). Adolescent maturity and the brain: The promise and pitfalls of neuroscience research in adolescent health policy. *The Journal of Adolescent Health: Official Publication of the Society for Adolescent Medicine*, 45(3), 216–221. https://doi.org/10.1016/j.jadohealth.2009.05.016

Kendi, I. X. (2019). *How to be an antiracist* (1st ed.). One World.

Kent, H. (2020, August 24). *Play! It's good for your family's health*. Mayo Clinic Health System. https://www.mayoclinichealthsystem.org/hometown-health/speaking-of-health/play-its-good-for-your-familys-health

Kesslak, J. P., So, V., Choi, J., Cotman, C. W., & Gomez-Pinilla, F. (1998). Learning upregulates brain-derived neurotrophic factor messenger ribonucleic acid: A mechanism to facilitate encoding and circuit maintenance? *Behavioral Neuroscience, 112*(4), 1012–1019. https://doi.org/10.1037/0735-7044.112.4.1012

Khalsa, S. B. (2004). Yoga as a therapeutic intervention: A bibliometric analysis of published research studies. *Indian Journal of Physiology and Pharmacology, 48*(3), 269–285. PMID: 15648399.

Kindness Rocks Project. (2022). *The kindness rocks project*. Available at https://www.thekindnessrocksproject.com/

Klein, C. (2015, July 17). *Disneyland's glitch-filled opening day*. History.com. https://www.history.com/news/disneylands-disastrous-opening-day-60-years-ago

Lazar, S., Bush, G., Gollub, R., Fricchione, G., Khalsa, G., & Benson, H. (2000). Functional brain mapping of the relaxation response and meditation. *Neuroreport, 11*.

Lee, M.-S., Lee, J., Park, B.-J., & Miyazaki, Y. (2015). Interaction with indoor plants may reduce psychological and physiological stress by suppressing autonomic nervous system activity in young adults: A randomized crossover study. *Journal of Physiological Anthropology, 34*(21). https://doi.org/10.1186/s40101-015-0060-8

Magnuson, C. D., & Barnett, L. A. (2013). The playful advantage: How playfulness enhances coping with stress. *Leisure Sciences, 35*(2), 129–144. https://doi.org/10.1080/01490400.2013.761905

Mar, R., Oatley, K., Hirsh, J., de la Paz, J., & Peterson, J. (2006). Bookworms versus nerds: Exposure to fiction versus non-fiction, divergent associations with social ability, and the simulation of fictional social worlds. *Journal of Research in Personality, 40*, 694–712. doi:10.1016/j.jrp.2005.08.002

Mayo Clinic. (2022). *Stress relief from laughter? It's no joke*. Available at https://www.mayoclinic.org/healthy-lifestyle/stress-management/in-depth/stress-relief/art-20044456

Mueller, S. M. (2009). The neuropsychology of the collector. In S. Satchell (Ed.), *Collectible investments for the high net worth investor* (pp. 31–51). Academic Press.

National Communication Association. (2013). *Flash memory: A history of flash mobs*. Available at https://www.natcom.org/communication-currents/flash-memory-history-flash-mobs

National Institute of Mental Health. (2022, January). *Prevalence of major depressive episode among adults*. Available at https://www.nimh.nih.gov/health/statistics/major-depression#part_155029

National Park Service. (2022). *Most famous national parks set visitation records in 2021*. Available at https://www.nps.gov/orgs/1207/most-famous-national-parks-set-visitation-records-in-2021.htm

Neumann, J. (2015). For disabled vets, playing team sports boosts quality of life. *Reuters Health*. Available at https://www.reuters.com/article/us-disabled-vets-sports-idUSKBN0MN2HI20150327

Newcombe, N., & Lerner, J. C. (1982). Britain between the wars: The historical context of Bowlby's theory of attachment. *Psychiatry*, *45*(1), 1–12. https://doi.org/10.1080/00332747.1982.11024127

Palmer, P. J. (2017). *The courage to teach: Exploring the inner landscape of a teacher's life* (20th anniversary ed.). Jossey-Bass.

Pang, A. (2016). *Rest: Why you get more done when you work less*. New York: Basic Books

Patel, A. V., Maliniak, M. L., Rees-Punia, E., Matthews, C. E., & Gapstur, S. (2018). Prolonged leisure time spent sitting in relation to cause-specific mortality in a large US cohort. *American Journal of Epidemiology, 187*(10), 2151–2158. https://doi.org/10.1093/aje/kwy125

Pellegrini, A. D., & Holmes, R. M. (2006). The role of recess in primary school. In D. G. Singer, R. M. Golinkoff, & K. Hirsh-Pasek (Eds.), *Play = learning: How play motivates and enhances children's cognitive and social-emotional growth* (pp. 36–53). Oxford University Press. https://doi.org/10.1093/acprof:oso/9780195304381.003.0003

Phillpotts, E. (1919). *A shadow passes*. New York: Macmillan.

Pink, D. (2009). *Drive: The surprising truth about what motivates us*. Penguin Random House.

PlayToday. (2022, July 29). *15 stats on mobile gaming demographics for 2021*. Available at https://playtoday.co/blog/stats/mobile-gaming-demographics/

Pollan, M. (2018). *How to change your mind: What the new science of psychedelics teaches us about consciousness, dying, addiction, depression, and transcendence*. Penguin Press.

Porte, J. (1984). *Emerson in his journals*. Belknap Press.

Powell, J. (2020). Music: How it affects your brain, changes your mood and helps you focus. *Science Focus*. Available at https://www.sciencefocus.com/the-human-body/music-science-brain-mood-focus/

Qiu, N., Ma, W., Fan, X., Zhang, Y., Li, Y., Yan, Y., Zhou, Z., Li, F., Gong, D., & Yao, D. (2018). Rapid improvement in visual selective attention related to action video gaming experience. *Frontiers in Human Neuroscience*, *12*. https://doi.org/10.3389/fnhum.2018.00047

Rao, S., & Dellabough, R.(2018). *An audience of one: Reclaiming creativity for its own sake*. Penguin Audio.

Raz, G. (2015, March 27). *How does play shape our development?* NPR TED Radio Hour. Available at https://www.npr.org/transcripts/395065944

Reynolds, P. H. (2004). *The dot*. Walker Books Ltd.

Rhea, D., Rivchen, A., & Pennings, J. (2013). The LiiNK Project®: Implementation of a recess and character development pilot study with grades K & 1 children. *Texas Association for Health, Physical Education, Recreation and Dance Journal (TAHPERD)*, 84 (Summer, 2), 14–35.

Rosenberg, H. (2020, December 1). The rise of yarn bombing. *UCSD Guardian*. Available at https://ucsdguardian.org/2020/12/01/the-rise-of-yarn-bombing/

Russ, S. W. (2003). Play and creativity: Developmental issues. *Scandinavian Journal of Educational Research*, *47*(3), 291–303. https://doi.org/10.1080/00313830308594

Ryan, R. M., Weinstein, N., Bernstein, J., Brown, K. W., Mistretta, L., & Gagné, M. (2010). Vitalizing effects of being outdoors and in nature. *Journal of Environmental Psychology, 30*(2), 159–168. https://doi.org/10.1016/j.jenvp.2009.10.009

Sapolsky, R. M. (2004). *Why zebras don't get ulcers*. Owl Books: Henry Holt & Company.

Savulich, G., Piercy, T., Fox, C., Suckling, J., Rowe, J. B., O'Brien, J. T., & Sahakian, B. J. (2017). Cognitive training using a novel memory game on an iPad in patients with amnestic mild cognitive impairment (aMCI). *International Journal of Neuropsychopharmacology, 20*(8), 624–633. https://doi.org/10.1093/ijnp/pyx040

Schmidt, R. C., Nie, L., Franco, A., & Richardson, M. J. (2014). Bodily synchronization underlying joke telling. *Frontiers in Human Neuroscience, 8*. Available at https://www.frontiersin.org/article/10.3389/fnhum.2014.00633

Schwantes, M. (2021, January 5). *Oprah Winfrey says her success comes down to mastering this daily routine. Inc.* https://www.inc.com/marcel-schwantes/oprah-winfrey-says-her-success-comes-down-to-mastering-this-daily-ritual.html

Siegel, D. J. (2012). *The developing mind: How relationships and the brain interact to shape who we are* (2nd ed.). Guilford Press.

Sifferlin, A. (2016, July). The healing power of nature. *Time*. Available at https://time.com/4405827/the-healing-power-of-nature/

Silverman, S. (1993). Student characteristics, practice, and achievement in physical education. *Journal of Educational Research, 21*(2), 141–157.

Sims Bishop, R. (1990). Mirrors, windows, and sliding glass doors. *Perspectives, 1*(3), ix–xi.

Stevenson, H. W., Lee, S.-Y., Chen, C., Stigler, J. W., Hsu, C.-C., Kitamura, S., & Hatano, G. (1990). Contexts of achievement: A study of American, Chinese, and Japanese children. *Monographs of the Society for Research in Child Development, 55*(1–2)(221), 123. https://doi.org/10.2307/1166090

Suliga, E., Cieśla, E., Rębak, D., Kozieł, D., and Głuszek, S. (2018, October). Relationship between sitting time, physical activity, and metabolic syndrome among adults depending on body mass index (BMI). *Medical Science Monitor, 24*, 7633–45. doi:10.12659/MSM.907582.

Taylor, M. (2022, March 16). *What really happens to your body when you stop going outside*. LIVESTRONG.COM. https://www.livestrong.com/article/13728588-effects-of-staying-inside/

Testoni, I., Wieser, M., Armenti, A., Ronconi, L., Guglielmin, M. S., Cottone, P., & Zamperini, A. (2016). Spontaneity as predictive factor for well-being. In C. Stadler, M. Wieser, & K. Kirk (Eds.), *Psychodrama. Empirical research and science, 2*, 11–23. Wiesbaden: Springer. https://doi.org/10.1007/978-3-658-13015-2_3#main-content

The grand opening of Disneyland. (n.d.). Designing Disney. https://www.designingdisney.com/parks/disneyland-resort/grand-opening-disneyland/

The Strong. (2021). *Stick*. https://www.museumofplay.org/toys/stick/

U.S. Department of Veterans Affairs. (2020). *The healing benefits of humor and laughter*. Available at https://www.va.gov/WHOLEHEALTHLIBRARY/tools/healing-benefits-humor-laughter.asp

van der Kolk, B. (2015). *The body keeps the score: Brain, mind, and body in the healing of trauma*. Penguin.

van der Kolk, B. A., Stone, L., West, J., Rhodes, A., Emerson, D., Suvak, M., & Spinazzola, J. (2014). Yoga as an adjunctive therapy for PTSD. *Journal of Clinical Psychiatry, 75*(6), 559–565.

Wallace, J. (2017, May 20). Why it's good for grown-ups to go play. *Washington Post*. https://www.washingtonpost.com/national/health-science/why-its-good-for-grown-ups-to-go-play/2017/05/19/99810292-fd1f-11e6-8ebe-6e0dbe4f2bca_story.html

Warburton, D. E. R., Nicol, C. W., & Bredin, S. S. D. (2006, March 14). Health benefits of physical activity: The evidence. *CMAJ, 174*(6), Canadian Medical Association, 801–809. doi:10.1503/cmaj.051351.

Ward-Wimmer, D. (2003). The healing potential of adults at play. In C. Schaeffer (Ed.), *Play therapy with adults* (p. 1–11). Wiley. Available at https://www.psychceu.com/Schaefer/intro.pdf

Williams, K. A., Petronis, J., Smith, D., Goodrich, D., Wu, J., Ravi, N., Doyle, E. J. Jr., Juckett, R. G., Kolar, M. M., Gross, R., & Steinberg, L. (2005). Effect of Iyengar yoga therapy for chronic low back pain. *Pain, 115*, 107–117.

Yarnal, C. M., & Qian, X. (2011). Developing and Validating Older Adult Playfulness Scale: An innovative construct and measurement for healthy aging research. *The American Journal of Play, 43*(1), 52–79.

Yenigun, S. (2014, August 6). *Play doesn't end with childhood: Why adults need recess too.* NPR. https://choice.npr.org/index.html?origin=https://www.npr.org/sections/ed/2014/08/06/336360521/play-doesnt-end-with-childhood-why-adults-need-recess-too

Yim, J. (2016). Therapeutic benefits of laughter in mental health: A theoretical review. *The Tohoku Journal of Experimental Medicine, 239*(3), 243–249. https://doi.org/10.1620/tjem.239.243

INDEX